INFECTION IN THE FEMALE

INFECTION IN THE FEMALE

WILLIAM J. LEDGER, M.D.

Professor and Chairman
Department of Obstetrics and Gynecology
Cornell Medical Center
New York, New York

Second Edition

LEA & FEBIGER   PHILADELPHIA

1986

Lea & Febiger
600 Washington Square
Philadelphia, PA 19106-4198
U.S.A.
(215)922-1330

First Edition, 1977

Library of Congress Cataloging in Publication Data

Ledger, William J., 1932-
    Infection in the female.

    Includes bibliographies and index.
    1. Generative organs, Female—Infections.
2. Communicable diseases in pregnancy. I. Title.
[DNLM: 1. Communicable Diseases—in pregnancy.
2. Genital Diseases, Female. 3. Pregnancy Complications,
Infectious.   WP 140 L473i]
RG218.L4   1985   618   85-6859
ISBN 0-8121-0992-9

PRINTED IN THE UNITED STATES OF AMERICA

Print No. 4   3   2   1

PREFACE

The preface for each edition of a medical book after the first seldom reflects reality. Usually, there are glowing references to the many advances in medicine that make this new update necessary. The fact of the matter is that the publishers, in this case Lea & Febiger, have to have sold enough copies of the first edition to make a second edition worthwhile, and the author has to believe the subject is important enough to invest the time and effort to make the necessary revisions for a new edition. These ingredients were present in 1983 when the revision began, and the stage was set for a second edition of *Infection in the Female.* In truth, what do we, the publishers and the author, hope to accomplish?

The first goal is to clarify some of the outdated information of the first edition. There has been remarkable progress in the treatment of women with infections since the first edition was published in 1977. Many therapeutic strategies mentioned as possibilities in 1977 have become a part of accepted clinical practice. For example, prophylactic antibiotics are widely used in obstetric and gynecologic operative procedures, a whole host of new antibiotics has been introduced, and there is increasing emphasis on an individual diagnostic and therapeutic approach to the patient with premature rupture of the membranes. These and many more new developments in diagnosis and treatment have rendered the 1977 edition obsolete.

The next goal is to modify some organizational shortcomings of the first book. The 1977 edition had too much emphasis upon laboratory microbiology and too little time devoted to clinical aspects of care. In this new edition I want to impart to the reader my philosophy of care of gynecologic-obstetric patients with an infection. To accomplish this, I've attempted to correlate laboratory findings with the clinical picture to help bridge the gaps between the sometimes confusing laboratory reports and their implications for the care of the sick patient. I have also tried to make the clinical comments more practical. I've included a new chapter on antibiotics, without a prolonged discussion of the site of action. Instead, there is an emphasis upon their pharmacokinetics, antimicrobial activity, and role in the care of women. In addition, I've split up the old Chapter 9 on community-acquired obstetric infections into two, one focused on fetal and newborn problems and the other emphasizing maternal care. I also deal with the problem patient with a factitious fever and attempt to provide the reader with the framework of a workup to distinguish types of infections that do versus those that do not require antibiotics for cure. My aim has been to provide greater clinical orientation in this volume.

Despite the extensive revisions, the philosophy of this new edition is the same as the previous edition. It is my attempt to provide a rational approach to the care of the woman with a gynecologic-obstetric infection. This is a personal view of the state of the art and represents a blend of my own experiences and my analysis of the information available in the literature. This view is colored by my own biases. I believe we are fortunate in obstetrics and gynecology because for the most part, we deal with young healthy women without serious underlying disease, and we have available to us a wide range of effective antimicrobials and other techniques to prevent or treat infections. Usually, we are successful. Our patients get better without complications. The focus of this book is not a gloom or doom analysis of the current state of practice nor an attempt to change every clinical strategy. The fact is, nearly all of our patients respond to our initial care. This book will give the reader some guidelines that should result in better care for women. As advocates for women, I hope obstetricians and gynecologists read this edition with enthusiasm.

New York, New York   William J. Ledger

CONTENTS

INFECTION IN THE FEMALE

Chapter 1
INFECTIONS IN OBSTETRIC AND GYNECOLOGIC PATIENTS

The subject of infection in women is no longer a stepchild of interest for the obstetrician-gynecologist. The past decade has been marked by the publication of several texts dealing either with infections in women or with the use of antibiotics in obstetrics and gynecology. The Infectious Disease Society of Obstetrics and Gynecology is vigorous and growing, and more emphasis has been placed upon problems of infections in postgraduate meetings for the practitioner.

The reasons for this renewed interest seem obvious. In the 1980s, problems of infection make up a significant proportion of clinical practice. Physicians make decisions about the care of infections in women on a daily basis, and they must stay abreast of the constant advances in technology, such as a plethora of new antibiotics for the treatment of bacterial infections, new diagnostic techniques including the ultrasound and CAT scan, plus the development of antiviral agents that can now be prescribed in clinical practice. All of these new approaches demand the physician's understanding before they can be properly employed.

In addition to these pressures, there is the spectre of malpractice haunting the practitioner. "Malpractice" is often a misnomer. The reality of the legal climate in the United States in the 1980s is that the doctor can expect a civil action if there has been a poor therapeutic result. Obstetrician-gynecologists should understand the societal pressure for such a system, since our specialty's record of policing itself is not above reproach. There is always the danger that the experts, in this case obstetrician-gynecologists, become so absorbed in specific aspects of the specialty that they neglect the needs and desires of the patient. In the current social environment, infections are a frequent source of litigation because of bad results. Infections may also be a cause of death directly, for example, group B beta-hemolytic *Streptococcus* sepsis and death in the newborn, or indirectly, as in aplastic anemia and death caused by the administration of chloramphenicol for a soft tissue pelvic infection. Alternatively, the bad result can be the morbidity of the pain and discomfort during the long hospital stay required for a patient with a pelvic abscess following either an emergency cesarean section or the insertion of an intrauterine contraceptive device in a young nulligravida.

The underlying question that will be asked in every one of these cases is whether or not the medical care met acceptable standards of practice. A recent evaluation of surgical and medical mishaps in the care of patients in the hospital identified common origins of physician error. The most important error of surgical judgment was unjustified optimism, which in cases of infection often takes the form of disregarding early signs of peritonitis.[1] Physicians with patient care responsibilities should also be aware that medicines are more likely to cause serious side effects in the most seriously ill patients (see Table 1–1).[2]

In any evaluation of infection complications, a distinction must be made between an error in judgment related to flawed reasoning and an error of negligence caused by inattention or lack of effort. The latter is an individual matter for correction that rests with the physician, but the former should be reduced by better understanding of the nature of infection in the female. Physicians with patient care responsibility want to be sure that appropriate diagnostic and therapeutic approaches have been followed in all cases of infection. These diverse pressures have led to an increased emphasis on infections in our specialty.

Any evaluation of infectious disease in obstetrics-gynecology requires historical perspective. As George Santayana observed, "Those who cannot remember the past are condemned to repeat it."[3] A review of the progress in the control and treatment of pelvic infection is necessary to understand the philosophies of care of the 1980s.

PREANTIBIOTIC MEDICAL CARE

Eighteenth and nineteenth century physicians accepted maternal death from sepsis as a natural phenomenon. In urban hospitals in the United States and Europe, the lack of recognition of the contributing role of dangerous medical practices contributed to this. The view of the inevitability of bad results was not limited to obstetricians. Surgeons viewed wound suppuration as a normal physiologic event, until Paré found it could be prevented when boiling oil was not introduced into fresh wounds. Obstetricians took solace in the biblical quote attributed to God: "I will greatly multiply your pain in childbearing; in pain you shall bring forth children. . . ."[4] In the 1850s, the magnitude of the problem of infection was reflected by a maternal death rate from sepsis exceeding 10% in some hospitals. Semmelweiss in Vienna and Holmes in Boston championed the theory of contagiousness. This interpretation was reached by Semmelweiss on the basis of postmortem dissection, while Holmes arrived at his conclusion by empirical reasoning. They were not the first, for Alexander Gordon of Aberdeen, Scotland, had reported similar conclusions in 1795.

The solution seemed simple. Hygienic measures should be employed to prevent the spread of infection from medical attendants to the patients. A remarkable

Table 1–1. Probabilities of Iatrogenic Complications Based on Data Obtained at Admission

Source of Admission	House Officer's Assessment	Probability of	
		Any Complication	Major Complication
Home or Housing Facility	Stable to good	0.25	0.04
	Fair	0.40	0.10
	Critical to poor	0.46	0.16
Other			
Hospital or Nursing Home	Stable to good	0.36	0.10
	Fair	0.52	0.20
	Critical to poor	0.57	0.31

feature of this era of history was the nearly total rejection of these ideas by the academic medical establishment. Klein, Semmelweiss' chief, dismissed him. Other prominent scientists voiced their opposition. Scanzoni refused to accept the ideas of Semmelweiss. In America, Meigs of Boston stated, "I remain incredulous as to the contagiousness of the malady."[5] The obstetric academic establishment of the nineteenth century was so absorbed in the study of the mechanics of childbirth that its members refused to acknowledge their own contribution to maternal sepsis.

Acceptance of the theory of contagiousness by the medical profession did not come until pioneers in research, such as Koch and Pasteur, established a microbiologic basis for infection. The identification of defined groups of organisms like the *Streptococcus* and the pneumococcus in the laboratory stimulated other investigators to recognize and document the organism recovered from various sites of infection and to relate this information to specific clinical syndromes. Physicians in the preantibiotic era justifiably prided themselves on their diagnostic acumen, for they were skilled in their descriptions of clinical entities. An example was the documentation by Ephraim McDowell of the first death from sepsis following ovariotomy: "The second day after the operation, she was affected with violent pain in the abdomen, together with an obstinate vomiting. On the third day she died. On examination after death, the uterus, contrary to expectation, appeared natural and inflamed, the right ovarium healthy, the silken cords were securely and properly fixed, and not in a situation likely to injure the adjoining parts. Her death had proceeded from peritoneal inflammation. This membrane throughout its whole extent, appeared greatly inflamed and the intestines largely inflated."[6] This woman probably died of a streptococcal infection, because McDowell's description matches the confirmed clinical picture of death caused by such an infection.

In the absence of effective systemic therapy, the basis for treatment was prevention. The prior cavalier attitude toward environmental and personal hygiene was replaced by an emphasis on meticulous sterile technique and infrequent examination of the genital tract. It was hoped that host defense mechanisms would prove adequate to deal with the bacteria introduced into operative sites during obstetric and gynecologic procedures. If there was clinical evidence of infection, the patient was strictly isolated from other normal patients to prevent the epidemic spread of bacterial infection.

In the twentieth century, before the introduction of antibiotics, obstetricians and gynecologists had an obvious interest in infection problems. Since these were a significant source of hospital mortality, the concern took many forms. Philip Williams of Philadelphia pioneered the concept of review committees of physicians who meticulously surveyed individual cases of maternal mortality. The committee members investigated physicians' errors of management in an attempt to upgrade future medical practice. The specialty also adopted a temperature definition of postpartum morbidity: an oral temperature of 100.4° F or higher on any two of the first 10 days post partum, excluding the first 24 hours. This guide could be applied to patients whose temperature was taken at least four times a day, and it became a standard of medical care. Patients meeting this temperature criterion were subjected to careful examination and isolated from afebrile patients. In addition, any review of the obstetric and gynecologic literature of the 1920s and 1930s reveals good utilization and understanding of microbiologic techniques by clinicians. There is evidence that these efforts had an impact, for there was a steady decline in the numbers of mothers dying from sepsis in the 1930s. What happened to the physicians' high level of interest?

ANTIBIOTIC ERA

The introduction of effective systemic antibiotics had two consequences for the practice of obstetrics and gynecology. The first was favorable—a major reduction in maternal mortality rates from sepsis. The downward trend in maternal mortality before the introduction of systemic chemotherapeutic agents was accelerated by the clinical availability of antibiotics. Few events in medical practive have had such a dramatic effect on patient mortality. Death from sepsis became a rarity on clinical services.

Few medical developments are completely free of adverse results, however, and there was an unfavorable side to the decline in sepsis. Obstetrics and gynecology, for a short period a leader in awareness and control of infectious disease, responded to the belief of general physicians that infection problems had been solved and no longer deserved academic attention or effort. Our specialty switched its priorities to endocrinology, infertility, control of reproduction, oncology, and perinatology and sought the same sort of dramatic breakthrough that came with the introduction of antibiotics to clinical practice. In fact, many academic clinical departments of obstetrics and gynecology changed their names to the department of Reproductive Biology, because they mistakenly believed all of the old challenges had been answered.

The limited clinical focus upon infectious disease is not just noted in obstetrics and gynecology. Today, this lack of concern begins with the medical student at the undergraduate level of medical education. Microbiologic research, spurred by the support of government, has changed from an almost purely descriptive science of the classification of microorganisms to one dealing with more basic biologic concepts of molecular and cellular biology. Within this framework, the interest and competence of the academic microbiologist have been directed more toward such problems as RNA replication in a strain of *Escherichia coli* than to the participation of microorganisms in infectious disease.

As a natural progression of the aforementioned trends, many medical school departments of microbiology have relinquished, in part or completely, the duties of teaching the relationship of microorganisms to disease. The teaching of these concepts has become the responsibility of clinical sections of infectious disease within the departments of internal medicine or pediatrics. Unfortunately, this major revision of curriculum too often is not acknowledged in schedule planning. Many recent graduates of medical schools have had spotty exposure to the concepts of clinical microbiology and infectious disease. It seems incongruous to me that some junior house officers in obstetrics and gynecology are more comfortable in their knowledge of events in the life cycle of the cell than in making decisions pertinent to the care of the patient with an infection.

The deficiencies in the competence of house officers have become increasingly difficult to correct because of the longer distance between the clinical microbiology laboratory and the patient's bedside. With the greater sophistication and expense of laboratory techniques, there has been a tendency nationwide to centralize laboratory facilities in order to increase the efficiency of personnel and equipment. In the care of obstetric and gynecologic patients with infections, this means that the small, satellite microbiology laboratories formerly under departmental control were closed and replaced by a large central laboratory often under the aegis of the pathology department. This arrangement has resulted in the virtual elimination of the daily contacts between physicans and laboratory personnel that formerly served to improve both the understanding and the quality of each group's function.

Concurrent with diminished physician competence in microbiologic confirmation of infectious disease has been an increasing dependence on routine administration of "cocktails" of new powerful systemic antibiotics for the care of the febrile patient, with no rationale other than "it works." The tenet that the optimal use of antimicrobial drugs requires a precise bacteriologic diagnosis, whenever possible, is honored too infrequently by practicing physicians. The usual excuse is that it costs the patient too much money, but the real saving is in physician effort. Our specialty's record in gynecologic patients is illustrative of this, for a survey of over 12,000 patients undergoing hysterectomies revealed that the majority of women who received systemic antibiotics during their hospitalization had not had cultures performed previously.[7] This is an unacceptable level of practice.

The increasing interest of physicians in the 1970s and 1980s in infections in obstetrics-gynecology has been stimulated by an increasing awareness of serious clinical problems caused by unfamiliar microorganisms. In the 1970s, the most dramatic new clinical development was the recognition of the importance of gram-negative anaerobic bacteria in serious pelvic infections. In the 1980s, there is a growing awareness of the significance of *Chlamydia,* plus the reality of an epidemic number of genital infections due to the herpes virus.

Technologic advances in medicine have established new practice patterns that have increased the risk of infection for women. The intrauterine device is associated with a higher rate of pelvic infections[8] than is found in women using oral contraceptives[9] or barrier methods of contraception.[10] The Dalkon shield, once widely promoted and used, is no longer available to the American public because of the risk of sepsis and death in the pregnant woman.[11] In obstetrics, the focus upon improved perinatal survival and the quality of the survivor's life have led to a dramatic increase in the cesarean section rate. When these women are compared with those who deliver vaginally, it is found that both the incidence[12] and severity[13] of postpartum uterine infections are increased. In gynecologic patients, indications for operations such as vaginal hysterectomy have extended to include younger premenopausal women, with an increased risk of more serious postoperative pelvic infections.[14] In oncology patients, therapeutic advances have included more extensive operative procedures such as radical hysterectomies, plus the extensive employment of systemic chemotherapeutic agents for the cure or control of malignancies of the genital tract. These treatment modalities have been popular because they cause remissions and prolonged life, but they have also been associated with an incidence of sepsis and death from the impairment of host defense mechanisms. Infections have again become an important issue for the obstetrician-gynecologist in the 1980s.

REFERENCES

1. Couch, N.P., Tilney, N.L., Rayner, A.A., and Moore, F.D.: The high cost of low-frequency events. N. Engl. J. Med., *304*:634, 1981.

2. Steel, K., Gertman, P.M., Crescenzi, C., and Anderson, J.: Iatrogenic illness on a general medical service at a university hospital. N. Engl. J. Med., *304*:638, 1981.
3. Santayana, G.: *The Life of Reason*. Vol. I. Reason in Common Sense. New York, Scribner, 1927.
4. Genesis 3:16. Holy Bible, Revised Standard Version.
5. Meigs, C.D.: Females and Their Diseases—A Series of Letters to His Class. Philadelphia, Lea and Blanchard, 1948.
6. McDowell, E.: Observations in diseased ovaria. Eclectic Repertory, *9*:546, 1819.
7. Ledger, W.J., and Child, M.A.: The hospital care of patients undergoing hysterectomy. An analysis of 12,026 patients from the Professional Activity Study. Am. J. Obstet. Gynecol., *117*:423, 1973.
8. Westrom, L., Bengtsson, L.P., and Mardh, P.A.: The risk of pelvic inflammatory disease in women using intrauterine contraceptive devices as compared to non-users. Lancet, *2*:221, 1976.
9. Osser, S., Liedholm, P., and Sjöberg, N.O.: Risk of pelvic inflammatory disease among users of intrauterine devices, irrespective of previous pregnancy. Am. J. Obstet. Gynecol., *138*:864, 1980.
10. Kelaghan, J., Rubin, G.L., Ory, H.W., and Layde, P.M.: Barrier method contraceptives and pelvic inflammatory disease. J.A.M.A., *248*:184, 1982.
11. Cates, W., Jr., Ory, H.W., Rochat, R.W., and Tyler, C.W., Jr.: Intrauterine device and deaths from spontaneous abortion. N. Engl. J. Med., *295*:1155, 1976.
12. Sweet, R.L., and Ledger, W.J.: Puerperal infectious morbidity. Am. J. Obstet. Gynecol., *117*:1093, 1973.
13. Ledger, W.J., Kriewall, T.J., and Gee, C.: The fever index. A technique for evaluating the clinical response to bacteremia. Obstet. Gynecol., *45*:603, 1975.
14. Livengood, C.H., III, and Addison, W.A.: Adnexal abscess as a delayed complication of vaginal hysterectomy. Am. J. Obstet. Gynecol., *143*:596, 1982.

Chapter 2

MICROORGANISMS THAT CAUSE INFECTION

All too often, physicians have a restricted vision of the role of microorganisms. The focus is on "pathogenic germs" or disease-causing organisms, whereas a much broader awareness is necessary. Microorganisms are everywhere: within and on the surface of our bodies, on inanimate objects in our living and working environments, and in the air we breathe and the liquids we drink. They are indispensable because they help to recycle the organic molecules of this world. The vast majority of microorganisms are innocuous and represent the necessary links in the cycle of change in our world. A few groups of bacteria, viruses, and fungi are dangerous to plants and humans. This microbiologic minority will be the major focus of this book, but it is important that we also acknowledge how dependent the quality of our lives is upon another tiny segment of the whole—the few hundred species of organisms out of the more then 100,000 that exist in nature that make products useful to mankind. Table 2–1 lists just a few of the microorganisms to which we are indebted.[1] Without their products, our lives would be barren. We need this added perspective before we address the problem of microorganisms that cause infection.

CLASSIFICATION OF MICROORGANISMS

It is important for the physician to have a system of classification of microorganisms in mind when evaluating a patient with a gynecologic infection. This will permit some discrimination in the selection of appropriate antibiotics. This is necessary, for the physician's therapeutic goal for the woman who needs antibiotics should be to select the least toxic agent with a likely chance to effect a clinical cure. A practical worklist of the bacteria that might be involved in these infections should eliminate the possibility of a physician's making an unthinking reflex response when an antibiotic prescription is written. Instead, there should be a rationale for every choice. Physician discipline is required for excellent care of the woman with an infection. This need for physicians in the 1980s is no different from the theme expressed three centuries B.C. by Euclid to Ptolemy I: "There is no royal road to geometry."[2] On every chart, inpatient or outpatient, the physician should make a commitment to the probable site of infection, the most likely microorganisms involved, the extent of the antibacterial activity of the antibiotics prescribed, and the toxic actions of the agents used (Table 2–2). Frequent repetition of this mental exercise will be most helpful in treatment of the patient who fails to respond to the initial choice of antibiotics or who has a

Table 2–1. Useful Products from Microorganisms

Organism	Type	Product
FOODS AND BEVERAGES		
Saccaromyces cerevisiae	Yeast	Baker's yeast, wine, ale, sake
Lactobacillus sanfrancisco	Bacterium	Sour french bread
Streptococcus thermophilus	Bacterium	Yogurt
Lactobacillus bulgaricus	Bacterium	Yogurt
Propionibacterium shermanii	Bacterium	Swiss cheese
Penicillium roquefortii	Mold	Blue-veined cheeses
Penicillium camembertii	Mold	Camembert and brie cheeses
VITAMINS		
Eremothecium ashbyi	Yeast	Riboflavin
Pseudomonas denitrificans	Bacterium	Vitamin B_{12}
Propionibacterium	Bacterium	Vitamin B_{12}
ENZYMES		
Aspergillus oryzae	Mold	Amylases
Kluyveromyces fragilis	Yeast	Lactase
Saccharomycopsis lipolytica	Yeast	Lipase
Bacillus	Bacterium	Proteases
POLYSACCHARIDES		
Leuconostoc mesenteroides	Bacterium	Dextran
PHARMACEUTICALS		
Penicillium chrysogenum	Mold	Penicillins
Cephalosporium acremonium	Mold	Cephalosporins
Streptomyces	Bacterium	Amphotericin B, kanamycins, neomycins, streptomycin, tetracycline, and others
ENTOMOPATHOGENIC BACTERIA		
Bacillus thuringiensis	Bacterium	Bioinsecticides
Bacillus popilliae	Bacterium	Bioinsecticides

(From Phaff, H.J.: Industrial micro-organisms. Sci. Am., *245*:77, 1981.)

toxic reaction to the drugs. When alternative antibiotics are selected in the first case, it will be important to pick an agent with different antibacterial coverage, while in the second case, antibiotics with similar antibacterial activity may be appropriate.

One practical system of classification of the microorganisms involved in disease is based upon their presence on body surfaces. In this scheme, organisms found on the skin or in the vagina or gastrointestinal tract of normal women are called endogenous, while those not normally present are called exogenous. A good example of the latter kind is *Neisseria gonorrhoeae.* This species is not part of the normal surface bacterial flora and has the potential to cause serious infections in women. The bacteriologic report of recovery of this organism should lead to antibiotic therapy to remove surface carriage.

Any view of normal surface bacterial flora in women must acknowledge the tremendous flux in the kinds and numbers of bacteria that can be recovered. These individual and group variations have been incompletely documented and the reasons for the changes have not been fully determined as yet. There are

Table 2–2. Checklist for Antibiotic Prescription

1. Probable site of infection, based upon clinical examination
2. Most likely microorganisms involved in the infection
3. Antibacterial spectrum of antibiotics prescribed
4. Possible toxic actions of antibiotics prescribed

many examples. No scientific information is available, surprisingly, about the effect of sexual intercourse on the bacterial flora of the vagina. Because of this, any documented changes of bacterial flora due to a changing endocrine status such as in premenopausal versus postmenopausal women contain no information describing the frequency of intercourse in these two different groups. Despite the absence of this and other vital data, some important microbiologic observations have been made.

It is known that lactobacilli are important components of the lower genital tract flora of women. They are most prevalent during the reproductive years, particularly during pregnancy, with the lowest incidence in population occurring before puberty and after menopause.[3-12] Anaerobes are important components of the normal vaginal flora, outnumbering aerobes by a factor of ten to one. The number of bacteria seems to be influenced by age of the host. Postmenopausal women have fewer anaerobic bacteria.[10] Normal bacterial flora also may be influenced by the patients' habitat prior to admission to a hospital. One recent study showed urinary tract infections among patients in a nursing home to be caused by more resistant bacteria.[13] Hospitalization and illness may influence surface flora population. In the respiratory tract, it has been reported that gram-negative aerobic colonization of the upper respiratory tract occurs with hospitalization.[14] Among house officers, similar findings occurred when they had a viral illness.[15] These changes in surface bacterial flora are not limited to the respiratory tract. The vaginal flora may be markedly influenced by hospitalization. Among nonpregnant women admitted for hysterectomy, it was found that there was a decrease in the number of lactobacilli and an increase in the number of *Escherichia coli* and *Bacteroides fragilis*.[8, 16] A dramatic impact upon the bacterial flora of women was caused by the systemic administration of antibiotics for five days. *Pseudomonas aeruginosa,* not found in the preoperative controls, was present in 20% of women who received this regimen.[16] Similar changes have been found in hospitalized postpartum women: a decrease in the number of lactobacilli and an increase in the isolation of *Bacteroides fragilis*.[9]

MECHANISMS OF DISEASE

There are a number of mechanisms by which bacteria of normal flora can cause disease. These are important concepts for the practitioner to understand, for there is often confusion about the significance of bacterial isolates from mucosal surfaces such as the vagina. There is a big difference between colonization in normal women and the isolation of organisms in disease. Outside of urinary tract specimens, there are few instances in which the isolation of either a specific species of bacteria or a critical number of bacteria can be correlated with disease. These surface organisms can cause problems. Stamey and his associates have postulated one way in which the normal bacterial flora can cause disease.[17] Certain gram-negative aerobic bacteria have an efficient mechanism whereby they attach to the vaginal mucosa near the urethra, multiply, and then invade the urinary tract, causing infection.

Actual bacterial invasion may not be necessary for some forms of disease. In toxic shock syndrome, coagulase-positive staphylococci, either present in the vagina or introduced from the patient's fingers with the insertion of a tampon, have their growth enhanced in some way by superabsorbent tampons and produce a toxin that results in a characteristic host response of fever, hypotension, skin rash, and eventual desquamation plus adverse effects on many other organ systems.[18] The problem in this instance is invariably the toxin produced and not the invasion of the bloodstream by the organism, for blood culture results in these seriously ill patients are rarely positive.

Recently, another possibility was raised by which normal flora bacteria may be involved in pelvic infection in the female. Toth and colleagues have demonstrated the efficiency of spermatozoa in carrying bacteria over distances in a moist environment.[19] Sperm deposited in the vagina at the time of intercourse may carry bacteria from an asymptomatic male carrier into the upper genital tract of the female, or bacteria in the vagina may attach to the spermatozoa and make their transit to the upper genital tract, resulting in salpingitis in some women. This proposed pathophysiology of salpingitis may account for the lowered incidence of this disease in women using either a barrier method of contraception[20] or oral contraceptives.[21] Both of these contraceptive techniques virtually eliminate the passage of spermatozoa to the upper genital tract.

In hospitalized patients on the obstetric and gynecologic service, a number of events occur that increase the risk of infection from bacteria of the normal flora. The insertion of foreign objects (a catheter) into a sterile body cavity (the bladder) may result in a urinary tract infection.[22] This risk of infection seems greater the longer the catheter is maintained in place.[23] Similarly, the long-term insertion of an intravenous line may result in an infection with normal skin bacteria as pathogens.[24] In addition, pelvic operative procedures can set the stage for the development of postoperative pelvic infections caused by bacteria normally present in the vagina. The crushing of tissue with clamps during a surgical procedure creates an environment conducive to the proliferation of facultative aerobes and anaerobes. Foreign materials used as suture ligatures increase the virulence of the surface bacteria contaminating the operative site.[25] Imperfect hemostasis will leave blood products at the operative site, and ferric ion enhances the virulence of gram-negative aerobes.[26]

A number of plans to lower the incidence of postoperative pelvic infections have demonstrated the importance of normal lower genital tract bacteria in the pathogenesis of these infections. Osborne and co-workers have shown that hot conization of the cervix just prior to hysterectomy reduces the postoperative pelvic infection rate.[27] This maneuver eliminates the endocervical source of bacterial contamination during the manipulation associated with hysterectomy. Swartz and Tanaree have demonstrated that postoperative closed suction drainage of the area between the vaginal cuff and peritoneum results in a lower postoperative infection rate.[28] This technique undoubtedly reduces the inoculum of bacteria and subsequent infection at the operative site. Intraoperative antibiotics either given systemically[29] or by lavage[30] reduce the incidence of postoperative site infection. Systemic antibiotics probably protect against tissue invasion by bacteria, and antibiotic lavage reduces the bacterial inoculum at the operative site while also achieving therapeutic serum levels by absorption.[31] These examples demonstrate the significance of normal bacterial flora in the subsequent development of infections.

BACTERIA THAT CAUSE INFECTION IN WOMEN

With the background knowledge that bacteria from normal flora can be implicated in infection, a classification will be helpful for physician reference. Familiarity with the organisms that can be recovered from the site of infection will influence the selection of antibiotics. One practical classification scheme categorizes bacteria as aerobes and anaerobes. This terminology requires explanation. Bacterial species such as *Escherichia coli* or the group B beta-hemolytic streptococci are called aerobes by this classification, but in reality they are facultative organisms, i.e., they can survive in the absence of oxygen. In fact, with the exception of *Pseudomonas,* all the bacterial species that clinicians call aerobes by this classification are facultative anaerobes.

Why bother, then, with this seeming charade of terminology? The classification has significance for the obstetrician-gynecologist because it identifies a wide range of organisms that have been implicated in soft tissue and urinary tract infections. These bacteria require no special techniques at the time of specimen collection to ensure their recovery and identification in the clinical microbiology laboratory. By contrast, the organisms we call anaerobes require special care and use of oxygen-free tubes or reduced media at the time of specimen collection to enhance their isolation by laboratory personnel. The anaerobic family of organisms has markedly different metabolic needs. Those needs vary from those of clostridia, which are relatively aerotolerant and may survive continued exposure to a low percentage of oxygen, to those of strains such as *Eubacterium aerofaciens,* which are very sensitive to any exposure to oxygen. The clinician's expertise in obtaining a specimen and the laboratory's commitment to excellent anaerobic techniques will be demonstrated by the lack of no growth reports from pelvic abscess specimens and the recovery of anaerobes other than clostridia. If no growth reports are frequently seen, both, the clinicians and the laboratory should reevaluate their procedures to improve shortcomings.

Another subclassification of bacteria is needed. These aerobes and anaerobes should be described as gram-positive and gram-negative. This is an important step in the deductive processes of the clinician. There is some correlation between the Gram stain findings and the antibiotic susceptibilities of these bacteria. For example, the major clinical impact of the aminoglycosides is upon gram-negative aerobic bacteria. This subclassification should be especially helpful in planning antibiotic treatment of seriously ill women in whom purulent material can be obtained from the infection site. This material, after Gram stain and microscopic examination, will give some clues as to the types of bacteria involved in these multibacterial infections. This, in turn, will provide some direction to the antibiotic strategy for this patient.

Since the Gram stain may be employed by the clinician to immediately classify the bacteria found in a purulent exudate, it is important that it be done properly. The steps necessary for accurate staining of these smears are described in Table 2–3.[32] Although the exact mechanism by which the Gram stain works is not known, it does differentiate bacteria on the basis of major variations in the cell wall. It is an appropriate starting point in the workup of the female patient with purulent material from a pelvic infection site.

Gram-Positive Aerobes

Gram-positive aerobes have distinctive morphologic and biologic characteristics. They have a thick cell wall in comparison with gram-negative aerobes, with a strong, rigid layer of mucopeptides.[33] The mucopeptides represent 60% or more of the cell wall and are entangled with teichoic acid and coated with magnesium

Table 2–3. Classification of Bacteria by Gram Stain

1. The cells are fixed by heat.
2. The cells are stained with the primary Gram stain, crystal violet, which is fixed to both gram-positive and gram-negative bacteria. The slide is usually flooded with dye for 1 minute and then washed with water.
3. An iodine-potassium iodide solution that forms an insoluble-in-water complex of primary stain and iodine is added.
4. A decolorizing agent, 70 to 100% alcohol, that extracts the dye from the gram-negative bacteria is applied. It usually requires 15 to 30 seconds until color stops running, and then the slide is again washed with water.
5. Safranin is applied for approximately 30 seconds to counterstain the gram-negative bacteria.
6. The slide is blotted dry or air-dried and examined under the oil-immersion objective.

ribonucleate. The osmotic pressure is 20 atm or higher (Figure 2–1). The gram-positive aerobes of significance for the obstetrician-gynecologist are listed in Table 2–4. The organisms in capital letters are not considered part of the normal flora of the lower genital tract.

AEROBIC STREPTOCOCCI

The gram-positive aerobic streptococci are easily isolated and identified in the clinical microbiology laboratory. They are facultative anaerobes, and growth in the laboratory is maintained in media enriched with blood and serum. They are distinguishable from pneumococci because they are not bile-soluble and from staphylococci because streptococci are catalase-negative. There are many streptococcal species, and the clinician should be familiar with the terminology of microbiology and know the clinical implications of the individual isolates.

Many clinicians are confused by the Greek letter terminology—alpha, beta, and gamma—used for streptococci. This classification describes the reaction of the streptococcal colonies on blood-agar plates.[34] The alpha reaction is a greening of the blood agar and not true hemolysis; the beta reaction is true hemolysis, with a clear area around the colonies; and the gamma response shows no reaction on the agar.

Confusion with terminology often stems from the fact that the major clinical concern with streptococci is with the Lancefield grouping, which employs letters of the alphabet based on the different cellular carbohydrates of the cell wall.[34] The Lancefield groups most frequently involved in infections in women are groups A, B, and D. It is easy to understand how the clinician might confuse group A with alpha hemolysis and group B with a beta hemolysis report. In fact, both group A and B streptococci usually show beta hemolysis on the sheep blood agar commonly used in clinical microbiology laboratories, while group D usually shows a gamma reaction (Table 2–5).[35] Sheep blood agar is the most commonly used blood agar in clinical laboratories because it does not support the growth of *Hemophilus influenzae;* therefore it is a helpful culture medium in the evaluation of specimens from the various upper respiratory tract infections. However, the sheep blood agar shows variable hemolytic responses for the important streptococci. Between 5 and 10% of the group A and B isolates will show alpha hemolysis, so it is important for the clinician to be sure that Lancefield group testing of the colonies showing alpha hemolysis is done in the clinical laboratory. These alpha strains are usually *Streptococcus viridans,* but they can be either group A or group B. Exact grouping of the streptococci can be performed by utilizing precipitate tests

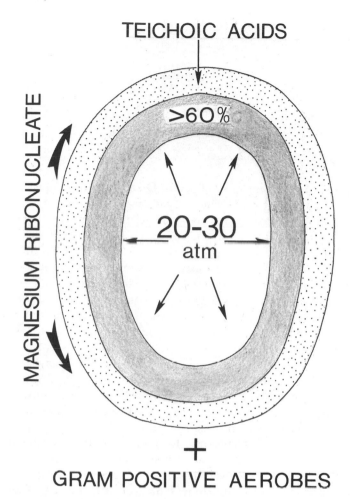

Fig. 2–1. A schematic view of gram-positive aerobes.

with acid-heat extracts of streptococcal cells tested against antisera. Most laboratories utilize bacitracin discs to distinguish group A organisms, a bile esculin slant to identify group D, and sodium hippurate to distinguish group B from *Streptococcus viridans.*

The recovery of these various streptococci may have great significance for the clinician. The group A beta-hemolytic *Streptococcus* is associated with serious life-threatening pelvic infections in postpartum patients[36] and in nonpregnant women who have an intrauterine device in place.[37] It is not part of the normal vaginal flora and is a highly contagious organism, but fortunately it remains highly susceptible to penicillin. The discovery of one case of a pelvic infection caused by this strain should be considered an epidemic, for the organism is easily spread from patient to patient or from physician carrier to patient.

The group B beta-hemolytic *Streptococcus* has been more frequently seen in postpartum uterine infections in recent years[38] and has been associated with fatal infection in the newborn.[39] It is part of the normal vaginal flora and remains highly susceptible to penicillin.

Table 2–4. Gram-Positive Aerobes

Gram-positive cocci
  1. *Streptococcus*
  2. *Staphylococcus*
  3. *PNEUMOCOCCUS*

Gram-positive bacilli
  1. Diphtheroids
  2. Lactobacilli
  3. *LISTERIA MONOCYTOGENES*

The clinical importance of group D streptococci in soft tissue pelvic infections is not known. Although frequently isolated from sites of infection and occasionally from the bloodstream, it was a rare cause of treatment failure in women with early postcesarean-section endomyometritis, for which an antibiotic regimen was employed (clindamycin-gentamicin) that is not effective in the laboratory against this organism.[40] These organisms can cause bacterial endocarditis. They are part of the normal vaginal flora and are the least sensitive of the aerobic streptococci to penicillin. For prophylaxis in patients with a cardiac lesion and for treatment of infections caused by these organisms, a combination of penicillin and an aminoglycoside is usually indicated. Included in the broad classification of group D streptococci is *Streptococcus bovis,* which is highly susceptible to penicillin alone.[41] The identification of group D in the laboratory may have increasing clinical significance as more and more of the second and third generation cephalosporins are prescribed. These antibiotics with a broad spectrum of activity are generally not effective against enterococci, and subsequent superinfections with these organisms may result. This has been especially true with moxalactam.[42]

Groups F and G streptococci have been isolated in infections in both obstetric and newborn patients.[43] They are susceptible to penicillin. *Streptococcus viridans* is not an important pathogen in soft tissue pelvic infections, since it has not been implicated in serious infections. However, it is a cause of endocarditis, is part of the normal vaginal flora, and is highly susceptible to penicillin.

AEROBIC STAPHYLOCOCCI

The recovery of aerobic *Staphylococcus* poses no problem in the clinical microbiology laboratory using sheep blood–agar plates. Individual colonies are often beta hemolytic, but in the laboratory they are easily differentiated from streptococci because they are catalase-positive.

Two strains of staphylococci are important to the clinician: *Staphylococcus aureus* and *Staphylococcus epidermidis.* They have markedly different pathogenicities for the

Table 2–5. Classification of Streptococcal Species Infecting Humans

Lancefield Group	Species	Usual Reaction on Blood Agar
Group A	*Streptococcus Pyogenes*	Beta
Group B	*Streptococcus agalactiae*	Beta
Group D	*Streptococcus faecalis*	Gamma
	Streptococcus faecium	
	Streptococcus bovis	
	Streptococcus equinus	

human host. Identification in the laboratory is simple, based upon the observations noted in Table 2–6.[44] Further subclassification of staphylococci can be done by bacteriophage typing. This testing is based upon the observation that strains of *Staphylococcus aureus* are lysogenic and the phage carried by one culture will be virulent for other cultures. A standard set of phages causes lysis and enables the laboratory to do phage typing. This procedure is rarely employed clinically and is usually done in investigations of a possible epidemic of *Staphylococcus aureus* infections in a hospital. Most clinical laboratories are not prepared to do this testing, and it is carried out either in state laboratories or those of the Centers for Disease Control (CDC).

The two strains of staphylococci *(S. aureus and S. epidermidis)* have a markedly different clinical impact upon patients. *Staphylococcus aureus* is associated with such serious hospital-acquired infections as postoperative abdominal wound abscess or postpartum breast infections, mastitis, or abscess. Generally, these organisms are not part of the surface flora when the patient enters the hospital and are acquired from the medical team's carriage of *S. aureus* on their skin, nares, hair, and so forth. These hospital-acquired organisms are usually resistant to penicillins and require alternate antibiotics, the semisynthetic penicillins, cephalosporins, or vancomycin. It is important to know the antibiotic susceptibility of hospital-acquired *Staphyloccous aureus.* This can vary from hospital to hospital and the choice of methicillin, appropriate in one setting, would not be appropriate in an institution where a significant number of the strains were resistant to the drug.[45] The recovery of coagulase-positive *Staphylococcus* from more than one blood culture bottle should be a source of clinical concern. These staphylococci have a propensity to attack intact heart valves,[46] and their recovery from the bloodstream dictates prolonged intravenous antibiotic therapy to prevent this serious problem. Recently, there has been an upsurge of community-acquired infections due to *Staphylococcus aureus*—the toxic shock syndrome.[18] Since these bacteria are acquired outside of the hospital, it is likely that these virulent organisms were part of the normal flora of the unfortunate victims. The strains causing toxic shock syndrome are usually not susceptible to penicillin and erythromycin but are responsive to semisynthetic penicillins, cephalosporins, and clindamycin.

Staphylococcus epidermidis is infrequently a serious concern in pelvic infections. It can cause superinfections in immunosuppressed patients who have been in the hospital for long periods of time and have had indwelling urinary or vascular

Table 2–6. Identification of *Staphylococcus*

Species	Colonies	Coagulase Production	Acid from Mannitol
Staphylococcus aureus	Often golden yellow (not a valid means of separating the two species)	+ + Delayed	+ − +
Staphylococcus epidermidis	Often white (not a valid means of separating the two species)	− −	− +

catheters. Fortunately, *Staphylococcus epidermidis* has low virulence. It is frequently part of the normal vaginal flora and has a pattern of antibiotic resistance similar to that of *Staphylococcus aureus.*

PNEUMOCOCCUS

The gram-positive coccus *Diplococcus pneumoniae* (pneumococcus) is classified as an aerobe. However, it is a facultative anaerobe, lacks cytochromes, and is related biochemically to the anaerobes. In the clinical microbiology laboratories, colonies will grow on sheep blood agar and a presumptive diagnosis can be made by a positive result of a bile solubility test or sensitivity to ethylhydrocupreine hydrochloride (Optochin). If exudate from the infection is available, these organisms can be diagnosed by the use of the quellung (Neufeld's) reaction. The quellung reaction is based upon the observation that pneumococci exposed to a homologous anticapsular serum have a capsular precipitin reaction in which the bacterial capsule appears refractile under the microscope. At least one clincial study showed this test to be more accurate than the Gram stain in making the initial diagnosis of pneumococcal pneumonia.[47]

Diplococcus pneumoniae is uncommonly encountered by the obstetrician-gynecologist. It is not considered part of the normal lower genital tract flora, and it is rarely recovered from either pelvic sites of infection or from the bloodstream. This organism is most frequently found in the patient with a community-acquired pneumonia.[48] Although it is quite susceptible to penicillin, a few strains have been isolated that are resistant to penicillin,[49] and there is increasing resistance in the laboratory to tetracycline.[50]

Gram-Positive Bacilli

Aerobic diphtheroids can be isolated on a blood-agar plate. The colonies are catalase-positive and a smear that is Gram stained and examined microscopically reveals clubbed, gram-positive bacilli that stain irregularly.

These aerobic diphtheroids do not have great clinical significance for the obstetrician-gynecologist. They are part of the normal vaginal flora of the lower genital tract, and are not considered pathogens.

Aerobic lactobacilli are frequently isolated from the lower genital tract of asymptomatic women. Although they have been recovered in surface cultures of the endocervix from women with pelvic infections, they are not thought to be pathogens.

Listeria monocytogenes thrives on sheep blood agar. The colonies produce beta hemolysis, are catalase-positive, and a smear will reveal gram-positive bacilli that are neither club-shaped nor pleomorphic. *L. monocytogenes* is an important pathogen for the obstetrician-gynecologist. These organisms should not be considered part of the normal vaginal flora. They have been isolated on occasion from pregnant patients at the time of a spontaneous abortion.[51] Although these bacteria are susceptible to penicillin, ampicillin, and tetracycline, one laboratory evaluation found greater bactericidal activity with combinations of penicillin and gentamicin, ampicillin and streptomycin, and ampicillin and gentamicin.[52] The clinical significance of this observation is not known.

Gram-Negative Aerobes

Gram-negative aerobes have unique anatomic characteristics. Their cell wall is far less rigid than that of gram-positive aerobes, containing less than 10% mucopeptides compared with the 60% or more mucopeptides of gram-positive aerobes (Figure 2–2).[33] The inner cell environment is different, because the intracellular osmotic pressure is less than 5 atm compared with 20 atm or greater with gram-positive aerobes.

This is one reason for the difference in general response to antibiotics of these two large groups of bacteria. Antibiotics like penicillin G, which act on the cell wall and result in rupture and dissolution of gram-positive bacteria, are less dramatically destructive with gram-negative aerobes because of their less rigid cell wall and lower intracellular pressure. The wide-spread use of penicillin in the 1960s was one factor in the increased occurrence of gram-negative aerobic infections in the hospital. This led to the extensive research efforts that yielded broader spectrum penicillins, the cephalosporins, and the newer aminoglycosides, all of which have more effective antibacterial activity against gram-negative aerobic organisms.

Gram-negative aerobes have varying degrees of clinical significance for the obstetrician-gynecologist. They are important when found in women with infections, since they are frequently isolated from specimens obtained from the urinary tract, the pelvis, and the bloodstream. Therefore, clinicians should know the antibiotic susceptibilities of the gram-negative aerobic isolates from their service in their own hospitals. These bacteria are generally not as resistant to multiple

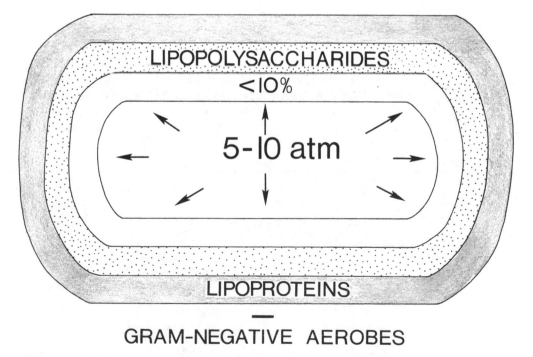

Fig. 2–2. A schematic view of gram-negative aerobes.

antibiotic therapy as are strains isolated from patients in medical or surgical care units or in a burn ward. The gram-negative aerobes do not seem to be as important as pathogens for the obstetrician-gynecologist in the 1980s as they were in the 1970s. One evaluation of bacteremia associated with postcesarean section endomyometritis had a low frequency of isolation of these organisms,[53] and there is no question that the number of patients with endotoxin shock from gram-negative aerobes is less now than in the decades of the 1960s and 1970s. Physician vigilance should be maintained. These bacteria can rapidly acquire resistance to antibiotics through the transference of extrachromosomal material, the (R) factor.[54] This transfer can occur among bacteria of different species. In addition, highly virulent gram-negative aerobes may be encountered in immunosuppressed oncology patients, and these life-threatening infections may require treatment with potentially toxic antibiotics for cure.

Clinicians should require that clinical microbiology laboratories have the capability to isolate and identify gram-negative aerobes. These organisms will grow on standard plates in the laboratory or on the multiple small medium discs that are commercially available to permit rapid speciation of the gram-negative aerobes. This expanded capability for speciation has led to a classification of these gram-negative aerobes as Enterobacteriaceae and other gram-negative aerobes.

Enterobacteriaceae

The members of this family of gram-negative aerobes have many common characteristics. They all are nonspore-forming and may be identified by the clinician on Gram stain as uniformly staining gram-negative rods that are usually extracellular. The individual species of this family of bacteria should be identified in the clinical microbiology laboratory and are listed in Table 2–7.

Escherichia coli is often encountered by the obstetrician-gynecologist. These organisms are part of the normal vaginal flora, and they are the most frequent isolates in urinary tract infections. Although at present they are less frequently isolated from soft tissue infection sites and the bloodstream than they were 10 years ago, they are important pathogens and should be considered in the antibiotic strategies for septic patients. In addition, they are a frequent cause of infection in the newborn, which seems to be brought about by a particular strain of *E. coli*

Table 2–7.   The Enterobacteriaceae

Organism	Genus and Species
1. Escherichieae	*Escherichia coli* *Shigella (dysenteriae, flexneri,* *boydii, sonnei)*
2. Klebsiella	*Klebsiella pneumoniae* *Enterobacter aerogenes* *Serratia marcescens*
3. Proteeae	*Proteus (mirabilis, vulgaris, normanii)* *Providencia (rettgeri, stuartii* *alcalifaciens)*
4. Salmonelleae	*Citrobacter (freundi, diversus)* *Salmonella (typhi, choleraesuis,* *paratyphi A)*

with a specific K_1 surface polysaccharide antigen.[55] The newer penicillins, cephalosporins, and aminoglycosides have all been used successfully to treat these infections.

Various members of the *Shigella* species are rarely encountered by the obstetrician-gynecologist. They are not part of the normal vaginal flora and are most frequently implicated in community-acquired diarrhea. They have also been isolated from the cervix of women with salpingo-oophoritis.[56] These strains are susceptible to treatment with trimethoprin-sulfamethoxazole.[57]

Klebsiella pneumoniae also has significance for the clinician. This species is part of the normal vaginal flora and has been isolated from patients with urinary tract and pelvic infections. In individual patients, this organism may be suspected by the presence of encapsulated gram-negative rods in the Gram stained specimen. In addition to individual patient infections, the physician should be alert to a cluster of patients developing infections caused by this organism. This problem of superinfection has been related to the widespread use of kanamycin on surgical services for treatment[58] or to prolonged use of ampicillin for prophylaxis[59] on a neurosurgical service. *Klebsiella pneumoniae* is usually resistant to ampicillin but is susceptible to both the newer aminoglycosides and to the second or third generation cephalosporins.

Enterobacter aerogenes is an important gram-negative rod for the clinician, even though it is infrequently involved in either urinary tract or pelvic infections. Its recovery almost invariably occurs in seriously ill patients who have major underlying disease. This species should not be considered part of the normal vaginal flora. Development of new penicillins, aminoglycosides, and cephalosporins has yielded antimicrobial agents that are effective against this organism.

Serratia marcescens has historical significance for the obstetrician-gynecologist because it demonstrates the transition of a strain of bacteria from a nonpathogen to a pathogen. In the 1940s and the 1950s, it was considered a nonpathogen for humans, and the organisms isolated from sites of infection were considered contaminants. As a result of this idea of a benign bacterial species, experiments were carried out by the government that consisted of spraying the surroundings of San Francisco Bay in "no risk" studies to measure the environmental spread of bacteria in case they were ever employed in biologic warfare. This insensitivity to public safety was not limited to government scientists. In medicine, this bacterial species was used as a "safe" biologic marker and was painted on the perineums of hospitalized patient "volunteers" in studies to determine the ascent of microorganisms into the bladder when an indwelling urethral catheter was in place.[60] Physicians' naivete about the safety of *Serratia* was replaced by considerable concern when this organism was implicated in life-threatening pneumonias in postoperative patients who had been treated with contaminated respirator equipment[61] and in cases of sepsis in burn unit patients.[62] Infections produced by these organisms are serious because of the resistance of this species to many of the frequently prescribed aminoglycosides[63] and the possibility of passive transfer of the organism from patient to patient by nonaseptic techniques of patient handling by hospital personnel. Fortunately for obstetrician-gynecologists, *Serratia marcescens* is rarely recovered from infection sites in patients, and it is not part of the normal vaginal flora. The only patients whom I have seen with this infection have been women with pelvic malignancies who have had prolonged hospitalization with long exposure to many systemic antibiotics and the use of an indwelling vascular line for hyperalimentation.

Members of the *Proteus* family have significance for the obstetrician-gynecologist. They are infrequently isolated from urinary tract infections or soft tissue pelvic infections, even though they are considered part of the normal vaginal flora. There are variations in the antibiotic susceptibilities of the various species of *Proteus,* as noted in Table 2–7, and it is important that the clinician check the susceptibility of the individual isolates. In general, these species are susceptible to the newer penicillins, the second and third generation cephalosporins, and the newer aminoglycosides.

The various *Providencia* species are rarely encountered in infections in obstetric-gynecologic patients. This is fortunate, because these organisms are resistant to many of the available aminoglycosides. *Providencia* is not part of the normal vaginal flora.

Members of the Salmonelleae family are rarely encountered in female patients. These organisms are not part of the normal vaginal flora. *Citrobacter* may be rarely recovered from patients with hospital-acquired infections. *Salmonella* is frequently involved in the bacterial gastroenteritis seen in patients who have visited or who reside in areas south of the United States. On an obstetric-gynecologic service with a large percentage of women from these areas, *Salmonella typhosa* infections may be seen in pregnant[64] and nonpregnant patients.[65] A careful history of gastroenteritis symptoms should be taken from women from these geographic areas who present with lower abdominal discomfort. In patients with *Salmonella typhosa* stool isolates, there has been an increase in the number of chloramphenicol-resistant strains,[66] and ampicillin is the drug of choice in these cases.

Other Gram-Negative Aerobic Organisms

These gram-negative organisms are distinct from the Enterobacteriaceae. They have many different microbiologic characteristics that will be noted when the individual members listed in Table 2–8 are discussed. They do have significance for the obstetrician-gynecologist because they are involved in recognizable infection entities in women and the newborn. With the exception of *Gardnerella vaginalis,* these gram-negative aerobes are not part of the normal vaginal flora.

Members of the *Pseudomonas* family, particularly *P. aeruginosa,* are rarely isolated from infections in obstetric-gynecologic patients. These organisms may be found in the patient who has been in the hospital for long periods of time and has received an antibiotic or antibiotics with a broad spectrum of antimicrobial activity.

Table 2–8.   Other Gram-Negative Organisms

Pseudomonas (aeruginosa, alcaligenes, cepacia, fluorescens, stutzeri, mallei)
Campylobacter fetus
Hemophilus influenzae
Gardnerella vaginalis
Hemophilus ducreyi
Calymmatobacterium granulomatis
Acinetobacter
Neisseria gonorrhoeae

In distinction to the Enterobacteriaceae, *Pseudomonas* requires oxygen for survival (i.e., it is not facultative), and it has polar flagella. There are many resistant strains among the species noted in Table 2–8. Treatment of a *Pseudomonas* infection outside of the urinary tract will probably require a combination of one of the newer penicillins or a third-generation cephalosporin, plus one of the newer amino-glycosides. Fortunately, these infections are rarely seen. If a *Pseudomonas* organism is isolated, the clinical laboratory should provide you with species identification as well as antibiotic susceptibility testing.

Campylobacter fetus is a comma-shaped, gram-negative aerobe that grows best in a microaerophilic environment. It is not considered part of the normal vaginal flora and has rarely been implicated in obstetric-gynecologic infections. The major concern has been its role in gastroenteritis. Recently, *Campylobacter fetus* has been associated with overwhelming intrauterine infection and fetal death in a pregnant woman with sepsis due to this organism.[67] This organism should be considered in the differential diagnosis of the pregnant patient with fever of unknown origin.

Hemophilus influenzae is rarely encountered by the obstetrician-gynecologist in infection. It is a rare isolate from the bloodstream of febrile postpartum patients[53, 65] and has been implicated in an occasional newborn patient with sepsis.[68] Recently, in our service at the New York Hospital-Cornell Medical Center, we had a death from sepsis in a premature newborn infant in the first 24 hours of life in which *Hemophilus influenzae* was isolated from the bloodstream of the baby and the genital tract of the mother. *Hemophilus influenzae* is a pleomorphic gram-negative rod, and it will not grow on sheep blood agar. Isolation in the laboratory requires the use of chocolate agar. One strain, with the type b capsular serotype, is involved in more than 90% of the serious infections due to this organism. In recent years, it has been noted that a few of the strains of *Hemophilus influenzae* produce a beta lactamase, making them resistant to ampicillin, formerly the drug of choice in these infections. If these strains are present, chloramphenicol is the drug of choice, although the cephalosporins, aminoglycosides, and trimethoprim-sulfamethoxazole also are effective.

Gardnerella vaginalis is a controversial organism for the obstetrician-gynecologist. On the one hand, its presence is implicated in the syndrome of nonspecific vaginitis,[69] while on the other hand some studies have shown its recovery from the vagina of asymptomatic women.[70] On occasion, it also has been recovered from the bloodstream of febrile postpartum patients.[65] It can be isolated from specimens placed in thioglycollate broth or in routine blood culture media, but optimal growth in the laboratory is achieved with Casman blood agar plus 5% fresh defibrinated rabbit blood and incubation in a CO_2-rich environment. If treatment is indicated, either ampicillin or metronidazole seems effective.

Hemophilus ducreyi is the causative organism of chancroid. It is not part of the normal vaginal flora. This gram-negative rod can be isolated on rabbit blood agar or chocolate agar. It is susceptible to tetracycline.

Calymmatobacterium granulomatis is the organism that results in the infection granuloma inguinale. It is not part of the normal vaginal flora. This gram-negative rod survives best in culture media with added egg yolk. It is susceptible to tetracycline.

Acinetobacter is rarely isolated from sites of pelvic infections. It is a gram-negative organism with a diplococcoid to coccobacillary form that is not part of the normal vaginal flora. Fortunately, these organisms are susceptible to aminoglycosides, cephalosporins, and the newer penicillins.

Neisseria gonorrhoeae is an important organism for the obstetrician-gynecologist. In the United States, it is frequently isolated from women with salpingitis and can cause eye infection in newborns. These gram-negative diplococci are not part of the normal flora of the vagina or endocervix. Laboratory recovery of this organism requires Thayer-Martin medium or a modification, with the culture plate maintained in a CO_2-rich environment. The colony growth, confirmation on Gram stain of gram-negative diplococci, and a positive oxidase reaction all combine to make a presumptive diagnosis of *Neisseria gonorrhoeae.* A correlation between virulence and colony types has been observed.[71,72] An additional laboratory variation has been the observation of opaque and transparent colonies that may be influenced by the presence of proteolytic enzymes in the female cervix.[73] This may have significance in the pathogenesis of gonococcal infections and the observed immune response. In the past, *Neisseria gonorrhoeae* has been susceptible to both penicillin and tetracycline, but in the past few years a new penicillin-resistant strain has been recovered with increasing frequency. Its presence can be suspected in the laboratory by the lack of inhibition of growth around the penicillin disc. This new fact of clinical practice has modified the recommendation of the Centers for Disease Control for the treatment of uncomplicated gonorrhea in women (Table 2–9).[74]

Anaerobes

A dramatic development in obstetrics-gynecology in the past 15 years has been the increasing awareness of the importance of anaerobic bacteria in pelvic infections. During the 1950s and the 1960s, it was common for clinicians to describe the smell of an abscess as a "typical *E. coli* odor" or to receive a report of nongrowth from the laboratory indicating a "sterile abscess," when in reality the major pathogens were anaerobic bacteria, present in huge numbers at the infection site. The low level of awareness of the significance of anaerobic bacteria in the 1960s is reflected in this description of a tuboovarian abscess: "Despite the fact that pus found in such surgical problems is probably gonococcal in origin and smells like *Escherichia coli,* the culture report is frequently sterile. It seems unwarranted to blame the bacteriologists for this, but it is a frequent and curious, if inexplicable finding."[75] In the 1980s, obstetrician-gynecologists know that *Neisseria gonorrhoeae*

Table 2–9.   Treatment of Uncomplicated Gonorrhea in Women

---

1. Amoxicillin 3.0 g or ampicillin 3.5 g with 1.0 g of probenecid by mouth
2. Aqueous procaine penicillin G 4.8 million U intramuscularly at 2 sites with 1.0 g of probenecid by mouth
3. Tetracycline 500 mg by mouth, 4 times a day for 7 days
   or
   Doxycycline cyclate 100 mg by mouth, twice a day for 7 days
4. A combined regimen to cover both gonorrhea and chlamydial infections utilizes regimens 1 and 3

For penicillinase-producing *Neisseria gonorrhoeae*:

1. Spectinomycin 2.0 g IM. Tetracycline may be added to treat coexisting chlamydial infections
2. Treatment failures with spectinomycin:
   Cefoxitin 2.0 g IM plus 1.0 g of probenecid by mouth, or cefotaxime 1.0 g in a single injection without probenecid

---

is rarely recovered from abscesses and that anaerobic bacteria are usually isolated in large numbers from these serious mixed bacterial infections.

There are a number of classifications of anaerobic bacteria that can be employed by the clinician. The classic system describes anaerobes on the basis of their Gram staining characteristics and their morphology (i.e., are they cocci, bacilli, or rods) and identifies individual numbers on the biochemical differences noted. As this technology advances, frequent changes in classification and names of individual species occur as well. Utilizing this classification, an enumeration of anaerobes found in pelvic infections or of importance to obstetrician-gynecologists is shown in Table 2–10. The new classification eliminates nearly all of the *Peptococcus* genus. They are now classified under peptostreptococci. Among the gram-negative rods, there has been further subdivision of *Bacteroides fragilis* and *melaninogenicus*.[76] Many of the species names noted under the various families are not familiar to the clinician, but they will be seen more frequently on laboratory reports as clinical laboratories become more sophisticated in their technology with anaerobic organisms.

An alternative classification is a much simpler one but can have more relevance for the clinician. By this method, anaerobes are subdivided on the basis of their susceptibility to penicillin G. Nearly all of the penicillin-resistant strains are gram-negative rods and include *Bacteroides (fragilis, bivius, disiens,* and *melaninogenicus)* plus a few strains of *Fusobacterium.* These species require alternative prescription patterns.

The clinician must have an understanding of the problems involved in the recovery and identification of anaerobic bacteria in the laboratory. Anaerobes generally grow slowly and they require special procedures, such as anaerobic jars or an anaerobic chamber for speciation. This inevitably means a longer wait for the generation of a laboratory report. The physician should demand an interim reporting system in which presumptive reports are given, based upon distinctive colony growth characteristics and the Gram stain microscopic appearance of the colonies. The preliminary report of a gram-positive anaerobic coccus can be an

Table 2–10. Anaerobes Recovered from Pelvic Infections in Women

I. Gram-positive cocci
   A. *Peptostreptococcus (anaerobius, parvulus, productus, species, assaccharolyticus, magnus, variabilis)*
   B. *Peptococcus*

II. Gram-positive bacilli
   A. Nonspore-forming
      1. *Actinomyces (israelii, naeslundii)*
      2. *Bifidobacterium (adolescentis, eriksonii)*
      3. *Eubacterium (alactolyticum, lentum, limosum)*
      4. *Lactobacillus (catenaforme)*
      5. *Propionibacterium acnes*
   B. Spore-forming
      1. *Clostridium*
         a. Histotoxic
         b. Nonhistotoxic

III. Gram-negative cocci
   A. *Acidaminococcus fermentans*
   B. *Megasphaeras elsdenii*
   C. *Veillonella (alcalescens, parvula)*

IV. Gram-negative rods
   A. *Bacteroides (bivius, disiens, fragilis, melaninogenicus, oralis, putredinis, ureolyticus)*
   B. *Fusobacterium (mortiferum, necrophorum, nucleatum, varium)*

important bit of information for the clinician who is trying to evaluate the clinical response of the patient with a serious pelvic infection.

GRAM-POSITIVE ANAEROBES

Gram-positive anaerobic cocci have distinctive microbiologic characteristics that distinguish them from other anaerobic species. Both the *Peptostreptococcus* (anaerobic streptococcus) and the *Peptococcus* (anaerobic staphylococcus) have similar growth patterns on a blood-agar plate. In the new classification (see Table 2–10), nearly all strains formerly called *Peptococcus* are now called *Peptostreptococcus*. The colonies have convex, gray to white growth, are opaque, and may have an alpha- or beta-hemolytic reaction. Definitive diagnosis is based upon the physiologic character-istics of these two groups of organisms. Speciation is based upon such tests as catalase, indole production, nitrate reduction, gelatin liquefaction, and the meas-urement of specific fermentation products. With wider employment of clinical laboratories with anaerobic microbiology capabilities, individual speciation of gram-positive anaerobic cocci is more widely available in the United States.

Anaerobic gram-positive cocci have great clinical significance for the obstetri-cian-gynecologist. They are part of the normal vaginal flora. At least one study of postpartum endomyometritis has cited them as the most frequent bacterial isolate,[77] and in an evaluation of blood cultures in patients with septic abortions they were the most frequent organisms isolated.[78] They can be recovered from women with salpingitis. In the patient with a fecal-smelling exudate from a pelvic infection source, the finding of gram-positive cocci on microscopic examination of the Gram stained specimen should suggest the diagnosis. The anaerobic cocci are not distinguishable from aerobic cocci on these microscopic evaluations. For-tunately for the physician, they remain susceptible to penicillin, and although frequently recovered, they have not been associated with serious pelvic infections. A few strains of *Peptostreptococcus* are not susceptible to clindamycin and metroni-dazole.

Gram-positive anaerobic bacilli constitute a diverse group of microorganisms for the obstetrician-gynecologist. The clinical microbiology laboratory can recover and identify the numerous individual species noted in Table 2–10. It is important that the physician have an awareness of their clinical significance.

Nonspore-forming gram-positive bacilli have a wide range of clinical signifi-cance for the obstetrician-gynecologist, particularly *Actinomyces israelii*. For reasons that are not yet apparent, the presence of an intrauterine device creates a genital tract environment in which these organisms can survive, colonize, and subse-quently cause serious pelvic infections.[79] The involvement of these organisms in a pelvic abscess can be suspected on microscopic examinations of the Gram stained tissue showing distinctive filamentous gram-positive bacilli. There is also a typical pathologic picture when material from a tuboovarian abscess is sectioned for microscopic slides; there are filamentous branches and the presence of sulfur granules. Such abscesses may require long-term therapy for cure, but fortunately these organisms are susceptible to penicillin and clindamycin. *Bifidobacterium* and *Eubacterium* are rarely isolated from pelvic infections. Both groups of organisms are susceptible to penicillin. The anaerobic lactobacilli and *Propionibacterium acnes* are part of the normal vaginal flora. They are not considered significant pathogens in pelvic infections.

The gram-positive spore-forming anaerobic bacilli are important pathogens for the obstetrician-gynecologist. They can usually be isolated in the hospital microbiology laboratory because they are more oxygen tolerant than other anaerobes. A good means of classification of clostridia is shown in Table 2–11.[80] Traditionally, infection with the histotoxic clostridia has had a serious prognosis in humans, for they have the ability to destroy tissue and blood cells. They can be involved in septic abortions and may cause overwhelming sepsis, intravascular hemolysis, renal failure, and death.[81] In critically ill patients with this clinical picture, laboratory confirmation of the diagnosis is important. *Clostridium perfringens* has a characteristic wide double zone of hemolysis on blood agar, and this species produces lecithinase on egg yolk agar. The other histotoxic species have specific characteristics or metabolic products that permit laboratory identification. Although these species may be associated with serious illness, their isolation in the laboratory does not confirm the presence of a serious infection. For example, *Clostridium perfringens* can be part of the normal vaginal flora in asymptomatic women. It has been recovered from the bloodstream of patients with infections cured by antibiotics alone,[65] and it has been isolated from the genital tract of women who have had a pelvic infection that is not serious.[82] These histotoxic strains are quite susceptible to penicillin and clindamycin. The nonhistotoxic strains of clostridia have taken on new importance in the past few years. Although these strains have been isolated from the bloodstream of patients with infections that responded rapidly to antibiotics, they were neither frequent nor serious problems. In recent years, one species of nonhistotoxic clostridia has assumed great importance for the obstetrician-gynecologist, *Clostridium difficile,* which is the causative agent in most cases of antibiotic-associated colitis.[83] The damage to the bowel is related to an enterotoxin produced by this species. Fortunately, it is susceptible to vancomycin and metronidazole.

GRAM-NEGATIVE ANAEROBES

Gram-negative anaerobic cocci are not frequently of concern to the obstetrician-gynecologist. They are rarely recovered from sites of infection, even though they are considered part of the normal vaginal flora. These organisms are sensitive to

Table 2–11.　Classification of Clostridia

Histotoxic Clostridia	Nonhistotoxic Clostridia
Clostridium perfringens	*Clostridium bifermentans*
C. septicum	C. butyricum
C. novyi	C. capilovale
C. tetani	C. cochlearium
C. botulinum	C. difficile
	C. fallax
	C. innocuum
	C. limosum
	C. multifermentans
	C. paraputrificum
	C. sordellii
	C. sphenoides
	C. sporogenes
	C. subterminale
	C. tertium
	CDC group P-1

exposure to oxygen, and I regard their isolation as a testimony to the competence of the clinical microbiology laboratory. In the laboratory, these organisms show nonhemolytic colony growth on blood agar. Speciation is accomplished by biochemical testing. These *Veillonella* have not been considered important pathogens in serious infections, and they are susceptible to penicillin.

Gram-negative nonspore–forming anaerobic rods are the most important groups of microorganisms for consideration in clinical therapeutic strategies in the 1980s. Although part of the normal vaginal flora, these organisms are invariably recovered from the most serious infection in women, the pelvic abscess that requires operative drainage or removal. In addition, many of these gram-negative anaerobic rods are not susceptible to the commonly employed antibiotic regimens for treatment of pelvic infection such as penicillin or a first generation cephalosporin in combination with an aminoglycoside. Alternative antibiotic strategies need to be employed.

The clinician should suspect involvement of these gram-negative anaerobic rods by the presence of clinical and laboratory signs. If a pelvic abscess is suspected or diagnosed, the index of suspicion should be high. In doing a microscopic examination of the Gram-stained foul-smelling purulent material, the presence of pleomorphic unevenly stained gram-negative rods, with many located within the white cells, should strongly suggest anaerobic pathogens.

A major focus of concern in the clinical microbiology laboratory should be the identification of the individual species of the anaerobic gram-negative rods. These organisms can be grown on blood-agar plates in an anaerobic jar or chamber. The individual species can then be identified by biochemical testing or by evaluation of carbohydrate fermentation products by gas chromatography. A few of the individual species in this group of gram-negative rods are of great importance to the clinician. *Bacteroides fragilis* is frequently involved in serious infections, and specific strains with a capsule are important in abscess formation.[84] Although generally susceptible to clindamycin, chloramphenicol, and metronidazole, recently a few strains of *Bacteroides fragilis* have been noted that are resistant to clindamycin.[85] Recent reports have noted the increasing frequency of isolation of strains of *Bacteroides bivius* and *Bacteroides disiens* from women with pelvic infections.[86,87] Since these species share the antibiotic susceptibilities of *B. fragilis,* similar antibiotic strategies should be employed when they are involved. *Bacteroides melaninogenicus* can be suspected in the laboratory by the appearance of a brown to black color of the colonies on blood agar. Formerly this species was uniformly susceptible to penicillin, but recently resistant strains have been noted.[88] This should be acknowledged in antibiotic prescription planning. *Fusobacterium* is sometimes recovered from pelvic abscesses. It should be considered a causative organism if the microscopic examination of exudate shows long filamentous branching forms. Some of the strains are resistant to penicillin but clindamycin, chloramphenicol, or metronidazole is appropriate.

Mycoplasma

Mycoplasma are unique organisms for the obstetrician-gynecologist. Microbiologically, they differ from bacteria in that they have no cell wall, and they are unlike viruses in that they have both DNA and RNA and can grow on cell-free media. They are part of the vaginal flora of asymptomatic women and have been recovered from the bloodstream of febrile postpartum patients[89] as well as from patients with salpingitis.[90] Despite these findings, the significance of this group of organisms in serious pelvic infections has not been established.

The recovery of *Mycoplasma hominis* and *Ureaplasma urealyticum* requires special culture techniques. The medium requires peptone enrichment with serum and yeast, and the subsequent growth yields colonies just visible to the naked eye. Under the lens of a dissecting microscope, these colonies have a "fried egg" appearance, with a dense central zone of growth and a peripheral zone with surface growth only. Both species of *Mycoplasma* are susceptible to tetracycline, but recently an increasing number of resistant strains have been noted.

Chlamydia

This group of organisms is the most exciting microbiologic entity for the obstetrician-gynecologist in the 1980s. It is apparent that *Chlamydia* has a great deal of importance in a number of infections in humans. In the male, it is responsible for nongonococcal urethritis,[91] while in the female it can cause cervicitis[92] and salpingitis[93] and has been implicated in adhesion formation after salpingitis.[94] In the newborn, it has been a cause of postdelivery conjunctivitis[95] and pneumonia.[96]

A major factor in this recent recognition of the clinical importance of *Chlamydia* is related to its specific nutritional needs in the laboratory. These organisms have both RNA and DNA but are obligate intracellular parasites. Their recovery in the laboratory can be achieved only if a tissue cell culture line and technicians familiar with tissue cell culture techniques are available. New testing with monoclonal antibodies may obviate this need. Fortunately for the physician, both tetracycline and erythromycin seem to be effective therapy.

Fungi

Medically important fungi are derived from the Class Deuteromyceyes and have asexual reproduction with no fusion of nuclei. The family members include *Aspergillus, Blastomyces, Candida, Coccidioides, Cryptococcus,* and *Histoplasma.* These yeast forms will grow after inoculation on Sabouraud glucose agar and can be identified on the basis of colony and microscopic characteristics.

For the obstetrician-gynecologist, *Candida* infections are frequently seen, whereas those caused by *Coccidioides* are rarely reported. *Candida albicans* can cause symptomatic vaginitis, and this can be treated with nystatin, miconazole, or clotrimazole. Untreated vaginal candidiasis in pregnancy may cause oral candidiasis (thrush) in the newborn. Disseminated adult infection has been seen in an immunocompromised host, particularly with a history of receiving broad-spectrum antibiotics. *Coccidioides immitis* infection is uncommon but can be found in the southwestern United States. Disseminated maternal infection and death have been reported.[97] Fortunately, in these rare cases, systemic therapy in the form of amphotericin B and ketoconazole is available.

Viruses

Although viruses are important pathogens for humans, they are a frequent source of confusion for the obstetrician-gynecologist. These obligate intracellular parasites have either DNA or RNA, but not both. Their special metabolic need in the laboratory, i.e., a tissue culture line, has seldom been met by clinical laboratories until recent years, so there is little familiarity with nomenclature of

Table 2–12. Classification of Viruses

I. DNA Viruses
   A. Parvoviridae   None are known to cause disease in humans
   B. Papovaviridae   Human wart virus
   C. Adenoviridae   Respiratory tract infections
   D. Herpetoviridae   1. Herpes
                            2. Varicella-zoster
                            3. Cytomegalovirus
                            4. Epstein-Barr virus
   E. Poxviridae   1. Vaccinia
                            2. Smallpox
                            3. Cowpox
                            4. Molluscum contagiosum

II. RNA Viruses
   A. Picornaviridae   1. Enteroviruses
                               a. Poliovirus
                               b. Coxsackievirus
                               c. Echovirus
                            2. Rhinovirus
   B. Togaviridae   1. Alphavirus (Eastern, Western, and Venezue-
                               lan equine encephalitis)
                            2. Flavivirus (St. Louis and Japanese B
                               encephalitis viruses, dengue)
                            3. Rubivirus (rubella)
   C. Reoviridae   Clinical significance not known
   D. Coronaviridae   Acute respiratory illnesses
   E. Orthomyxoviridae   Influenza A, B, C
   F. Retroviridae
      Oncoviridae   (Leukemia and sarcoma viruses of animals)
   G. Arenaviridae   1. Lymphocytic choriomeningitis virus
                            2. Astrovirus
   H. Rhabdoviridae   Rabies
   I. Paramyxoviridae   1. Parainfluenza
                            2. Measles
                            3. Mumps
                            4. Respiratory syncytial virus

the various agents. In addition, most physicians are not familiar with the various tests of immunologic response that determine past or recent infections. The growing awareness of the significance of viruses in human infection has led to wider availability of laboratory facilities as well as to increased knowledge among physicians about the diagnosis of viral infections. A classification of viruses with clinical significance for the obstetrician-gynecologist is listed in Table 2–12. These viruses cause a diverse number of infections in humans. The DNA viruses include agents that cause genital warts as well as some of the individual TORCH agents including cytomegalovirus and herpesvirus. The RNA viruses cause a wide range of clinical syndromes, including the rubella of the TORCH syndrome, and there is evidence that the cytopathic retrovirus (HTLV-III) related to AIDS is an RNA virus.[98]

REFERENCES

1. Phaff, H.J.: Industrial micro-organisms. Sci. Am., *245*:77, 1981.
2. Euclid to Ptolemy I from Proclus, Commentary on Euclid. Prologue. Bartlett, J.: Familiar Quotations. 15th ed. Boston, Little, Brown and Co., 1980.
3. Weinstein, L., and Howard, J.H.: The effect of estrogenic hormone on the H-ion concentration and the bacterial content of the human vagina with special reference to the "Doderlein bacillus." Am. J. Obstet. Gynecol., *37*:698, 1937.

4. Weinstein, L., Bogin, M., Howard, J.H., and Finkelstone, B.B.: A survey of the vaginal flora at various ages with special reference to the Doderlein bacillus. Am. J. Obstet. Gynecol., *32*:211, 1936.
5. Cruickshank, R., and Sharman, A.: The biology of the vagina in the human subject. II. The bacterial flora and secretion of the vagina at various age periods, and their relations to glycogen in the vaginal epithelium. J. Obstet. Gynecol. Br. Emp., *41*:208, 1934.
6. Bartlett, J.G., Onderdonk, A.B., Drude, E., Goldstein, C., Anderka, M., Alpert, S., and McCormack, W.M.: Quantitative bacteriology of the vaginal flora. J. Infect. Dis., *136*:271, 1977.
7. Hammerschlag, M.R., Alpert, S., Onderdonk, A.B., Thurston, P., Drude, E., McCormack, W.M., and Bartlett, J.G.: Anaerobic microflora of the vagina in children. Am. J. Obstet. Gynecol., *131*:853, 1978.
8. Ohm, M.J., and Galask, R.P.: Bacterial flora of the cervix from 100 pre-hysterectomy patients. Am. J. Obstet. Gynecol., *122*:683, 1975.
9. Goplerud, C.P., Ohm, M.J., and Galask, R.P.: Aerobic and anaerobic flora of the cervix during pregnancy and the puerperium. Am. J. Obstet. Gynecol., *126*:858, 1976.
10. Larsen, B., Goplerud, C.P., Petzold, C.R., Ohm-Smith, M.J., and Galask, R.P: Effect of estrogen treatment on the genital tract flora of post-menopausal women. Obstet. Gynecol., *60*:20, 1982.
11. Tashjian, J.H., Coulam, C.B., and Washington, J.A., II: Vaginal flora in asymptomatic women. Mayo Clin. Proc., *51*:557, 1976.
12. Larsen, B., and Galask, R.P.: Vaginal microbial flora: Composition and influences of host physiology. Ann. Intern. Med., *96*:926, 1982.
13. Garibaldi, R.A., Brodine, S., and Matsumiya, S.: Infections among patients in nursing homes. N. Engl. J. Med., *305*:731, 1981.
14. Johanson, W.G., Pierce, A.K., and Sanford, J.P.: Changing pharyngeal bacterial flora of hospitalized patients. N. Engl. J. Med., *281*:1137, 1969.
15. Ramirez-Ronda, C.H., Fuxench-Lopez, Z., and Nevarez, M.: Increased pharyngeal bacterial colonization during viral illness. Arch. Intern. Med., *141*:1599, 1981.
16. Ohm, M.J., and Galask, R.P.: The effect of antibiotic prophylaxis on patients undergoing total abdominal hysterectomy. Alterations of the microbial flora. Am. J. Obstet. Gynecol., *125*:448, 1976.
17. Stamey, T.A., and Condy, M.: The diffusion and concentration of trimethoprim in human vaginal fluid. J. Infect. Dis., *131*:261, 1975.
18. Tofte, R.W., and Williams, D.N.: Clinical and laboratory manifestations of toxic shock syndrome. Ann. Intern. Med., *96*:843, 1982.
19. Toth, A., O'Leary, W.M., and Ledger, W.J.: Evidence for microbial transfer by spermatozoa. Obstet. Gynecol., *59*:556, 1982.
20. Kelaghan, J., Rubin, G.L., Ory, H.W., and Layde, P.M.: Barrier method contraceptives and pelvic inflammatory disease. J.A.M.A., *248*:184, 1982.
21. Osser, S., Gullberg, N.B., Liedholm, P., and Sjoberg, N.D.: Risk of pelvic inflammatory disease among intrauterine users irrespective of previous pregnancy. Lancet, *1*:386, 1980.
22. Givens, C.D., and Wenzel, R.P.: Catheter associated urinary tract infections in surgical patients. A controlled study on the excess morbidity and costs. J. Urol., *124*:646, 1980.
23. Burke, J.P., Garibaldi, R.A., Britt, M.R., Jacobson, J.A., Conti, M., and Alling, D.W.: Prevention of catheter associated urinary tract infections. Am. J. Med., *70*:655, 1981.
24. Altemeier, W.A., McDonough, J.J., and Fullen, W.D.: Third day surgical fever. Arch. Surg., *103*:158, 1971.
25. Georgiade, N.G., King, E.H., Harris, W.A., Tenery, J.H., and Schlech, B.A.: Effect of three proteinaceous foreign materials on infected and subinfected wound models. Surgery, *77*:569, 1975.
26. Bullen, J.J., Rogers, H.J., and Griffiths, S.E.: Role of iron in bacterial infection. Curr. Top. Microbiol. Immunol., *80*:1, 1978.
27. Osborne, N.G., Wright, R.C., and Dubay, M.: Pre-operative hot conization of the cervix. Am. J. Obstet. Gynecol., *133*:374, 1979.
28. Swartz, W.H., and Tanaree, P.: T-tube suction drainage and/or prophylactic antibiotics. Obstet. Gynecol., *47*:665, 1976.
29. Young, R., Platt, L., and Ledger, W.J.: Prophylactic cefoxitin in cesarean section. Surg. Gynecol. Obstet., *157*:11, 1983.
30. Rudd, E.G., Long, W.H., and Dillon, M.B.: Febrile morbidity following cefamandole nafate intrauterine irrigation during cesarean section. Am. J. Obstet. Gynecol., *141*:12, 1981.
31. Duff, P., Gibbs, R.S., Jorgensen, J.H., and Alexander, G.: The pharmacokinetics of prophylactic antibiotics administered by intraoperative irrigation at the time of cesarean section. Obstet. Gynecol., *60*:409, 1982.
32. Bartholomew, J.W., and Mittwer, T.: The Gram stain. Bacteriol. Rev., *16*:1, 1952.
33. Lorian, V.: The mode of action of antibiotics on gram negative bacilli. Arch. Intern. Med., *128*:623, 1971.

34. Brown, J.H.: The use of blood agar for the study of streptococci. Monograph No. 9. New York, The Rockefeller Institute for Medical Research, 1919.
35. Weinstein, L. (ed.): Streptococcal Disease. Kalamazoo, Michigan, Upjohn, 1974.
36. Ledger, W.J., and Headington, J. T.: Group A beta-hemolytic streptococcus: An important cause of serious infection in obstetrics and gynecology. Obstet. Gynecol., *39*:474, 1972.
37. Marshall, B.R., Hepler, J.K., and Jingugi, M.S.: Fatal *Streptococcus pyogenes* septicemia associated with an intrauterine device. Obstet. Gynecol., *41*:83, 1973.
38. Faro, S.: Group B beta-hemolytic streptococci and puerperal infections. Am. J. Obstet. Gynecol., *139*:686, 1981.
39. Baker, C.J.: Summary of the workshop in perinatal infections due to group B streptococcus. J. Infect. Dis., *136*:137, 1977.
40. DiZerega, G., Yonekura, L., Roy, S., Nakamura, R.M., and Ledger, W.J.: A comparison of clindamycin-gentamicin and penicillin-gentamicin in the treatment of post cesarean section endomyometritis. Am. J. Obstet. Gynecol., *134*:238, 1979.
41. Moellering, R.C., Jr., Watson, B.K., and Kunz, L.J.: Endocarditis due to Group D streptococci: Comparison of disease caused by *Streptococcus bovis* with that produced by enterococci. Am. J. Med., *57*:239, 1974.
42. Moellering, R.C., Jr.: Enterococcal infections in patients treated with moxalactam. Rev. Infect. Dis., *4*:S708, 1982.
43. Shlaes, D.M., Lerner, P.I., Wolinsky, E., and Gopalakrishna, K.V.: Infections due to Lancefield group F and related streptococci (*S. milleri, S. anginosus*). Medicine, *60*:197, 1981.
44. Ivler, D.: Staphylococcus. *In* Manual of Clinical Microbiology. Edited by J. E. Blair, E. H. Lenette, and J. P. Truant. Baltimore, Williams & Wilkins Co., 1970, chapter 5.
45. Haley, R.W., Hightower, A.W., Khabbaz, R.F., Thornsberry, C., Marstone, W.J., Allen, J.R., and Hughes, J.M.: Methicillin-resistant *Staphylococcus aureus* infection in United States hospitals. Ann. Intern. Med., *97*:297, 1982.
46. Mirimanoff, R.O., and Glauser, M.P.: "Endocarditis during *Staphylococcus aureus* septicemia in a population of non-drug addicts. Arch. Intern. Med., *142*:1311, 1982.
47. Merrill, C.W., Gwaltney, J.M., Jr., Hendley, J.O., and Sande, M.A.: Rapid identification of pneumococci. N. Engl. J. Med., *288*:510, 1973.
48. Benedetti, T.J., Valle, R., and Ledger, W.J.: Antepartum pneumonia in pregnancy. Am. J. Obstet. Gynecol., *144*:413, 1982.
49. Jacobs, M.R., Koornhof, H.J., Robins-Browne, R.M., Stevenson, C.M., Vermaak, Z.A., Freiman, I., Miller, G.B., Witcomb, M.A., Isaacson, M., Ward, J.I., and Austrian, R.: Emergence of multiply resistant pneumococci. N. Engl. J. Med., *299*:735, 1978.
50. Finland, M.: Changing patterns of susceptibility of common bacterial pathogens to antimicrobial agents. Ann. Intern. Med., *76*:1009, 1972.
51. Rappaport, F., Rabinovitz, M., Toaff, F., and Krochik, N.: Genital listerosis as a cause of repeated abortion. Lancet, *1*:1273, 1960.
52. Moellering, R.C., Jr., Medoff, G., Leech, I., Wennersten, C., and Kunz, L.J.: Antibiotic synergism against *Listeria monocytogenes*. Antimicrob. Agents Chemother., *1*:30, 1972.
53. DiZerega, G.S., Yonekura, M.L., Keegan, K., Roy, S., Nakamura, R., and Ledger, W.J.: Bacteremia in post-cesarean section endomyometritis: Differential response to therapy. Obstet. Gynecol., *55*:587, 1980.
54. Smith, H.W.: Transfer of antibiotic resistance from animal and human strains of *Escherichia coli* to resident *E. coli* in the alimentary tract of man. Vet. Rec., *85*:31, 1969.
55. Robbins, J.B., McCracken, G.H., Jr., Gotschlich, E.C., Orskov, F., Orskov, I., and Hanson, L.A.: *Escherichia coli* K$_1$ capsular polysaccharide associated with neonatal meningitis. N. Engl. J. Med. *290*:1216, 1974.
56. Amstey, M.S., and Gandell, D.L.: Salpingitis-perihepatitis in a patient with cervical *Shigella sonnei*. Obstet. Gynecol., *55*:70S, 1980.
57. Barada, F.A., Jr., and Guerrant, R.L.: Sulfamethoxazole-trimethoprim versus ampicillin in treatment of acute invasive diarrhea in adults. Antimicrob. Agents Chemother., *17*:961, 1980.
58. Gardner, P., and Smith, A.H.: Studies on the epidemiology of resistance (R) factors. Ann. Intern. Med., *71*:1, 1969.
59. Price, D.J.E., and Sleigh, J.D.: Control of infection due to *Klebsiella aerogenes* in a neurosurgical unit by withdrawal of all antibiotics. Lancet, *2*:1213, 1970.
60. Kass, E.H., and Schneiderman, L.F.: Entry of bacteria into the urinary tracts of patients with inlying catheters. N. Engl. J. Med., *256*:556, 1957.
61. Cabrera, H.A.: An outbreak of *Serratia marcescens* and its control. Arch. Intern. Med., *123*:650, 1969.
62. Yu, V.L.: *Serratia marcescens*. N. Engl. J. Med., *300*:887, 1979.
63. John, J.F., Jr., and McNeill, W.F.: Characteristics of *Serratia marcescens* containing a plasmid coding for gentamicin resistance in nosocomial infections. J. Infect. Dis., *143*:810, 1981.
64. Duff, P., and Engelsgjerd, B.: Typhoid fever on an obstetric-gynecology service. Am. J. Obstet. Gynecol., *145*:113, 1983.

65. Ledger, W.J., Norman, M., Gee, C., and Lewis, W.: Bacteremia on an obstetric-gynecologic service. Am. J. Obstet. Gynecol., *121*:205, 1975.
66. Overturf, G., Marton, K.I., and Mathies, A.W., Jr.: Antibiotic resistance in typhoid fever. N. Engl. J. Med., *289*:463, 1973.
67. Gribble, M.J., Salit, I.E., Isaac-Renton, J., and Chow, A.W.: Campylobacter infections in pregnancy. Am. J. Obstet. Gynecol., *140*:423, 1981.
68. Wallace, R.J., Baker, C.J., Quinones, F.J., Hollis, D.G., Weaver, R.E., and Wiss, K.: Nontypable *Hemophilis influenzae* (biotype 4) as a neonatal, maternal and genital pathogen. Rev. Infect. Dis., *5*:123, 1983.
69. Gardner, H.L., and Dukes, C.D.: *Hemophilus vaginalis* vaginitis. Am. J. Obstet. Gynecol., *69*:962, 1955.
70. McCormack, W.M., Hayes, C.H., Rossner, B., Errand, J.R., Crockett, V.A., Alpert, S., and Zinner, S.H.: Vaginal colonization with *Corynebacterium vaginale* (*Hemophilus vaginalis*). J. Infect. Dis., *136*:740, 1977.
71. Kellogg, D.S., Jr., Peacock, W.L., Jr., and Deacon, W.E.: *Neisseria gonorrhoeae.* I. Virulence genetically linked to clonal variations. J. Bacteriol., *85*:1274, 1963.
72. Kellogg, D.S., Jr., Cohne, I.R., and Norin, L.C.: *Neisseria gonorrhoeae.* II. Clonal variation and pathogenicity during 35 months in vitro. J. Bacteriol., *96*:596, 1968.
73. James, J.F., and Swanson, J.: Studies on gonococcus infection: XIII. Occurrence of color opacity colonial variants in clinical cultures. Infect. Immun., *19*:332, 1978.
74. Centers for Disease Control: Morbidity and Mortality Weekly Report Supplement. Sexually transmitted diseases. Treatment guideline 1982. *31*:335, 1982.
75. Novak, E.R., and Woodruff, J.D.: Novak's Gynecologic and Obstetric Pathology. 6th ed., Philadelphia, W.B. Saunders, 1967.
76. Bergey's Manual of Determinative Bacteriology. 8th ed., Baltimore, Williams & Wilkins, 1983.
77. Gibbs, R.S., O'Dell, T.N., MacGregor, R.R., Schwarz, R.H., and Morton, H.: Puerperal endometritis: A prospective microbiologic study. Am. J. Obstet. Gynecol., *121*:919, 1975.
78. Rotheram, E.B., and Schick, F.S.: Nonclostridial anaerobic bacteria in septic abortion. Am. J. Med., *46*:80, 1969.
79. Hager, W.D., and Majmudar, B.: Pelvic actinomycosis in women using intrauterine contraceptive devices. Am. J. Obstet. Gynecol., *133*:60, 1979.
80. Alpern, R.J., and Dowell, V.R., Jr.: Nonhistotoxic clostridial bacteremia. Am. J. Clin. Pathol., *55*:717, 1971.
81. Decker, W.H., and Hall, W.: Treatment of abortions infected with *Clostridium welchi.* Am. J. Obstet. Gynecol., *95*:394, 1966.
82. Ledger, W.J., and Hackett, K.: Significance of clostridia in female reproductive tract. Obstet. Gynecol., *41*:525, 1973.
83. Yonekura, M.L., and diZerega, G.S.: Antibiotic associated colitis. Obstet. Gynecol. Surv., *35*:743, 1980.
84. Onderdonk, A.B., Kasper, D.L., Cisneros, R.L., and Bartlett, J. G.: The capsular polysaccharide of *B. fragilis* as a virulence factor: Comparison of the pathogenic potential of encapsulated and unencapsulated strains. J. Infect. Dis., *136*:82, 1977.
85. Tally, F.P., Cuchural, G.J., Jacobus, N.V., Gorbach, S.L., Aldridge, K.E., Cleary, T.J., Finegold, S.M., Hill, G.B., Iannini, P.B., McCloskey, R.V., O'Keefe, J.P., and Pierson, C.L.: Susceptibility of the *Bacteroides fragilis* group in the United States in 1981. Antimicrob. Agents Chemother., *23*:536, 1983.
86. Sweet, R.L., Yonekura, M.S., Hill, G., Gibbs, R.S., and Eschenbach, D.A.: Appropriate use of antibiotics in serious obstetric and gynecologic infections. Am. J. Obstet. Gynecol., *146*:719, 1983.
87. Gall, S.A., Kohan, A.P., Ayers, O.M., Hughes, C.E., Addison, W.A., and Hill, G.B.: Intravenous metronidazole or clindamycin with tobramycin for therapy of pelvic infections. Obstet. Gynecol., *57*:51, 1981.
88. Finegold, S.M.: Pathogenic anaerobes. Arch. Intern. Med., *142*:1988, 1982.
89. McCormack, W.M., Lee, Y.H., Rosner, B., Rankin, J.S., and Lin, J.S.: Isolation of genital mycoplasma from blood obtained shortly after vaginal delivery. Lancet, *1*:596, 1975.
90. Eschenbach, D.A., Buchanan, T.M., Pollock, H.M., Forsyth, P.S., Alexander, E.R., Lin, J.-S., Wang, S.-P., Wentworth, B.B., McCormack, W.M., and Holmes, K.K.: Polymicrobial etiology of acute pelvic inflammatory disease. N. Engl. J. Med., *293*:166, 1975.
91. Bowie, W.R., Alexander, E.R., and Holmes, K.K.: Etiologies of post-gonococcal urethritis in homosexual and heterosexual men: Roles of *Chlamydia trachomatis* and *Ureaplasma urealyticum.* Sex. Transm. Dis., *5*:151, 1978.
92. Ripa, T., Svensson, L., Mardh, P.-A., and Westrom, L.: *Chlamydia trachomatis*-cervicitis in gynecologic outpatients. Obstet. Gynecol., *52*:698, 1978.
93. Mardh, P.-A., Ripa, T., Svensson, L., and Westrom, L.: *Chlamydia trachomatis* infection in patients with acute salpingitis. N. Engl. J. Med., *296*:1377, 1977.
94. Henry-Suchet, J., Catalan, F., Loffredo, V., Serfaty, D., Siboulet, A., Perol, Y., Sanson, M.J.,

Debache, C., Pigeau, F., Coppin, R., DeBrux, J., and Poynard, T.: Microbiology of specimens obtained by laparoscopy from control patients with pelvic inflammatory disease or infertility with tubal obstruction. *Chlamydia trachomatis* and Ureaplasma urealyticum. Am. J. Obstet. Gynecol., *138*:1022, 1980.

95. Schachter, J., Grossman, M., Holt, J., Sweet, R., and Spector, S.: Infection with *Chlamydia trachomatis:* Involvement of multiple anatomic sites in neonates. J. Infect. Dis., *139*:232, 1979.

96. Tipple, M.A., Beem, M.O., and Sexon, E.M.: Clinical characteristics of the afebrile pneumonia associated with *Chlamydia trachomatis* infection in infants less than 6 months of age. Pediatrics, *63*:192, 1979.

97. Smale, L.E., and Walchter, K.G.: Dissemination of coccidioidomycosis in pregnancy. Am. J. Obstet. Gynecol., *107*:356, 1970.

98. Vilmer, E., Rouzioux, C., Venizet Brun, F., Fisher, A., Chermann, J.C., Barre-Sinoussi, F., Gazengel, C., Dauguet, C., Manigne, P., Griscelli, C., and Montagnier, L.: Isolation of new lymphotropic retrovirus from two siblings with haemophilia B, one with AIDS. Lancet, *1*:753, 1984.

Chapter 3
PROPER COLLECTION OF MICROBIOLOGIC SPECIMENS

In obstetrics and gynecology, the widest gap between expectation and reality is illustrated by the contact of clinicians with personnel of the hospital microbiology laboratory. The frustrations are apparent in each of the two camps. Attending physicians are aware that bacteriology data may not be helpful because of lack of correlation with the clinical picture of the patient. One such example is a culture report of pus with no bacterial growth obtained from a specimen of a patient with sepsis. Microbiologists have daily reminders that clinicians either do not think proper specimen collection is important for patient care or do not understand basic medical microbiology. A dried-out endocervical swab submitted in a sterile tube after weekend storage in an emergency room refrigerator will not yield a growth of *Neisseria gonorrhoeae* even if this organism was present in the endocervix of the patient when the physician obtained the specimen. In this case, the failure to isolate *Neisseria gonorrhoeae* was not the fault of the laboratory.

Too frequently, incomplete knowledge of microbiology leads to the unacceptable physician practice of omitting specimen collection prior to antibiotic prescription. Fortunately for the patient and the physician, most women in whom this diagnostic step is eliminated will be cured with the initial choice of antibiotics. The most frequently given physician justification for the failure to order a culture is concern about the medical costs of unnecessary laboratory tests. This rationale is confusing, for these same doctors are frequently the ones who will order unnecessary and expensive diagnostic tests such as an ultrasonogram or a CAT scan in a woman with an acute abdomen who should undergo an immediate laparotomy. All too frequently, these tests delay the decision of the physician to operate and often the results do not influence his or her choice.

Alternatively, the physician with an incomplete understanding of microbiology sometimes will emphasize form and not substance in the bacteriologic evaluation of a patient with an infection. For these practitioners, the diagnostic goal is the defensive practice posture that produces a culture report of a specimen obtained in whatever manner prior to antibiotic prescription. No thought is associated with this maneuver, and these inaccurate reports have little or no impact on subsequent patient care. Too often, a patient attendant such as a nurse on the evening shift will be ordered over the phone by these physicians to blindly insert a swab into the patient's vagina and to send this specimen to the laboratory before antibiotics are administered to the patient. The microbiology report generated for the chart will reflect surface bacterial flora that frequently bear no relationship to the bacteria causing disease at the site of infection. No pretreatment physical examination has been done, and the evolution of the infection has been modified by systemic antibiotics. In those patients who fail to respond to the initial antibiotics, this lack of valid clinical and microbiologic information will complicate patient care. One study from Iowa demonstrated that prior administration of antibiotics made it difficult to determine the exact site of infection on clinical grounds.[1] Even more important in these patients who fail to respond is that no useful microbiologic information has been generated from the initial assessment to aid in the choice of new antibiotics.

There is another reason for the importance of a good microbiologic examination. Bacteria causing infections in obstetric-gynecologic patients may vary from hospital to hospital. Information on the range of bacteria isolated and their antibiotic susceptibilities can be generated from periodic cumulative reporting of the output of the microbiology laboratory. If cultures are not obtained, this grouped data will not be available. The unacceptable medical practice of incomplete or inaccurate microbiology data collection can be avoided. The starting point in the evaluation of the patient with an infection is to obtain comprehensive microbiologic information so that the best patient care can be provided.

SPECIMEN COLLECTION

The collection of an adequate specimen requires physician familiarity with the principles of microbiology so that appropriate procedures are followed. Unlike the blood chemistry laboratory, where a single blood specimen will suffice for a battery of accurate, useful tests, a variety of different techniques may be necessary to obtain meaningful microbiologic data. During the clinical examination, the physician should be differentiating in his mind the organisms that may be implicated in the infection. This is important because different culture techniques may be necessary for different types of organisms. For example, the operative drainage of a pelvic abscess with an overwhelming fecal odor should place anaerobes at the top of the physician's differential diagnosis list. In the evaluation of a patient with acute salpingitis, major bacteriologic concerns should be *Chlamydia trachomatis* and *Neisseria gonorrhoeae.* The identification of these diverse bacteria by the laboratory will require a variety of samples and culture techniques. In addition, the clinician should know the normal surface bacteria, so that the sampling techniques employed will differentiate contaminants from bacterial pathogens. Specific collection techniques will be discussed further on in this chapter.

RESPIRATORY TRACT

Upper Respiratory Tract

The obstetrician-gynecologist infrequently needs to get upper respiratory tract specimens. The most common situation is in the pregnant antepartum patient with a sore throat that is clearly inflamed on examination. The major bacterial concern for the clinician in this situation is the group A beta-hemolytic *Streptococcus.* It has been estimated that 95% of all acute episodes of pharyngitis are viral, but in patients with a sore throat of bacterial etiology, the group A beta-hemolytic *Streptococcus* is the most common offender.[2] The best microbiologic approach to confirm the diagnosis of a streptococcal pharyngitis is to obtain material from the posterior oral pharynx on a sterile swab and then to place this swab in a transport tube with sterile liquid to keep it moist. These specimens should be transported to the laboratory that same day so the swab can be plated on sheep blood agar plates. If group A beta-hemolytic streptococci are present on the swab, they will be isolated and then identified in the laboratory.

One other group of patients with pharyngitis requires special diagnostic techniques. This population may or may not present with an irritated or sore throat, but patients will give a history of having practiced fellatio. They sometimes have an inflamed throat with an exudate on examination. A swab should be utilized to get a sample of the pharyngeal secretions and then be placed in a transport tube with a liquid medium to maintain its moisture. These should be transported to the laboratory the same day, where the swab will be plated on a specific medium to enhance the growth of the probable causative organism, *Neisseria gonorrhoeae.*

Lower Respiratory Tract

Many obstetrician-gynecologists are unfamiliar with the proper diagnostic approaches to the patient with pneumonia, and most of these patients are referred to the care of internists. However, pregnant women and postoperative patients can develop pneumonia. In each of these situations, the obstetrician-gynecologist is the primary responsible physician and should have a systematic approach to specimen collection.

In the pregnant patient who presents with clinical evidence of pneumonia, the major bacterial concern should be *Streptococcus pneumoniae.* The physician will want to evaluate the infected secretions from the lower respiratory tract but must be aware of the abundance and diversity of the bacteria of the pharynx and mouth, where anaerobic flora outnumber aerobes by a factor of five to one. To confirm the presence of *Streptococcus pneumoniae* requires rapid evaluation of a sputum specimen collected under direct physician observation. Upper tract contamination of the sputum is impossible to avoid, but rapid processing will diminish this problem. The specimen should be visually examined immediately by the physician, and mucopurulent material should be selected for Gram staining and culture. The quality of the specimen collection can be judged by the presence of polymorphonuclear leukocytes and the absence of epithelial cells on the microscopic examination of the Gram stained cells. One recent study indicated that expectorated sputum is of poor quality and too contaminated for meaningful cultures to be obtained if it contains more than 10 squamous epithelial cells and fewer than 25 leukocytes per low-power microscopic field.[3]

The presence of lancet-shaped gram-positive diplococci on Gram staining is highly suggestive of the diagnosis of pneumococcal pneumonia. Care is needed in the processing of the purulent sputum for culture. Pneumococci are very susceptible to drying, and the material should be delivered to the laboratory in a tube containing Amies' modification of Stuart's medium. The impact of drying on the recovery of pneumococci is reflected in the experiment noted in Table 3–1.[4] All the swabs were saturated with an equivalent quantity of *Streptococcus pneumoniae.* In patients suspected of having a pneumococcal pneumonia, it is important to obtain blood cultures prior to the onset of therapy. If positive, these

Table 3–1. Recovery of *Streptococcus pneumoniae*

Hours at Room Temperature	Dry	Amies Transport Media
0	1×10^5	
2	0	2×10^4
4	0	2×10^4
24	0	9×10^3

(From Barry, A.L., Fay, G.D., and Sauer, R.L.: Efficiency of a transport medium for the recovery of aerobic and anaerobic bacteria from applicator swabs. Appl. Microbiol., *24*:31, 1972.)

confirm the diagnosis and the positive cultures will identify the most seriously ill patients.

Similar microbiologic specimens should be obtained in patients with other types of community-acquired pneumonias. In the patient with an influenza type A infection, the physician should be aware of the possibility of an associated *Staphylococcus aureus* pneumonia. In less critically ill patients with pneumonia, one differential diagnosis should be for *Mycoplasma pneumoniae* pneumonia, and a portion of the sputum should be sent for *Mycoplasma* culture on special media. The clinician should be aware that primary isolation may take from two to three weeks. Included in the differential diagnosis of seriously ill patients is viral pneumonia, but the same specimen samples should be obtained. In the past five years, seriously ill patients with Legionnaires' disease have been seen. These patients have a pneumonia with *Legionella pneumophila* as the pathogen, and Gram staining of the pulmonary secretions reveals few polymorphonuclear leukocytes and no bacteria.[5] Diagnosis by culture is difficult because the organism grows so slowly.

Aspiration pneumonia is usually caused by the abundant anaerobic bacterial flora of the pharynx and mouth. It may be difficult to differentiate surface flora from bacterial pathogens on a sputum specimen. In these patients, transtracheal aspiration should be considered. Fortunately for the obstetrician-gynecologists, these patients are rarely seen on our service. However, in the drug or alcohol abuser or the woman with an uncontrolled seizure disorder, this possibility should be considered. Transtracheal aspiration is not without complications, and one death has been reported with this procedure.[6] As a result, the decision to perform the procedure should rest in the hands of the infectious disease consultant.

Hospital-acquired pneumonias in postoperative and postpartum patients should elicit different microbiologic concerns from the responsible clinician. Hospitalized patients have been noted to have their upper respiratory tracts colonized by gram-negative bacteria,[7] and these may be the pathogens in the patient with a hospital-acquired pneumonia.[8] In these patients, careful microscopic examination of a good Gram stained sputum specimen will provide the first clue to the possible pathogens, which can then be confirmed by sputum or blood culture or both. Aspiration pneumonia occasionally does occur in hospitalized patients and is usually associated with general anesthesia. In addition to the concern about gram-negative aerobes, anaerobes may be involved. Here again, a decision about transtracheal aspiration should be made by the consultant. If it is done, a portion of the specimen should be placed in an oxygen-free tube for transport to the laboratory for anaerobic culture and isolation. The microscopic examination of the Gram stained sputum may strongly suggest anaerobic involvement because of the filamentous pleomorphic appearance of some of the gram-negative anaerobes that are frequently involved in these infections above the diaphragm.

URINARY TRACT

The understanding of techniques for the proper collection of urine specimens for microbiologic evaluation is important. For the obstetrician-gynecologist, infections of the urinary tract are among the most common seen in both office and hospital practice. In addition, the detection of asymptomatic bacteriuria is a necessary aspect of prenatal care. These practice considerations demand clinician knowledge about proper specimen collection.

The sine qua non for the diagnosis of asymptomatic bacteriuria or a urinary tract infection is a positive culture of properly collected and processed urine specimens, free of contamination by lower genital tract bacteria. Alternate techniques with some correlation with positive cultures may also be employed. The microscopic examination of urinary sediment avoids the 24 to 48 hour delay of the culture results, but there are shortcomings to the method. The presence of pyuria alone (five to ten leukocytes per high-power field) is not a reliable sign of infection. These white cells may be present in women with no urinary tract infection, for example in normal postpartum patients, while they may not be present in 50% of women with significant bacteriuria. There is a much better correlation between the presence of bacteria in the microscopic examination of uncentrifuged urine and a positive bacterial culture. All of these immediate microscopic evaluations should be confirmed by results of a urine culture. In addition to confirmation, the culture permits both identification of the organism and antibiotic susceptibility testing.

A number of techniques have been proposed for urine collection for culture. All have their advantages and disadvantages. A traditional method that yields an uncontaminated sample is transurethral catheterization. It avoids surface contamination but does carry with it a 1 to 2% chance of resulting bacteriuria in patients previously free of infection.[9] Direct needle aspiration of the bladder has been advocated by some investigators, either transvaginally[10] or by suprapubic aspiration.[11] Most clinicians are not enthusiastic about these invasive techniques. The time involved and the potential for complications are big factors in the decision to use other approaches. In the vast majority of cases, physicians will opt for a clean voided urine sample to obtain culture data.

Reliance upon clean voided urine samples and significant colony counts requires physician understanding of the principles advocated by Kass.[12] All obstetricians-gynecologists should be aware that urine is an excellent culture medium for bacteria. Poor cleansing of the introitus before voiding or poor collection techniques will increase the contamination of the urine specimen by lower genital tract bacteria. Physicians' responsibility for proper specimen collection does not end here. If the urine specimen cannot be transported to the laboratory immediately, storage at room temperature permits multiplication of bacteria and results in significantly higher bacterial colony counts. The major concern should be the false-positive culture result, for the urine showing no growth in a patient who is not receiving antibiotics accurately reflects the status of the urinary tract. One clean voided specimen of urine with a colony count of 100,000 or higher has an 80% chance of accuracy. That is, four out of five samples will reflect genuine urinary tract bacterial colonization, whereas one out of five will indicate specimen contamination. Two consecutive clean voided urine specimens with recovery of the same organism have a 91% chance of indicating urinary tract infection, and three consecutive specimens are 96% accurate.[13] All of these criteria show positive correlation between the colony counts of voided urine and bladder bacteria in women with asymptomatic bacteriuria. Some recent studies indicate that less than 10^5 bacteria correlates with the presence of bladder bacteria in women with dysuria[14] and is indicative of subsequent infection in hospitalized patients with an indwelling catheter.[15]

Careful evaluation of the microbiologic report of the urine sample will often indicate whether or not the specimen was properly collected and processed. In screening women for asymptomatic bacteriuria or in the evaluation of the patient with pyelonephritis, the recovery of significant numbers of many different species of bacteria almost always means specimen contamination. Patients in these categories usually have only a single species of bacteria involved. One exception is the woman with dysuria in whom more than one species may be isolated from a voided urine specimen,[14] while another is the rare patient on an ob-gyn service with some form of obstructive uropathy and a chronic urinary tract infection. In the past, the recovery of gram-positive aerobic cocci in women was thought to be a possible sign of contamination because of the infrequency with which these organisms were recovered from the urinary tract (Table 3–2).[13] On our service it is apparent that these gram-positive organisms are more frequently recovered from urine cultures, and this has been documented by Mead and Harris in San Antonio and Vermont (Table 3–3).[16]

The aforementioned base of knowledge provides guidelines for the microbiologic evaluation of women with suspected urinary tract infections. Patients should be categorized as outpatient or inpatient, since the two groups present with different problems of diagnosis.

Evaluation of the Urine of Ambulatory Patients

All pregnant women should be evaluated in the antepartum period for asymptomatic bacteriuria. Since more than 90% of the antepartum population does not have bacteriuria and transurethral catheterization carries a small risk of subsequent urinary tract infection, the specimen utilized should be from clean voided urine. A number of screening techniques can be used with this sample. Inexpensive but accurate tests are the major focus for these screening procedures. Two major types of tests are widely employed. The Greiss test measures the reduction of nitrate to nitrite in the urine caused by the presence of a significant number of en-

Table 3–2. Occurrence of Bacterial Species in Asymptomatic Bacteriuria of Pregnancy*

Genus	%
Escherichia coli	76
Klebsiella-Enterobacter	16
Proteus species	5
Pseudomonas and other gram-negative rods	1
Staphylococcus species	1
Streptococcus faecalis	1

* From Kass, E.H.: The role of asymptomatic bacteriuria in the pathogenesis of pyelonephritis. *In* Biology of Pyelonephritis. Edited by Quinn, E., and E. H. Kass. Boston, Little Brown & Co., 1960, pp. 399–412.

Table 3–3. Incidence of Group B Beta-Hemolytic Streptococcal Urinary Tract Infections in Antepartum Patients

Diagnosis	Total	Patients with Group B Infections	
		Number	(%)
Asymptomatic bacteriuria	236	11	4.7
Cystitis	68	5	7.4
Pyelonephritis	67	3	4.5
Totals	371	19	5.1

(From Mead, P.J., and Harris, R.E.: Incidence of group B beta hemolytic streptococcus in antepartum urinary tract infections. Obstet. Gynecol., *51:*412, 1978.)

terobacteria.[17] The major shortcomings of the test are that it does not yield positive results in some women with significant bacteriuria, particularly when gram-positive aerobes are involved, and some incubation time in the bladder is needed. The best specimen for this test is the first-voided urine in the morning, to achieve the incubation time needed for nitrate reduction. This was best illustrated in a study from the University of Southern California in which first-voided urine specimens were not employed, and there was a poor pickup of women with significant bacilliuria on the basis of a positive nitrite test.[18] As a result, the positive test has significance, but a negative test does not rule out the possibility of significant bacteriuria. As an alternative to the Greiss test, a number of small culture kits have been developed that the clinician can use in the office to detect significant bacterial growth.[19] When either of these types of screening tests is positive, another clean voided urine sample should be obtained for regular culture in the laboratory. This will more strongly confirm the presence or absence of significant bacteriuria (two positive tests is 91% accuracy) and also allow the laboratory to identify the microorganisms and provide antibiotic susceptibilities.

The patient who presents with symptoms of cystitis requires careful specimen collection. A major concern should be that an infection other than a bladder infection is the source of the symptoms. Women with vaginitis or urethritis may present with symptoms of frequency of and burning on urination. The vaginal secretions should be microscopically examined for the presence of yeast, trichomonads, or a nonspecific cause, and cervical swabs should be obtained and cultured on specific media for *Neisseria gonorrhoeae*. The majority of these acutely dysuric women will have urinary tract infections. A carefully obtained clean voided urine specimen is needed for the diagnosis, and it is important that the clinician and the laboratory work together with the new diagnostic criteria for the patient. Recent studies using careful methods of microbiologic confirmation indicate that only 51% of these dysuric women with coliforms in bladder urine had equal to or greater than 10^5 bacteria per ml of midstream urine.[14] The most predictive test for these patients is a count of coliform bacteria equal to or greater than 10^2 per ml of urine. The clinician should have an understanding with the clinical laboratory that in all clean voided urine specimens from women with dysuria, coliform bacteria in quantities of 10^2 or greater will be identified and antibiotic susceptibilities obtained. In addition, many of these women will have more than one organism isolated from the midstream specimen (Table 3–4).[14] The isolation of multiple bacteria in these cases should not represent specimen contamination.

Table 3–4. Percentage of Midstream Urine Specimens Containing Mixed Growth (More than One Organism Isolated) by Colony Count Among Patients with Coliform Bladder Infections

Colony Count	Number with Mixed Growth / Total Number of Specimen
Coliforms per ml	
$\geq 10^5$	16 of 50 (32%)
10^4	14 of 19 (74%)
10^3	6 of 10 (60%)
10^2	11 of 14 (79%)
10^1	4 of 5 (80%)

(From Stamm, W.E., Counts, G.W., Running, K.R., Fihn, S., Turck, M., and Holmes, K.K.: Diagnosis of coliform infection in acutely dysuric women. N. Engl. J. Med., *307:*463, 1982. Reprinted by permission of the New England Journal of Medicine.)

Evaluation of the Urine of Hospitalized Patients

For the responsible physician, the microbiologic evaluation of urine from hospitalized patients usually presents a different set of circumstances. Screening procedures for asymptomatic bacteriuria make up a smaller percentage of the total number of urine tests. When screening is done on preoperative patients, reliance upon a clean voided technique and the criteria of Kass seems appropriate. For most hospitalized patients, the urine evaluation is done for women with symptoms of urinary tract infection or as part of the workup of febrile postoperative or postpartum patients. The patient with a community-acquired urinary tract infection or with pyelonephritis who requires hospital admission presents minimal diagnostic problems. The clinical picture is almost always clear-cut. In most cases, a clean voided urine sample can be obtained for urinalysis and culture. Occasionally, these febrile patients will have difficulty voiding and providing an uncontaminated specimen, and in such symptomatic women, it is appropriate to obtain a urine sample by transurethral catheterization.

The complete workup of a febrile hospitalized postoperative or postpartum patient is another matter. In these patients, one possible site of infection is the urinary tract. In some, an indwelling transurethral or suprapubic catheter will be in place at the time of evaluation, and a urine sample for culture can be obtained from these conduits. In all postoperative and postpartum patients who require an indwelling catheter, it is a prudent move to routinely send a portion of the last collected urine for culture when the catheter is removed. If the patient subsequently becomes febrile, this culture report may be helpful in the evaluation.

There can be problems in obtaining an adequate urine specimen in febrile hospitalized patients. Many of these women have varying degrees of voiding difficulties, which may be attributable to perineal discomfort from an episiotomy or colporrhaphy incision or abdominal discomfort from an incision site. Although it may require close physician or nursing supervision, most of these patients are able to provide a clean voided urine sample for microscopic examination and culture. Occasionally, on immediate microscopic examination of the specimen by the physician, it will be obvious that it is contaminated. In this circumstance, alternate invasive sampling techniques should be employed. These include transurethral catheterization, which is the most popular method but carries with it a low percentage possibility that women free of urinary tract problems may develop an infection from the catheterization.[9] As alternatives, transvaginal[10] and transabdominal aspiration[11] also can be employed. These have never achieved great popularity because they are invasive techniques and must be performed by the physician. The same principles of specimen collection should be applied to hospitalized women being treated for bacteriuria or urinary tract infection who are being tested for cure. Rarely is a specimen obtained by catheterization necessary.

LOWER GENITAL TRACT

Evaluation of the Asymptomatic Antepartum Patient

Over the past two decades, a wide range of microbiologic screening surveys have been done in asymptomatic pregnant women. Studies have demonstrated a poorer outcome for the newborn in pregnant women with lower genital tract carriage of group B beta-hemolytic *Streptococcus*,[20] *Neisseria gonorrhoeae*,[21] *Mycoplasma*,[22] and *Chlamydia*.[23] Although the relationship between maternal vaginal colonization and infection in the neonate has statistical significance, to date no study has demonstrated a cause and effect relationship. Studies of antibiotic intervention in the mother resulting in elimination of surface bacteria have not achieved better clinical results. Although it may not be cost-effective, an antepartum endocervical culture for *Neisseria gonorrhoeae* will identify women whose infants are at risk for infection.

Some high-risk antepartum patients should have a microbiologic evaluation. A lower genital tract culture for the presence of *Listeria monocytogenes* should be obtained in women with a history of either one or more midtrimester pregnancy losses or the delivery of an infant who subsequently develops a *Listeria monocytogenes* infection.[24] The endocervical swab should be placed in a liquid transport medium to be subsequently plated in the laboratory. The laboratory request should specifically ask for *Listeria monocytogenes* identification. Awareness of this diagnostic priority may help lab technicians avoid the hasty assumption that aerobic gram-positive bacilli are diphtheroids, as on this assumption they would fail to do the specific tests to identify *Listeria.* In the woman with a history of genital herpes during pregnancy who is asymptomatic, an endocervical culture for the virus should be obtained at 36 weeks' gestation and repeated at weekly intervals until the patient delivers.[25] The swab should be placed in a viral transport medium to be taken to the laboratory. If the culture is positive in a woman with no visible lesions, it should be repeated in one week. If the patient has perineal lesions or complains of prodromal perineal discomfort without visible lesions, a perineal culture should be obtained as well. In those with premature rupture of the membranes, three separate swabs should be obtained at the time of sterile speculum examination. One is placed in a standard transport medium for subsequent culture for group B *Streptococcus* and *Listeria monocytogenes;* one is placed in a special transport medium for the culture of *Neisseria gonorrhoeae;* and the third is placed in a special transport medium for *Chlamydia* culture. Although *Chlamydia* is grown on cell culture, as are viruses, the transport media may be different from some of the tetracycline-containing transport media for viruses, which will inhibit the recovery of *Chlamydia.* The new monoclonal antibody tests for *Chlamydia* will eliminate the necessity for cell culture in most laboratories.

Evaluation of the Symptomatic Patient—Vulvar Lesions

The physician evaluating patients with vulvar lesions must understand the underlying fear and concern of women about genital herpes simplex. The heavy publicity of the lay press, combined with the reality of the disease, has had an impact on the psyche of sexually active women. A careful history should be obtained from these patients, and at the time of physical examination they should be asked to point out the exact site of perineal discomfort. If the patient is seen early in the course of the illness, small, clear vesicles may be present; sometimes they will be gone by the time the patient is seen by the physician. Since the diagnosis of herpes is most reliable by culture, all physicians should have transport media available for the transfer of the specimen to the hospital or state laboratory for culture. A sterile swab should be used to abrade the lesion and to obtain as much of the secretions as possible for culture. It is the responsibility of the physician to ensure that the hospital or state laboratories provide this viral culture service, for blood antibody testing does not define the activity of herpes simplex infection.

There are a number of less common lesions that will be seen in the vulva. Any ulcer, particularly a painless one, should be evaluated by dark-field microscopic examination. Most hospitals have facilities and personnel available to do the test. The presence of spirochetes in the microscopic examination confirms the diagnosis of primary syphilis. Raised wartlike lesions are usually diagnosed as condyloma acuminatum. A small biopsy specimen will confirm the diagnosis and rule out the much less common condyloma latum due to syphilis. In older postmenopausal women, a small break in the skin at the introitus may cause discomfort during intercourse. Although this usually results from a lack of estrogen, a biopsy is helpful to avoid overlooking a malignancy.

There are also more rarely encountered lesions of the vulva in gynecologic patients. These are often long-standing and involve fistula formation. The clinical evaluation of these lesions requires a biopsy for pathologic confirmation and appropriate microbiologic cultures. The most common etiologic agents in these rare cases are *Chlamydia* (the pathogen in *lymphogranuloma venereum*), the gram-negative rod *Hemophilus ducreyi* (which causes chancroid), the gram-negative aerobe *Donovania granulomatis* (which causes granuloma inguinale), and *Mycobacterium tuberculosis* (which causes cutaneous tuberculosis). Specific microbiologic tests can be employed to help confirm the diagnosis. A portion of the sample should be placed in an appropriate transport medium to support the growth of *Chlamydia*. If material can be aspirated from fluctuant inguinal nodes, it should be plated on either rabbit blood agar or chocolate agar to isolate *Hemophilus ducreyi*. The vulvar lesions should be scraped and the Giemsa stain applied. The presence of small encapsulated bodies in mononuclear cells—Donovan's bodies—confirms the diagnosis of granuloma inguinale. A portion of the biopsy should be incubated anaerobically in a medium containing egg yolk to isolate the organism. An additional portion of the biopsy should be sent for culture for tuberculosis. These patients are rare cases and will be an infrequent concern for the gynecologist-obstetrician. All the various microbiologic transport media should be ready in advance of the biopsy so that all the appropriate tests can be done at one time.

Evaluation of the Symptomatic Patient—Vaginal Disease

An inappropriate physician evaluation may delay the accurate diagnosis of the patient with a symptomatic vaginal discharge. So much emphasis has been placed on the gross appearance of the major categories of vaginal infections that too often the busy outpatient physician forgoes immediate microscopic examination of vaginal secretions. In addition, many physicians will request a bacterial culture of the secretions to guide their therapy, particularly in the patient who fails to respond to the first course of therapy. A wide variety of vaginal aerobic and anaerobic bacteria have been recovered from both asymptomatic and symptomatic patients.[26] No study to date has demonstrated that the isolation of a specific bacterial species, such as *Escherichia coli* or the group D *Streptococcus,* has been associated with any vaginal disease.[27] Because of this, bacterial culture screening in symptomatic women should be avoided. It wastes the patient's money and too frequently leads to inappropriate antibiotic therapy that does not eliminate symptoms and in fact may worsen them.

An important starting point in the evaluation of symptomatic women with vaginal discharge is physician recognition that all lubricating jellies contain substances that may either inhibit the growth of or kill many microorganisms. Jellies should be avoided when the speculum is inserted in these patients so that the vaginal secretions can be obtained for microscopic examination and culture if indicated.

An immediate microscopic examination of the vaginal secretions should be performed by the physician in every case. One part of secretions obtained by a swab should be transferred to a slide containing a drop of saline at room temperature and a coverslip applied, and a second portion should be placed on a second slide with a drop of 10% potassium hydroxide. The resulting mixture on the second slide should be smelled by the physician for a fishlike odor, and then a coverslip applied. Each of these specimens should then be examined microscopically. In the saline specimen, the diagnosis of the protozoan *Trichomonas vaginalis* is made by the presence of the active, flagellated single-celled organism. Mycelia may be present in the saline suspension but more often are confirmed in the microscopic examination of the KOH preparation. Although the presence of "clue" cells—stippled epithelial cells whose cytoplasm is filled with gram-negative rods—has been touted as the most distinctive diagnostic feature of nonspecific vaginitis,[28] the diagnostic specificity of these cells has not been proved.[29] I believe that the most specific diagnostic test for nonspecific vaginitis is the presence of a fishlike odor when vaginal secretions are added to the KOH on the slide. All of these immediate microscopic examinations will suffice for diagnosis of over 90% of women seen with vaginitis.

In these symptomatic patients, culture for *Neisseria gonorrhoeae* should frequently be obtained. In an evaluation of those presenting to an emergency room with symptoms of vaginitis, significantly more had positive culture results for *Neisseria gonorrhoeae.*[30] In addition, symptomatic women who have been sexually active with more than one partner or whose male partner has been sexually active with more than one woman should have a culture done for the presence of *Neisseria gonorrhoeae.*

The recovery of the pathogen *Neisseria gonorrhoeae* from the lower genital tract requires knowledge of the special growth requirements of this microorganism. This gram-negative diplococci, which survives so well in the mucous membranes of an intact male or female host, does not compete well in the laboratory with the bacterial representatives of the abundant normal flora of the lower genital tract of sexually active women. To encourage growth of the organism, a medium enriched with glutamine and carboxylase should be placed in a carbon dioxide–

rich environment. The most popular media have been modifications of the original medium of Thayer and Martin, which contains the antibiotics vancomycin and colistimethate plus the antifungal agent nystatin; these are added to the agar to inhibit the growth of competing organisms.[31]

A number of surveys have been performed to determine the anatomic sites of *Neisseria gonorrhoeae* with the highest yield of positive results.[32] A few patients had positive culture results with rectal specimens when the results of endocervical cultures were negative, but the most important time for routine utilization of the rectal site for culture is after antibiotic treatment of a patient who previously had a positive culture to determine if the organism has been eliminated. The routine sampling of this site led to discovery of more than one third of treatment failures that would have been missed by endocervical sampling alone.[33] The traditional microscopic examination of a Gram-stained endocervical smear for the presence of gram-negative intracellular diplococci is not diagnostic, because it has major shortcomings: These diplococci are often not seen in the smear of a patient with a positive culture, and other *Neisseria,* not *Neisseria gonorrhoeae,* may be present in patients whose culture results are negative.

With this as background, cultures for *Neisseria gonorrhoeae* can be obtained and there is an excellent chance for recovery of the organism if it is present in the endocervix. When these patients are first seen, a swab should be placed in the endocervical canal and kept there for at least 15 seconds; it should then be processed immediately. A number of commercial kits are available that will recover *Neisseria gonorrhoeae* and also allow the oxidase test to be performed to confirm the diagnosis. This can be done within the office setting. An alternative approach has been to utilize transport media to maintain the viability of the *Neisseria gonorrhoeae* on the specimen swab until primary plating can be done in the laboratory. There are much better techniques than the alternative of a dry swab in a sterile tube (Table 3–5).[4] Both Stuart's and Amies' transport media are commercially available, but the recovery of *Neisseria gonorrhoeae* drops with time, and significant losses can be demonstrated after 24 hours.[4] With the increase in the number of cases of penicillin-resistant gonorrhea being isolated in the United States, all positive cultures for *Neisseria gonorrhoeae* should be tested for penicillin resistance. This will be obvious in the lack of growth inhibition around the penicillin disc, and specific tests for the presence of beta-lactamase can be performed.

Table 3–5. Effect of a Transport Medium on the Recovery of *Neisseria gonorrhoeae* from Two Types of Swabs

Swab	Hours at Room Temperature	Dry	Amies Transport
Cotton	0	7×10^5 (700,000)	—
	2	2×10^2 (200)	1×10^4 (4000)
	4	0	3×10^3 (900)
	24	0	10
Calcium alginate	0	1×10^6 (1,000,000)	—
	2	0	5×10^3 (5000)
	4	0	2×10^3 (2000)
	24	0	0

(From Barry, A.L., Fay, G.D., and Sauer, R.L.: Efficiency of a transport medium for the recovery of aerobic and anaerobic bacteria from applicator swabs. Appl. Microbiol., *24:*31, 1972.)

Special microbiologic studies should be done in some women with symptoms of vaginitis. In the patient with a discharge but no abnormal findings at the time of the initial microbiologic examination by the physician, a culture should be carried out for *Candida albicans*. A swab with vaginal secretions should be placed on Sabouraud's medium, or one of the commercial kits to grow *Candida* that are available for office practice should be used. For the patient with *Trichomonas* infection who is a treatment failure and not a reinfection case, the CDC should be contacted so that appropriate culture media can be obtained that will permit growth of *Trichomonas vaginalis* and subsequent analysis for susceptibility to metronidazole. In the patient with a discharge who has a normal microscopic examination, no yeast growth on culture, and who clinically has a cervicitis, endocervical cultures should be obtained for *Chlamydia*. The endocervical swab should be placed in a transport medium and sent to the laboratory for culture on cells. In the patient wearing an intrauterine device who has a "dirty" Pap smear with clumps of debris,[34] an endocervical swab should be placed in an oxygen-free tube and sent to the lab for culture to confirm the presence of *Actinomycosis bovis*. There is still controversy about the diagnostic significance of the recovery of *Gardnerella vaginalis* from vaginal secretions, because it can be found in asymptomatic women.[35] At present, the fishy odor of vaginal secretions with the addition of 10% KOH seems diagnostic for nonspecific vaginitis, and cultures for *Gardnerella vaginalis* are not recommended as a test for cure.

Recovery of Anaerobic Bacteria from Clinical Sites

Proper specimen collection of anaerobic bacteria in pelvic infections requires physician awareness of the normal bacterial flora of the lower genital tract and knowledge of the capabilities of clinical laboratories in processing material for anaerobic bacteria. There is an abundant anaerobic flora in the vagina and endocervix. When women develop a pelvic infection, such as postpartum endomyometritis or salpingitis, the lower genital tract is utilized by the physician for examination and culture. Any attempt to sample either the endometrium through the endocervix or the peritoneal cavity through the vagina must be made with the awareness of this surface contamination. In addition, anaerobic culture techniques in the clinical laboratory have not been quantified as they have for aerobes in urine specimens. A swab of the endometrium brought through the contaminated endocervix cannot be evaluated for significant numbers of pathogenic anaerobes as opposed to small numbers of normal surface flora. A significant colony count for anaerobic bacteria cannot be generated in clinical microbiologic laboratories. Because of this, it makes no sense to submit a vaginal swab or an endocervical swab for anaerobic bacterial isolation in a patient with a pelvic infection. This practice is expensive and does not contribute to the therapeutic decisions of the responsible physician.

There are specific sampling techniques for anaerobes that should be utilized whenever possible. Every attempt should be made to eliminate the surface contamination of the lower genital tract and then to sample the site of infection. In patients with a suspected anaerobic uterine infection after either abortion or delivery, a number of double-lumen sheathed techniques have been devised to eliminate surface contamination.[36, 37] To date, however, there has not been great enthusiasm for these techniques, for two reasons. (1) There is concern that surface contamination has not been eliminated with these new instruments, and (2) the procedure does require the physician to perform a pelvic examination, often during the hours of the evening (for this is the time when the first temperature elevation occurs). Alternative sampling sites have been employed in these women with suspected uterine infections. An attempt at direct aspiration of the uterine cavity through the abdominal wall has been reported.[38] This eliminates the surface contamination of the lower genital tract, but the yield of positive cultures has been low. Alternatively, needle culdocentesis of the peritoneal cavity in women with a postpartum endomyometritis has been done.[39] The yield of positive anaerobic cultures was much higher, but the extent of surface vaginal contamination is not known. Neither of those methods has achieved any clinical popularity, and they are not in current use in this country.

In antepartum women with premature labor[40] or premature rupture of the membranes,[41] transabdominal amniocentesis has been performed to obtain amniotic fluid for microscopic examination and culture. Anaerobic bacteria have been recovered from these samples. In women with salpingitis, great stress has been placed on the peritoneal fluid obtained by needle culdocentesis for anaerobic culture.[42] This method does not eliminate the concern about surface contamination, however, and in one study there was poor correlation between organisms in the peritoneal fluid and those obtained directly from tubal fluid aspiration.[43] Recently, there has been interest expressed in the sheathed double-lumen endometrial aspiration in women with salpingitis to detect the presence of *Chlamydia*.[44]

Specimens for anaerobic culture most likely to be free of surface contamination are those obtained from the infection site at the time of operation. Amniotic fluid obtained at the time of cesarean section, purulent material aspirated directly from a pelvic abscess, or a portion of an abscess wall itself eliminates the concern about surface contamination, and the material usually has large numbers of organisms present. These purulent collections can be placed in a glass syringe and the needle capped with a rubber stopper. The glass is better than a plastic syringe because it is not permeable to the air, but the huge numbers of anaerobes present in most purulent specimens do not make the availability of glass syringes a critical element in specimen collection.

Along with an awareness of the problems of surface contamination, there are a number of other important concerns in the anaerobic specimen to be processed in the laboratory. An aspirate of infected material is always preferable to a swab. A frequently repeated error of specimen collection occurs in the operating room during the incision and drainage of a pelvic abscess. The pus is carried by suction to a cannister on the wall, and a barely moist swab is sent to the laboratory in a sterile tube. In situations in which purulent material can be obtained, a sample of the pus is always preferable to a swab.

After obtaining an appropriate specimen, the most critical factor in the isolation of anaerobic organisms in the laboratory is the length of time the collected specimen is exposed to atmospheric oxygen. The longer the interval of exposure before plating in the laboratory, the less likely it is that anaerobic bacteria will be isolated. A number of good transport systems have been devised and are currently in use in many institutions. One prototype is oxygen-free tubes for transport to the laboratory. The clinician should be aware that these tubes need to be held upright when the specimen is inserted so that atmospheric oxygen will not enter the system, since the carbon dioxide used to fill the tubes is heavier than air. These oxygen-free tubes markedly increase the length of time that anaerobes remain alive on the clinical specimen. Despite this, the oxygen-free tubes require 24-hour coverage within the laboratory so that the specimen can be processed immediately to ensure the growth of anaerobes. This immediate processing is particularly important if a swab specimen has been obtained. If a quantity of pus has been collected in an oxygen-free tube, a few hours of delay will not interfere with the recovery of anaerobes.

An alternative to oxygen-free tubes for transport is bedside plating of the specimen by the clinician, utilizing a portable anaerobic jar. Although this is an effective method,[45] it has not proved to be popular on clinical services except for research.

Another method for the handling of specimens for recovery of anaerobes is a transport medium. This is an inferior method for a number of reasons. The recovery of anaerobes with this technique is less successful than with other techniques. Nearly all the organisms we call aerobes are facultative anaerobes and will successfully compete with anaerobes for the nutrients in the transport broth; therefore the anaerobes may be overgrown. In addition, identification of individual anaerobes may be slower because recognition of bacterial growth in the broth requires subculture and two or three more days of incubation before the preliminary anaerobic identification can be done. Despite these disadvantages, this technique is widely used because it has the advantage of simplicity and easy incorporation into existing laboratory procedures that do not provide 24-hour coverage.

Pelvic Examination for Patients with a Soft-Tissue Pelvic Infection

Significant specimens can be obtained during the pelvic examination and prior to antibiotic therapy; these may be of great help in the subsequent management of patients. Clinicians should require that the materials needed for culture are available in the hospital in which they work. A complete microscopic data base should be obtained on all patients.

Infections Resulting from Abortions

A number of specimens will be important for the evaluation of the patient with an infection after an abortion. Aerobic endocervical cultures should be obtained, particularly to screen for the presence of group A beta-hemolytic *Streptococcus*. Special care should be used to obtain an endocervical swab culture that will grow *Neisseria gonorrhoeae* if present. This is an important microbiology test, for one study from Baltimore showed a higher infection rate after termination of pregnancy in women whose cultures were positive for this organism.[46] If a double-lumen sheathed endometrial sampling system is available, endometrial cultures should be obtained for aerobes and anaerobes. One recent study implicates *Chlamydia* in postabortion infections;[47] therefore a protected specimen should be cultured for this organism if the laboratory is capable of doing the test. Aspiration through the cul-de-sac to obtain peritoneal fluid for aerobic and anaerobic cultures is a helpful test in the seriously ill patient. The endocervical culture should not be used as a test for microbiologic cure in patients with a postabortion infection because of the abundant surface flora that may persist despite antibiotic therapy. Repeat endocervical cultures for *Neisseria gonorrhoeae* are necessary in the patient with a pretreatment culture that was positive for this organism.

Salpingo-oophoritis

The number of microscopic tests performed on women with salpingitis should be influenced by the microbiologic data collected to date. An endocervical swab should be obtained for aerobic culture to grow *Neisseria gonorrhoeae* if present. Testing should not stop here, however, for there is little correlation between the organisms recovered from this sample and those in the infected fallopian tubes.[48] There is controversy about the use of culdocentesis aspiration for culture. Monif and colleagues have championed this test as the biologic marker in their classification of salpingitis as endometritis-salpingitis-peritonitis,[42] while Sweet and associates have questioned its value because of the poor microbiologic correlation between peritoneal bacteria and those bacteria isolated from the fallopian tube secretions of patients with salpingitis at laparoscopy.[43] Despite these concerns, the test is very helpful to the physician in the evaluation of the afebrile patient suspected of having salpingitis. The presence of bacteria on the immediate Gram stained peritoneal fluid makes the diagnosis more secure. Attempts to recover *Chlamydia* from peritoneal fluid have rarely met with success. As an alternative diagnostic step, there is evidence that *Chlamydia* can be isolated from endometrial biopsies utilizing a double-lumen technique.[44]

Antepartum Patients with Premature Labor or Premature Rupture of the Membranes

A clean examination with a sterile speculum should be performed in women with premature labor and premature rupture of the membranes. The physician's major concern is to identify organisms that might have an adverse effect on the newborn. Two swabs should be obtained from the surface of the cervix, one for aerobic cultures and one for the isolation of *Neisseria gonorrhoeae*. The important aerobic isolates are the group A and B beta-hemolytic streptococci, *Escherichia coli*, and *Listeria monocytogenes*. In addition, a viral culture should be done for herpes simplex. In these patients, there should also be awareness that bacterial contamination of the amniotic fluid may precede the clinical events of premature labor or premature rupture of the membranes.[40, 41] This sequence occurs infrequently, so there should be careful case selection before a transabdominal amniocentesis is performed to obtain an uncontaminated sample of amniotic fluid.[49] In patients with premature labor, amniocentesis should be reserved for the mother to be who requires a second course with intravenous tocolytic agents. If induction is not planned in women with premature rupture of the membranes at less than 34 weeks' gestation, the amniocentesis should be performed on the patient who has both demonstrable amniotic fluid on ultrasonography, and a uterine window free of placenta for the procedure.[50] The fluid should be submitted for aerobic and anaerobic cultures, and an immediate microscopic examination of Gram stained uncentrifuged fluid should be performed. There is correlation between the presence of bacteria on the microscopic examination and growth of bacteria on culture.[40, 49]

Intrapartum Patient with Chorioamnionitis

In the febrile patient in labor suspected of having chorioamnionitis, an uncontaminated specimen of amniotic fluid should be obtained for microscopic study and for aerobic and anaerobic cultures. A simple but effective technique utilizes an intrauterine catheter. If not already in place, a catheter should be inserted to monitor the progress of labor in these women because of the high cesarean section rate for "failure to progress." Seven ml of fluid should be withdrawn and discarded to clear the line, and then a fresh sample should be obtained with a clean syringe.[40] The amniotic fluid should be subjected to microscopic examination and aerobic and anaerobic cultures. In these women in labor, the best correlation between the microscopic examination and bacterial isolation is the presence of bacteria on an unspun specimen. White blood cells are frequently seen in amniotic fluid of women in labor who have no clinical evidence of infection[50] (Figure 3–1); therefore their presence is not diagnostic.

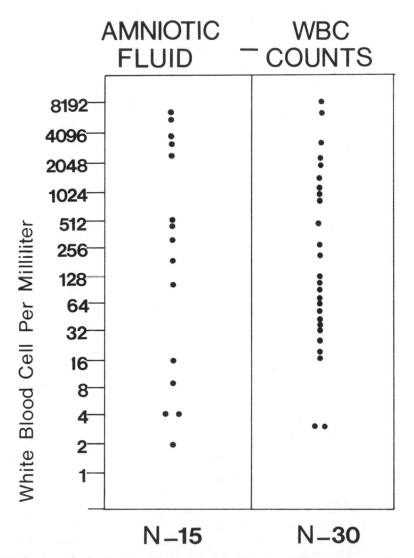

Fig. 3–1. Amniotic fluid white blood cell counts from patients in labor. The 15 patients in the left column developed an infection, while the 30 patients in the right column did not.
(From Bobitt, J.R., and Ledger, W.J.: Amniotic fluid analysis. Obstet. Gynecol., *51:*56, 1978.)

The Postpartum Patient

Postpartum patients with infections should have a careful pelvic examination performed. Aerobic cultures for the group A and group B beta-hemolytic strep- tococci should be done, as well as the special techniques needed to isolate *Neisseria gonorrhoeae*. Anaerobic cultures should not be employed unless surface bacterial contamination can be avoided by the utilization of a double lumen for specimen collection. In patients with a late developing postpartum infection after discharge from the hospital, an endometrial culture using the sheathed technique should be done for the possible isolation of *Chlamydia*.[51]

Intraoperative Cultures in Gynecologic Operative Procedures

Any surgical patient with an active infection or an abscess should have direct aspiration of the material to test for aerobic and anaerobic organisms. In addition, women having tubal reconstructive operations with lysis of pelvic adhesions should have a sample of those adhesions sent for chlamydial culture, because of the strong possibility of recovering these organisms in this situation.[52] A specimen of the adhesions should be placed in a liquid transport medium to be processed in the laboratory for the presence of *Chlamydia*.

The Febrile Postoperative Gynecologic Patient

A pelvic examination should be performed as part of the fever workup of every postoperative gynecologic patient. If the uterus is still in place, a needle culdo- centesis may be appropriate when a soft-tissue pelvic infection is suspected. The aspirated material should be examined microscopically and aerobic and anaerobic cultures should be performed. In the patient who has had a hysterectomy, the vaginal cuff should be carefully assessed. If a collection is suspected on exami- nation, it should be aspirated with a needle-syringe and the fluid evaluated with Gram stain and sent for aerobic and anaerobic cultures. The author has rarely been able to aspirate fluid in this clinical situation, and instead a swab of the cuff material may be sent in the appropriate transport tubes. If the febrile patient has an abdominal incision, this should be examined. If there is drainage from the wound, it should be opened in its entirety in order to evaluate the integrity of the fascia as well as to collect purulent material for Gram staining and aerobic and anaerobic cultures. If the febrile patient has had a transverse abdominal incision and no grossly purulent material is present on exposure of the subcu- taneous tissue, a needle aspirate of the subfascial space should be performed to be sure that purulent material is not present there.

Cultures of Rectal Material

In addition to women who will need cultures of rectal samples for *Neisseria gonorrhoeae* as a test for cure, there are two separate groups of patients who require such cultures as part of their cure. The huge influx of Asian and Caribbean refugees into the United States in the past few years has increased the pool of women with parasitic intestinal disease being seen by the obstetrician-gynecologist. In those suspected of having these diseases, a fresh stool sample should be obtained and submitted for ova and parasite examination.[53] The other population to be examined includes women who develop diarrhea—five or more bowel movements in a 24-hour period—while on antibiotics. Although clindamycin is the antibiotic that immediately comes to mind, this problem can be seen with all systemic antibiotics prescribed for hospitalized patients. The patient should be examined and a rectal swab left in place for at least 15 seconds and then placed in an oxygen-free tube to be cultured for *Clostridium difficili*. Many laboratories are now capable of identifying the toxin produced by this organism if it is present in a stool specimen.[54]

Blood Cultures

The blood culture is the single most important microbiologic assessment of the hospitalized febrile patient on the obstetric-gynecologic service. Surface veins are more accessible to the clinician than deep pelvic structures, and surface contamination by the bacterial skin flora is more easily avoided than contamination by the normal flora of the vagina and endocervix when pelvic structures are sampled. A positive blood culture result helps the clinician to focus on the most invasive of the bacteria in these multibacterial pelvic infections. In the past, we have assumed that patients with bacteremia are our most seriously ill,[55] but with modern aggressive antibiotic coverage, this does not seem to be true of the obstetric patient.[56] There is a wide variation in the number of women sampled who subsequently have positive blood cultures. Rotheram and Schick recovered microorganisms from the blood of 34 of 56 (60.7%) patients who had had septic abortions.[57] Our sampling of obstetric and gynecologic patients at the Los Angeles County-University of Southern California Medical Center yielded a lower percentage of positive cultures, 139 of 1410 patients or 9.9%.[55] The yield of positive blood cultures is much higher in postpartum patients. In an evaluation of febrile patients with endomyometritis following cesarean section, 48 of 200 or 24% had positive blood cultures.[58]

Great care should be exercised in the collection of blood for culture. The fluid culture system that receives the blood is designed to promote the growth of the few organisms that may be in the bloodstream. It should be obvious to the clinician that the system is equally capable of growing a few organisms from surface contamination if care has not been taken in the sample collection. Steps to avoid skin contamination should be followed in every patient. The skin site for specimen collection should be degreased by vigorous cleansing with alcohol sponges. Following this, an antiseptic solution with iodine should be applied to the site, and it should be allowed to dry. The blood sample should be obtained without palpation of the vein after the antiseptic solution has been applied. When the blood sample has been collected, the needle should be discarded and a fresh needle used to inoculate the bottle containing the medium. Most microbiology laboratories provide an anaerobic and an aerobic bottle, with the latter vented so that atmospheric oxygen will be added to the system at the time of inoculation. Ideally, two separate skin sites should be employed at the time of the initial evaluation, so that four bottles will be available for study in the laboratory. Although repeated blood culture samples at half-hour intervals are important in the workup of the patient suspected of having subacute bacterial endocarditis, they have not been routinely done in the workup of the febrile hospitalized patient on the obstetric-gynecologic service. Washington has suggested that three sets of blood cultures over a 24-hour period will yield a higher percentage of positive cultures.[59] This hypothesis needs to be tested in obstetric-gynecologic patients. Organisms of low pathogenicity that are part of the normal bacterial flora should usually be regarded as contaminants when recovered in a blood culture. For example, it is normally prudent to disregard the isolation of the coagulase-negative staphylococci, *Bacillus* species, diphtheroids, and *Propionibacterium acnes*. However, in a debilitated febrile oncology patient undergoing chemotherapy, the recovery of coagulase-negative staphylococci may be significant. In one recent study, 5.8% of the organisms isolated in patients with positive blood cultures were thought to be contaminants.[55] On some services, the differentiation between skin contamination and bloodstream sampling has been based on the criterion that more than one of the blood culture bottles must produce positive results. However, MacGregor and Beatty report that by following this criterion, there are still 11% of contaminated specimens that would be incorrectly read as positive.[60]

Some obstetric-gynecologic patients will require special considerations when blood for culture is obtained. Patients on systemic antibiotics may have a secondary temperature elevation. Since the blood specimen bottles are usually large (100 ml) and are designed to enhance the growth of a few organisms, the more blood added to the bottle, the higher the concentration of antibiotic in the culture medium. Instead of 10 ml of blood, only 2 ml should be inoculated in these cases. An additional clinical concern is the debilitated patient who develops fungemia after prolonged antibiotic treatment and long periods of hyperalimentation.[61] This differential diagnosis should be considered in every septic patient undergoing this therapy. Blood cultures can yield the diagnosis, but Hoschal has shown good correlation between positive results from blood cultures in these women and the presence of fungal forms in the urine.[62] If these fungal forms are seen in the urine, the intravenous line should be removed immediately.

REFERENCES

1. Ohm, M.J., and Galask, R.P.: The effect of antibiotic prophylaxis on patients undergoing total abdominal hysterectomy. I. Effect on morbidity. Am. J. Obstet. Gynecol., *125*:442, 1976.
2. Infectious Disease. Kalamazoo, Michigan, The Upjohn Company, 1974.
3. Geckler, R.W., Gremillion, D.H., McAllister, C.K., and Ellenbogen, C.: Microscopic and bacteriological comparison of paired sputa and transtracheal aspirates. J. Clin. Microbiol., *6*:396, 1977.
4. Barry, A.L., Fay, G.D., and Sauer, R.L.: Efficiency of a transport medium for the recovery of aerobic and anaerobic bacteria from applicator swabs. Appl. Microbiol., *24*:31, 1972.
5. Meyer, R.D., and Finegold, S.M.: Legionnaire's disease. Ann. Rev. Med., *31*:219, 1980.
6. Ries, K., Levison, M.E., and Kaye, D.: Transtracheal aspiration in pulmonary infection. Arch. Intern. Med., *133*:453, 1974.
7. Johanson, W.G., Pierce, A.K., Sanford, J.P., and Thomas, G.D.: Nosocomial respiratory infections with gram negative bacilli. Ann. Intern. Med., *77*:701, 1972.
8. George, W.L., and Finegold, S.M.: Bacterial infections of the lung. Chest, *81*:502, 1982.
9. Jackson, G.G., Arana-Sialer, J.A., Anderson, B.R., Grieble, H.G., and McCabe, W.R.: Profiles of pyelonephritis. Ann. Intern. Med., *110*:663, 1962.
10. Simpson, J.W., McCracken, A.W., and Radwin, H.M.: Transvaginal aspiration of bladder in screening for bacteriuria. Obstet. Gynecol., *43*:215, 1974.
11. Dove, G.A., and Gower, P.E.: Suprapubic aspiration in general practice. Lancet, *2*:304, 1977.
12. Kass, E.H.: Bacteriuria and the diagnosis of infections of the urinary tract. Arch. Intern. Med., *100*:709, 1957.
13. Kass, E.H.: The role of asymptomatic bacteriuria in the pathogenesis of pyelonephritis. *In* Biology of Pyelonephritis. Edited by E. Quinn and E.H. Kass. Boston, Little, Brown & Co., 1960, pp. 399–412.
14. Stamm, W.E., Counts, G.W., Running, K.R., Fihn, S., Turck, M., and Holmes, K.K.: Diagnosis of coliform infection in acutely dysuric women. N. Engl. J. Med., *307*:463, 1982.
15. Stark, R.P., and Maki, D.G.: Bacteriuria in the catheterized patient. What quantitative level of bacteriuria is relevant? N. Engl. J. Med., *311*:560, 1984.

16. Mead, P.J., and Harris, R.E.: Incidence of group B beta hemolytic streptococcus in antepartum urinary tract infections. Obstet. Gynecol., *51*:412, 1978.
17. Czerwinski, A.W., Wilkerson, R.G., Merrill, J.A., Braden, B., and Colmore, J.P.: Further evaluation of the Greiss test to detect significant bacteriuria. Am. J. Obstet. Gynecol., *110*:677, 1971.
18. Lenke, R.R., and Von Dorsten, J.P.: The efficacy of the nitrite test and microscopic urinalysis in predicting urine culture results. Am. J. Obstet. Gynecol., *140*:427, 1981.
19. Kunin, C.M., and DeGroot, J.E.: Self screening for significant bacteriuria. Evaluation of Dip-Strip combination nitrate/culture test. J.A.M.A., *231*:1349, 1975.
20. Regan, J.A., Chao, S., and James, L.S.: Premature rupture of membranes, preterm delivery, and group B streptococcal colonization of mothers. Am. J. Obstet. Gynecol., *141*:184, 1981.
21. Handsfield, H.H., Hodson, W.A., and Holmes, K.K.: Neonatal gonococcal infection. I. Orogastric contamination with *Neisseria gonorrhoeae*. J.A.M.A., *225*:697, 1973.
22. Braun, P., Lea, Y., Klein, J.O., Marcy, S.M., Klein, T.A., Charles, D., Levy, P., and Kass, E.H.: Birth weight and genital mycoplasmas in pregnancy. N. Engl. J. Med., *284*:167, 1971.
23. Martin, D.H., Koutsky, L., Eschenbach, D.A., Daling, J.R., Alexander, E.R., Benedetti, J.K., and Holmes, K.K.: Prematurity and perinatal mortality in pregnancies complicated by maternal *Chlamydia trachomatis* infections. J.A.M.A., *247*:1585, 1982.
24. Petrilli, E.S., D'Ablaing, G., and Ledger, W.J.: *Listeria monocytogenes* chorioamnionitis: Diagnosis by transabdominal amniocentesis. Obstet. Gynecol., *55*:5S, 1980.
25. Grossman, J.H., III, Wallen, W.C., and Sever, J.L.: Management of genital herpes simplex virus infection during pregnancy. Obstet. Gynecol., *58*:1, 1981.
26. Larsen, B., and Galask, R.P.: Vaginal microbial flora: Composition and influences of host physiology. Ann. Intern. Med., *96*:926, 1982.
27. Osborne, N.G., Grubin, L., and Pratson, L.: Vaginitis in sexually active women: Relationship to nine sexually transmitted organisms. Am. J. Obstet. Gynecol., *142*:962, 1982.
28. Gardner, H.L.: *Haemophilus vaginalis* vaginitis after twenty-five years. Am. J. Obstet. Gynecol., *137*:385, 1980.
29. Mardh, P-A., and Westrom, L.: Adherence of bacteria to vaginal epithelial cells. Infect. Immunol., *13*:661, 1976.
30. Curran, J.W., Rendtorff, R.C., Chandler, R.W., Wiser, W.L., and Robinson, H.: Relationship of female gonorrhea to abnormal uterine bleeding, urinary tract symptoms, and cervicitis. Obstet. Gynecol., *45*:195, 1975.
31. Thayer, J.D., and Martin, J.E.: Improved medium selective for cultivation of *N. gonorrhoeae* and *N. meningitis*. Public Health Rep., *81*:559, 1966.
32. Schroeter, A.L., and Lucas, J.B.: Gonorrhea—diagnosis and treatment. Obstet. Gynecol., *39*:274, 1972.
33. Schroeter, A.L., and Reynolds, G.: The rectal culture as a test of cure of gonorrhea in the female. J. Infect. Dis., *125*:499, 1972.
34. Gupta, P.K., Hollander, D.H., and Frost, J.K.: Actinomycetes in cervicovaginal smears: An association with IUD usage. Acta Cytol., *20*:295, 1976.
35. McCormack, W.H., Hayes, C.H., Rosner, B., Evrand, J.R., Crockett, V.A., Alpert, S., and Zinner, S.H.: Vaginal colonization with *Corynebacterium vaginale* (*Hemophilus vaginalis*). J. Infect. Dis., *136*:740, 1977.
36. Gibbs, R.S., Jones, P.M., and Wilder, C.J.: Antibiotic therapy of endometritis following cesarean section; treatment successes and failures. Obstet. Gynecol., *52*:31, 1978.
37. Gravett, M.G., Watkins, H., and Eschenbach, D.A.: Endometrial cultures obtained by a triple lumen transcervical method and cervical cultures in postpartum endometritis. Abstract 17. Annual Meeting Infectious Disease Society Obstetrics-Gynecology, 1983.
38. Ledger, W.J., Gee, C., Pollin, P., Lewis, W.P., Sutter, V.L., and Finegold, S.M.: A new approach to patients with suspected anaerobic post-partum pelvic infections. Trans-abdominal uterine aspiration for culture and metronidozole for treatment. Am. J. Obstet. Gynecol., *126*:1, 1976.
39. Platt, L.D., Yonekura, M.L., and Ledger, W.J.: The role of anaerobic bacteria in post-partum endomyometritis. Am. J. Obstet. Gynecol., *135*:814, 1979.
40. Bobitt, J.R., Hayslip, C.C., and Damato, J.D.: Amniotic fluid infection as determined by transabdominal amniocentesis in patients with intact membranes in premature labor. Am. J. Obstet. Gynecol., *140*:947, 1981.
41. Garite, T.J., Freeman, R.K., Linzey, E.M., and Braly, P.: The use of amniocentesis in patients with premature rupture of membranes. Obstet. Gynecol., *54*:226, 1979.
42. Monif, G.R.G.: Significance of polymicrobial bacterial superinfection in the therapy of gonococcal endometritis-salpingitis-peritonitis. Obstet. Gynecol., *55*:154S, 1980.
43. Sweet, R.L., Mills, J., Hadley, K.W., Blumenstock, E., Schachter, J., Robbie, M.O., and Draper, D.L.: Use of laparoscopy to determine the microbial etiology of acute salpingitis. Am. J. Obstet. Gynecol., *134*:68, 1979.

44. Mardh, P.A., Moller, B.R., Ingerselv, H.J., Nussler, E., Westrom, L., and Wolner-Hanssen, P.: Endometritis caused by *Chlamydia trachomatis*. Br. J. Vener. Dis., *57*:191, 1981.
45. Ledger, W.J., Gee, C.L., Pollin, P., Nakamura, R.M., and Lewis, W.P.: The use of pre-reduced media and portable jars for the collection of anaerobic organisms from clinical sites. Am. J. Obstet. Gynecol., *125*:677, 1976.
46. Burkman, R.T., Tonascia, J.A., Atienza, M.F., and King, T.M.: Untreated endocervical gonorrhea and endometritis following elective abortion. Am. J. Obstet. Gynecol., *126*:648, 1976.
47. Moller, B.R., Ahrons, S., Laurin, J., and Mardh, P.A.: Pelvic infection after elective abortion associated with *Chlamydia trachomatis*. Obstet. Gynecol., *59*:210, 1982.
48. Lip, J., and Burgoyne, X.: Cervical and peritoneal bacterial flora associated with salpingitis. Obstet. Gynecol., *28*:561, 1966.
49. Miller, J.M., Jr., Pupkin, M.J., and Hill, G.B.: Bacterial colonization of amniotic fluid from intact fetal membranes. Am. J. Obstet. Gynecol., *136*:796, 1980.
50. Bobitt, J.R., and Ledger, W.J.: Amniotic fluid analysis. Obstet. Gynecol., *51*:56, 1978.
51. Wager, G.P., Martin, D.H., Koutsky, L., Eschenbach, D.A., Daling, J.R., Chiang, W.J., Alexander, E.R., and Holmes, K.K.: Puerperal infectious morbidity: Relationship to route of delivery and to antepartum *Chlamydia trachomatis* infection. Am. J. Obstet. Gynecol., *138*:1028, 1980.
52. Suchet, J.H., Catalan, F., Loffredo, V., Serfaty, D., Siboulet, A., Perol, Y., Sanson, M.J., Debache, C., Pigeau, F., Coppin, R., deBrux, J., and Poynard, T.: Microbiology of specimens obtained by laparoscopy from controls and from patients with pelvic inflammatory disease or infertility with tubal obstruction: *Chlamydia trachomatis* and *Ureaplasma urealyticum*. Am. J. Obstet. Gynecol., *138*:1022, 1980.
53. Most, H.: Treatment of parasitic infections of travelers and immigrants. N. Engl. J. Med., *310*:298, 1984.
54. George, W.L., Sutter, V.L., and Finegold, S.M.: Antibiotic agent-induced diarrhea—a bacterial disease. J. Infect. Dis., *136*:822, 1977.
55. Ledger, W.J., Norman, M., Gee, C., and Lewis, W.P.: Bacteremia on an obstetric-gynecologic service. Am. J. Obstet. Gynecol., *121*:205, 1975.
56. Blanco, J.D., Gibbs, R.S., and Castaneda, Y.S.: Bacteremia in obstetrics: Clinical course. Obstet. Gynecol., *58*:621, 1981.
57. Rotheram, E.B., Jr., and Schick, S.F.: Nonclostridial anaerobic bacteria in septic abortion. Am. J. Med., *46*:80, 1969.
58. DiZerega, G., Yonekura, L., Roy, S., Nakamura, R.M., and Ledger, W.J.: A comparison of clindamycin-gentamicin and penicillin-gentamicin in the treatment of post cesarean section endomyometritis. Am. J. Obstet. Gynecol., *134*:238, 1979.
59. Washington, J.A., II: Blood cultures; principles and techniques. Mayo Clin. Proc., *50*:91, 1975.
60. MacGregor, R.R., and Beaty, H.N.: Evaluation of positive blood cultures. Arch. Intern. Med., *130*:84, 1972.
61. Montgomerie, J.Z., and Edwards, J.E.: Association of infection due to *Candida albicans* with intravenous hyperalimentation. J. Infect. Dis., *137*:197, 1978.
62. Hoschal, V.L., Jr.: Intravenous catheters and infection. Surg. Clin. North Am., *52*:1407, 1972.

Chapter 4
LABORATORY TESTING OF ANTIBIOTICS

Physician confusion about antibiotic susceptibility testing leads to many irrational decisions about the prescription of antibiotics. Based upon disc susceptibility testing, currently prescribed antibiotics will frequently be discontinued and new ones administered without regard for either the site of the infection or the clinical response of the patient. Physicians should be aware of the limitations of antibiotic susceptibility testing. A patient with a pelvic abscess may not respond to systemic antibiotic therapy even though in the laboratory the anaerobic bacteria causing the infection are susceptible to these antibiotics. Antibiotics alone will not cure this patient; operative intervention in conjunction with drugs will be effective. In contrast, a woman with a urinary tract infection may be cured by an antibiotic even though the organism is resistant to that drug in the laboratory because of the interaction of host defense mechanisms and the high concentration of antibiotic in the urine. Interpretation of antibiotic susceptibility testing requires understanding of the type of infection and the limitations of this laboratory test system.

DISC SUSCEPTIBILITY TESTS

The most commonly used evaluation of antibiotics in clinical microbiology laboratories is disc susceptibility testing. This test is performed on bacterial isolates from specimens supplied by clinicians. The laboratory reports the bacteria isolated to be resistant, intermediate, or susceptible to a wide range of antibiotics. Proper integration of these test results into the therapeutic strategy of the physician requires understanding of both the mechanics of and the scientific basis for the test.

Disc susceptibility testing was designed to be employed in all clinical microbiology laboratories, no matter what the size of the hospital. Although the zone diameters of inhibition around the discs have been correlated with the minimal inhibitory concentrations of antibiotics by tube dilution testing, it was obvious to everyone in clinical microbiology laboratories that tube dilution testing was too time-consuming for technicians to be routinely employed for all isolates.

The techniques for disc susceptibility testing are simple and straightforward. A few colonies of bacteria on primary isolation plates are transferred to a test tube containing trypticase soy yeast broth, emulsified, and incubated for two to six hours. The turbidity of the suspension is compared with a barium sulfate turbidity standard and diluted with water if necessary to avoid too heavy a bacterial inoculum. A sterile swab is dipped in this suspension and then stroked in overlapping directions on a large plate (150 mm in diameter) containing Mueller-Hinton agar. In addition to this traditional approach, a number of alternative techniques have been devised to achieve uniform growth on the plate surface. The large plates have been dried for at least 30 minutes before inoculation, and all should be used within four days for preparation so that accurate reproducible results are achieved. Antibiotic discs are pressed firmly on the plate and the plate is then incubated overnight at 37° C. The plates are reevaluated the next working day, and calipers are employed to measure the diameter of the growth inhibition zone in millimeters. The susceptibility of the organism is determined by comparison to a zone-size interpretation chart.[1] Each of these steps is dependent upon several test assumptions, and these may not be valid in every test performed by a clinical microbiology laboratory. Awareness of potential shortcomings will aid physician interpretation.

Accurate disc susceptibility testing depends upon the interaction of many variables. The paper disc, saturated with a known quantity of antibiotic, has been designed to release the antibiotic into the agar with a resulting circular diffusion gradient of antimicrobial agent around the disc. If diffusion proceeds normally, there should be a higher concentration of antibiotic next to the disc, which diminishes as the distance from the disc increases. This diffusion of antibiotic is the basis for interpretation of antibiotic susceptibility by zone size (Table 4–1).[2] Thus, it is possible that a microorganism will be reported to the clinician as resistant even if there is a small zone of inhibition of bacterial growth adjacent to an antibiotic disc, because the therapeutic administration of antibiotics to a patient will not achieve levels in the human equivalent to those next to the disc. A zone of inhibition that is reported as intermediate susceptibility requires the most careful evaluation by the physician. It is frequently possible to get high concentrations of antibiotics in the urinary tract, so that the intermediately susceptible organisms in this site are more likely to be eliminated than these same bacteria in other pelvic soft tissue sites.

Variations in the amount of antibiotic that diffuses from the disc can influence zone size. Although the Federal Drug Administration (FDA) regulates the antibiotic content of standard discs, the required acceptable range is between 67 to 150% of the labeled value. It should be obvious that this standard permits an over twofold variation in antibiotics in these discs. In addition to this accepted difference, the antibiotic potency of the discs can deteriorate. Standard laboratory practice includes storage of discs in a refrigerator when not in use and discarding of batches of discs if the expiration date has been reached or passed. Some of the individual discs present problems. Methicillin discs are known to deteriorate rapidly, with smaller inhibitory zone size seen in the laboratory after 48 hours of incubation when compared to the 24-hour reading. Some antibiotics such as colistin, bacitracin, and vancomycin diffuse poorly from the disc into the Mueller-Hinton agar. The result is that inhibition zones indicating susceptibility to these agents are smaller than those of other classes of antibiotics. Some substances may be added to the Mueller-Hinton media, for example sheep blood for streptococci, or the environment may be altered with the addition of carbon dioxide for *Neisseria gonorrhoeae.* These substances may interfere with the antimicrobial activity of individual antibiotics in this test system (Table 4–2).[2] Another factor may induce

Table 4-1. Zone Size Interpretative Chart

Antibiotic or Chemotherapeutic Agent	Disc Potency	Diameter of Zone of Inhibition (mm)		
		Resistant[a]	Intermediate	Susceptible[b]
	μg			
Amikacin	10	≤ 11	12–13	≥ 14
Ampicillin when testing:				
gram-negative enteric organisms and enterococci	10	≤ 11	12–13	≥ 14
staphylococci and penicillin G–susceptible organisms	10	≤ 20	21–28	≥ 29
Hemophilis species[c]	10	≤ 19		≥ 20
Bacitracin	10 U	≤ 8	9–12	≥ 13
Carbenicillin when testing:				
Proteus spp. and *Escherichia coli*	100	≤ 17	18–22	≥ 23
Pseudomonas aeruginosa	100	≤ 13	14–16	≥ 17
Cefamandole	30	≤ 16	15–17	≥ 18
Cefoxitin	30	≤ 16	15–17	≥ 18
Cephalothin[d]	30	≤ 14	15–17	≥ 18
Chloramphenicol	30	≤ 12	13–17	≥ 18
Clindamycin	2	≤ 14	15–16	≥ 17
Colistin	10	≤ 8	9–10	≥ 11
Erythromycin	15	≤ 13	14–17	≥ 18
Gentamicin	10	≤ 12	13–14	≥ 15
Kanamycin	30	≤ 13	14–17	≥ 18
Methicillin	5	≤ 9	10–13	≥ 14
Nalidixic acid	30	≤ 13	14–18	≥ 19
Neomycin	30	≤ 12	13–16	≥ 17
Nitrofurantoin	300	≤ 14	15–16	≥ 17
Penicillin G when testing:				
staphylococci	10 U	≤ 20	21–28	≥ 29
other organisms	10 U	≤ 11	12–21	≥ 22
Polymyxin B	300 U	≤ 8	9–11	≥ 12
Streptomycin	10	≤ 11	12–14	≥ 15
Sulfonamides	300	≤ 12	13–16	≥ 17
Tetracycline	30	≤ 14	15–18	≥ 19
Trimethoprim-sulfamethoxazole	1.25 23.75	≤ 10	11–15	≥ 16
Tobramycin	10	≤ 11	12–13	≥ 14
Vancomycin	30	≤ 9	10–11	≥ 12

[a] Resistant size or smaller.
[b] Susceptible size or larger.
[c] For testing *Hemophilis,* use Mueller-Hinton agar plates supplemented with 1% hemoglobin and 1% Isovitalex (BBL). Prepare inoculum by suspending growth from a 24-hour chocolate agar plate in Mueller-Hinton broth to the density of a 0.5 McFarland standard.
[d] The cephalothin disc is used for testing susceptibility to all cephalosporin type antibiotics except for cefoxitin and cefamandole. This includes cephaloridine, cephalexin, cefazolin, and cephapirin. *Staphylococcus aureus* exhibiting resistance to methicillin discs should be reported as resistant to cephalosporin type antibiotics regardless of zone size.
Note: Complete Standard ASM-2 is available from the National Committee for Clinical Laboratory Standards, Villanova, PA 19085.
(From Acar, J.F.: The disc susceptibility test. *In* Antibiotics in Laboratory Medicine. Edited by V. Lorian. Baltimore, Williams & Wilkins, 1980. Copyright 1980, the Williams & Wilkins Co., Baltimore.)

variation in the results of antibiotic disc susceptibility testing. Thickness of the agar in the Mueller-Hinton plates is important. One study demonstrated an increase in the size of zones as thickness of the medium decreased.[3] Since the size of the zone of inhibition is the critical factor in the interpretation of disc susceptibility tests, laboratories should use media that are approximately 4 mm in depth. All clinical microbiology laboratories must have an ongoing program of quality control testing to be sure that these potential variances are not influencing test results.

Table 4-2. Substances that Interfere with Antimicrobial Activity

Substances	Antibiotics
Defibrinated blood	Sulfonamides
Chocolatized agar	Sulfonamides
	Trimethoprim
	Aminosidic antibiotics
Carbon dioxide (CO_2)	Aminosidic antibiotics
	Erythromycin group
	Lincomycin
	Tetracyclines
	Novobiocin

(From Acar, J.F.: The disc susceptibility test. *In* Antibiotics in Laboratory Medicine. Edited by V. Lorian. Baltimore, Williams & Wilkins, 1980. Copyright 1980, the Williams & Wilkins Co., Baltimore.)

In critically ill patients with sepsis, there is a clinical need for more rapid antibiotic susceptibility testing to help guide critical prescription decisions. There is a five-hour rapid method that has been reported to be comparable to the Kirby-Bauer method.[4] This requires prewarming of the plates to 37° C, modification of the inoculum turbidity, addition of blood for gram-positive organisms, and different criteria for zone size diameters that indicate susceptibility.

The results of disc susceptibility testing must be interpreted by the physician who has the primary responsibility for the care of the patient. It is not an acceptable clinical practice to alter antibiotic therapy solely because the laboratory reports an organism that is resistant to the antibiotics now prescribed for the patient. Clinician interpretation should be more sophisticated and not a reflex action. The laboratory environment that yielded the resistant report may not be comparable to that of the human host. The antibiotic discs have been designed to release antibiotic into the agar in concentrations that are ordinarily achieved in the human with standard therapeutic regimens. Lack of correlation may reflect higher levels of antibiotic in the urinary tract, or the profound local factors of protein binding, pH, and the metabolic state of the bacteria, or release of substances that prevent the action of antibiotics in the human host. In some cases, operative intervention and not the prescription of new antibiotics will be necessary for cure. Finally, a poorly collected specimen may yield surface bacteria that are not involved in the clinical evolution of the infection. All these possibilities must be considered by the clinician before any alterations in antibiotic therapy are made.

AGAR DILUTION TESTING

For the clinical laboratory, the most reproducible antibiotic susceptibility testing for anaerobic bacteria is the agar dilution technique.[5] Commercial kits are available, and the results of these tests seem the most easily read by laboratory personnel whose primary interest is not directed toward anaerobes. This testing should be available for the clinician responsible for the inpatient care of seriously ill patients with anaerobic infections.

TUBE DILUTION TESTS

Tube dilution tests are much more accurate than disc susceptibility tests. The variability in the amount of antibiotic added to the tubes is much less than with antibiotic discs. With tubes, the lowest drug concentration that shows no visible growth is reported as the Minimum Inhibitory Concentration (MIC).

Despite the accuracy of the tube dilution tests, they are infrequently employed in clinical microbiology laboratories. Obviously, they are time-consuming and expensive because of the laboratory personnel required. Fortunately, disc susceptibility tests have been based upon tube dilution testing standards. There are a few situations in which tube dilution testing may be very important in the care of a patient. For the patient with subacute bacterial endocarditis, tube dilution testing may be a better way to determine the best combination of antibiotics. In addition, a gram-negative anaerobic rod recovered from a patient with a serious pelvic infection that is responding slowly to antibiotics is more appropriately tested for susceptibility by either the agar diffusion or tube dilution test. These indications for tube dilution testing are rarely seen on most clinical services, but every clinical microbiology laboratory should have this capability.

In addition to the MIC, the clinician will hear the terminology of minimal bactericidal concentration (MBC). This refers to the level of antibiotic needed to achieve a "killing" effect on the organisms, and it is frequently referred to in the description of the actions of new antibiotics. For the obstetrician-gynecologist, this testing is seldom needed for patient care. In clinical medicine it is rarely employed in cases of bacterial endocarditis, in which only a bactericidal agent will achieve a cure.

ANTIBIOTIC SUSCEPTIBILITY TESTS FOR ANAEROBES

Microbiologic technology has not reached the point where routine antibiotic susceptibility testing of anaerobic organisms can be accurately performed in a clinical microbiology laboratory. There are a number of reasons for this. To date, an accurate reproducible method for disc susceptibility testing of anaerobes that can be put in effect in all clinical microbiology laboratories has not been devised. In the various techniques used to achieve an anaerobic environment in the laboratory, changes in pH or CO_2 may markedly influence the impact of some antibiotic discs on anaerobic bacterial growth (see Table 4–2). Also, anaerobes tend to grow more slowly in the laboratory than aerobic bacteria. Frequently, there will not be confluent growth on the agar plate after transfer from the broth.[6] Some anaerobes, such as *Clostridium perfringens,* grow more rapidly than others and may have small zones of inhibition with discs even though they are antibiotic-susceptible.[6] In addition, there may be irregular growth of organisms, i.e., cloudy zones or zones of growth next to the antibiotic discs that make interpretation very difficult. To date, these problems have not been overcome to the point that clinicians should feel confident with the results of disc susceptibility testing in clinical laboratories. With the known shortcomings of the disc method, the report of *Bacteroides fragilis* that is resistant to clindamycin may not accurately reflect the actual impact of this antibiotic upon this important pathogen.

There is an alternative approach to the processing of anaerobic bacteria in the clinical laboratory. The major concerns for the clinician for antibiotic resistance in anaerobic bacteria are the gram-negative isolates. The first priority for the laboratory should be accurate identification of the individual bacterial species. The technology to do this is available, and all clinical laboratories can perform this service. Recent studies have demonstrated the isolation of a small number of these gram-negative anaerobes that are resistant to clindamycin as well as to the newer cephalosporins and penicillins.[7] Recently, chloramphenicol resistance has been reported in the Philippines, a phenomenon not seen in the United States.[8] Since these antibiotics are widely prescribed for soft tissue pelvic infections, the isolation of a gram-negative anaerobic rod from a patient with a soft tissue pelvic infection should be an indication for antibiotic susceptibility testing, using the agar dilution technique.

DETERMINATION OF ANTIBIOTIC LEVELS

There are a number of important reasons for determining antibiotic levels in the blood. The most frequent indication for this testing is in antibiotic research and development. Important components of study of any new antibiotic are the blood levels achieved with various routes of administration and dosage levels and the loss of the antibiotic from the body as a serum half-life is determined. Although these measurements are important for the clinician so that he may expand his understanding of the pharmacodynamics of new antibiotic regimens, they are not ordinarily required in daily clinical practice. However, there are situations in which the measurement of antibiotic levels may be of great importance for the clinician. Philipson has shown repeatedly that all antibiotics studied, whether given orally or systemically, achieve lower levels in pregnant patients than in nonpregnant controls.[9] This observation may not be of significance if antibiotics are given with a wide safety margin, for example if high doses are safely prescribed with the penicillins and cephalosporins. But it may be of critical importance when aminoglycosides are prescribed with a narrow dosage margin because of the concern about achieving toxic levels. Studies in young healthy obstetric[10] and gynecologic[11] patients have shown lower than expected blood values of aminoglycosides because of excellent renal function and rapid clearance of the antibiotic. In these women, it is imperative to monitor blood levels of the aminoglycosides.

A number of tests have been employed to measure the level of antibiotics in body fluids. Until the last few years, most have utilized a biologic test system. An aliquot of blood serum is added to a disc and placed on a culture plate that has a confluent growth of a test organism such as *Sarcina lutea.* After incubation overnight, the zone of inhibition around the disc is measured and the level of antibiotic in the blood is calculated from a table relating the size of the inhibition zone to various antibiotic concentrations. This table has been prepared from previous experiments with different concentrations of the antibiotic in question. The major drawbacks to the system are the difficulties in measuring antibiotics in patients receiving more than one antibiotic and all the problems associated with the maintenance of an accurate biologic test system. For example, the laboratory must be geared to keeping a stock of test organisms, and all evaluations should be done in triplicate to diminish the chance of method error. This biologic assay system will produce valuable data for the analysis of new antibiotics but is not available in clinical microbiology laboratories.

A recent breakthrough in laboratory technology has been the development of accurate radioimmunoassay tests for aminoglycosides.[12, 13] This has been a needed addition to standard clinical microbiology laboratories because it circumvents all of the problems with a biologic test system. Once in place, it is a simpler test to perform, it produces results that can be replicated from one laboratory to another, and antibiotic levels measured are not influenced by the administration of more than one antibiotic to the patient. Most important for the clinician, it permits accurate measurement of aminoglycoside levels in obstetric-gynecologic patients who, in the majority of cases, because of their young age and excellent renal function, may not achieve therapeutic levels of the drug. Also, lower serum levels of gentamicin have been reported in febrile patients.[14] Other women will require this assay to be performed to avoid toxicity. Very obese women may require decreased doses of aminoglycosides because of higher serum levels achieved with the standard administration formula based on weight.[15] Similarly, debilitated elderly patients[16] or women with acute pyelonephritis[17] may have diminished renal function and have the potential of achieving toxic levels of antibiotics with standard dosage regimens. In the past, there has been dependence on formulas to calculate dosage intervals for aminoglycosides[18] or on the use of a computer program with multiple variables entered to compute doses for the next 24 hours.[19] Although these formulas are helpful as a guide to avoid toxicity and may be accurate for many patients, they all depend upon a number of assumptions for the total population that will not be met in every individual patient to whom the formula has been applied. This is particularly true when administering gentamicin and tobramycin.

Because of this, there should be this standard of practice for obstetrician-gynecologists who are prescribing aminoglycosides. If the hospitalized patient is sick enough to warrant prescription of these potentially toxic agents, radioimmunoassay of blood levels of the aminoglycosides prescribed should be done after 24 hours of therapy. The results of the tests, whether performed in the hospital microbiology laboratory or a commercial laboratory, should be available to the clinician within 24 hours so that appropriate dosage changes can be accomplished. Readings of peak and trough levels of the aminoglycosides should be done in every case. The peak level is obtained 30 minutes after intravenous administration of the antibiotic. A trough level should be obtained just before the next administered dose. The desired peak levels for gentamicin-tobramycin are 4 to 6 ng/ml, and the trough levels should be less than 2 ng/ml. If the levels are normal and serum creatinine values remain unchanged, peak and trough levels can be repeated in two to four days. If they are abnormal, the prescription should be modified and daily tests repeated until normal levels are achieved. If this measurement of aminoglycosides is not available to the obstetrician-gynecologist, aminoglycosides should not be prescribed unless the clinician feels this is the only antibiotic that will achieve a cure in an individual patient. In this situation, the greater predictability of achieved blood levels with kanamycin or amikacin would make their selection more appealing.

REFERENCES

1. Bauer, A.W., Kirby, W.M.M., Sherris, J.C., and Turck, M.: Antibiotic susceptibility testing by a standardized disc method. Am. J. Clin. Pathol., 45:493, 1966.
2. Acar, J.F.: The disc susceptibility test. *In* Antibiotics in Laboratory Medicine. Edited by V. Lorian. Baltimore, Williams & Wilkins, 1980.
3. Barry, A.L., and Fay, G.D.: The amount of agar in antimicrobic disc susceptibility test plates. Am. J. Clin. Pathol., 59:196, 1973.
4. Barry, A.L., Joyce, L.J., Adams, A.P., and Benner, E.J.: Rapid determination of antimicrobial susceptibility for urgent clinical situations. Am. J. Clin. Pathol., 59:693, 1973.

5. Hauser, K.J., Johnston, J.A., and Zabransky, R.J.: Economic agar dilution technique for susceptibility testing of anaerobes. Antimicrob. Agents Chemother. *7*:712, 1975.
6. Wilkins, T.D.: Antibiotic susceptibility testing of anaerobic bacteria. *In* Anaerobic Bacteria: Role in Disease. Edited by A. Balows et al. Springfield, Ill., Charles C. Thomas, 1974.
7. Tally, F.P., Cuchural, G.T., Jacobus, N.V., Gorbach, S.L., Aldridge, K.E., Cleary, T.J., Finegold, S.M., Hill, G.B., Iannini, P.B., McCloskey, R.V., O'Keefe, J.P., and Pierson, C.L.: Susceptibility of the *Bacteroides fragilis* group in the United States in 1981. Antimicrob. Agents Chemother. *23*:536, 1983.
8. Limson, B.M.: Unpublished observations.
9. Philipson, A.E.L.: Pharmacokinetics of antibiotics in the pregnant woman. *In* Antibiotics in Obstetrics and Gynecology. Edited by W.J. Ledger. The Hague, Martinus Nijhoff, 1982.
10. Zaske, D.E., Cipolle, R.J., Strate, R.G., Malo, J.W., and Koszalkas, M.F., Jr.: Rapid gentamicin elimination in obstetric patients. Obstet. Gynecol., *56*:559, 1980.
11. Zaske, D.E., Cipolle, R.J., Strate, R.G., and Dickes, W.F.: Increased gentamicin dosage requirements: Rapid elimination in 249 gynecology patients. Am. J. Obstet. Gynecol., *139*:896, 1981.
12. Sabath, L.D.: A simple rapid microassay for nephrotoxic antibiotics. Scope Monograph. Kalamazoo, Michigan, Upjohn Co., 1972.
13. Lewis, J.E., Nelson, J.C. and Elder, H.A.: Radioimmunoassay of an antibiotic: Gentamicin. Nature, *239*:214, 1972.
14. Pennington, J.E., Dale, D.C., Reynolds, H.Y., and MacLowry, J.D.: Gentamicin sulfate pharmacokinetics: Lower levels of gentamicin in blood during fever. J. Infect. Dis., *132*:270, 1975.
15. Schwartz, S.N., Pazin, G.J., Lyon, J.A., Ho, M., and Pasculle, A.E.: A controlled investigation of the pharmacokinetics of gentamicin and tobramycin in obese patients. J. Infect. Dis., *138*:499, 1978.
16. Zaske, D.E., Sawchuk, R.J., Gerding, D.N., and Strate, R.G.: Increased dosage requirements of gentamicin in burn patients. J. Trauma, *16*:824, 1976.
17. Whalley, P.J., Cunningham, F.G., and Martin, F.G.: Transient renal dysfunction associated in the acute pyelonephritis of pregnancy. Obstet. Gynecol., *46*:174, 1975.
18. McHenry, M.C., Gavan, T.L., Gifford, R.W., Jr., Geurkink, N.A., Van Ommen, R.A., and Wagner, J.G.: Gentamicin dosages for renal insufficiency. Ann. Intern. Med., *74*:192, 1971.
19. Jelliffe, R.W.: New developments in drug dosage regimens. J. Mond. Pharm., *1*:15, 1972.

Chapter 5

HOST RESPONSE TO INFECTION—LABORATORY EVALUATION

Understanding the many mechanisms of the host response to infection is important for the obstetrician-gynecologist. It keeps in perspective the wide variety of clinical responses seen in women with infections that would seem to have the same prognosis based upon laboratory and microbiologic data. For example, the woman under age 25 with salpingitis is far less likely to have the residual of blocked tubes after treatment than the woman over age 30 with a similar infection.[1] In addition, specific diseases can occur as a result of deficiencies in the immune system. The most publicized recent example has been increased frequency of Kaposi's sarcoma in male homosexuals with acquired immune deficiency syndrome (AIDS).[2] Finally, and most important, knowledge of the host response to infection is necessary for the interpretation of the laboratory tests that are utilized with great frequency by clinicians. If the mechanisms of the host response are understood, then the laboratory results can be correctly interpreted and appropriate clinical decisions made. This is an area of frequent confusion for the clinician. The potential for error is best exemplified by the evaluation of a group of women who mistakenly received live rubella virus as a vaccine during pregnancy.[3] A number of these women received the immunization even though the available laboratory data indicated that they were immune, with detectable blood antibody levels as a result of past exposure to the wild virus. This therapeutic mistake was potentially dangerous to the fetus because of live virus exposure, and it was totally avoidable. The therapeutic maxim for all clinicians must be *"primum non nocere,"* first of all, do no harm. This chapter will attempt to provide an outline of the host response with illustrations of the clinical states associated with various deficiencies.

MECHANICAL BARRIERS

The skin is the first line of defense for the human host. The epidermis, the superficial skin layer, provides a protective barrier over the entire body surface. There are antimicrobial substances on the surface of the skin that in most people will prevent colonization with virulent organisms having the potential to adhere, invade, and then cause disease. There are a number of examples in which alteration of this barrier can result in clinical infection. The most dramatic is seen in patients with extensive body burns. These burned areas become colonized with pathogenic bacteria that invade the bloodstream, resulting in sepsis and death.[4] An example more frequently observed by the obstetrician-gynecologist is the increased abdominal wound infection rate seen in women who have been prepped by shaving the evening before operation compared with the rate in those whose hair has been removed by electric clippers in the operating room just prior to the operative procedure.[5] Shaving with a razor on the prior evening evidently produces many small breaks in the skin surface, permitting overgrowth by a large number of bacteria that in turn results in a higher abdominal wound infection rate.

The mucous membranes are also important elements in host defense. Studies of these local mechanisms have been more detailed in the respiratory and the gastrointestinal tracts. The combination of active cilia and the production of mucus that contains antibacterial factors such as secretory immunoglobulin A (IgA), lysozyme, lactoferrin, and alpha-antitrypsin acts to protect the human host against bacterial invasion.[6] A respiratory virus, influenza, impedes this mucociliary transport, and the result is a high incidence of superinfection in the form of bacterial pneumonia.[7] The mucosal barrier of the gastrointestinal tract is similar to that of the respiratory tract and is aided by gastrointestinal motility, which clears the tract of large numbers of bacteria. If motility is interrupted or slowed by tumor growth or ileus, there can be an overgrowth of bacteria and the potential arises for invasive infection.[8] A therapeutic mandate should be to avoid the symptomatic treatment of gastrointestinal problems. The use of pharmacologic agents that diminish gastrointestinal motility in the presence of bacterial infection of the gastrointestinal tract is usually contraindicated. For example, the prescription of antiperistaltic agents in the antibiotic-associated pseudo-membranous enterocolitis due to *Clostridium difficile* may prolong the disease process and increase its severity by interfering with a physiologic mechanism (diarrhea) that will clear the gastrointestinal tract of these anaerobic pathogens.[9] If the mucosal barrier of the gastrointestinal tract is damaged by cytotoxic therapy for neoplastic disease, serious bacterial infections can result.[10]

Less is known about the mucosal barrier of the lower genital tract. Clearly some local defense mechanism exists. For example, although *Neisseria gonorrhoeae* can be recovered from the endocervical cultures of 5 to 10% of some urban pregnant populations, gonococcal salpingitis rarely occurs in pregnancy. This failure of development of salpingitis is not related to the inability of these strains of *Neisseria gonorrhoeae* to invade and behave as pathogens, since the most common bacterial agent of infectious arthritis in pregnancy is *Neisseria gonorrhoeae*,[11] and this is a blood-borne infection. Studies of the cervix have shown the local secretion of immunoglobulins, particularly immunoglobulin A (IgA) with specific activity against viral and bacterial antigens, as well as of lysozymes with antibacterial activity against gram-positive aerobes. In nonpregnant women, the most virulent transparent *Neisseria gonorrhoeae* colonies can be found after contact with the cells of the ectocervix of young women.[12] This may account in part for the higher infection rate of gonococcal salpingitis in women under the age of 24 compared with women over the age of 30.[13]

In addition to the protection given the human host by the various mucous membranes, there is good evidence that one body fluid, amniotic fluid, contains many potent antibacterial factors. Different investigators found lysozyme in amniotic fluid,[14, 15] with concentrations that were usually higher than in the maternal serum. This enzyme is bactericidal for some gram-positive aerobic bacteria, and it can act in concert with antibody and complement against gram-negative aerobic bacteria. Beta-lysin, a bactericidal factor, has been identified in the amniotic fluid of women at term.[16] Bactericidin was present in 17% of amniotic fluid samples obtained near term.[17] This substance is bactericidal to gram-positive organisms and can work together with lysozymes, antibodies, and complement against gram-negative bacteria. Transferrin is present in amniotic fluid.[18] This is an important substance in host defense, because it chelates iron and makes it unavailable for assimilation by replicating bacteria. Immunoglobulins are also found in the amniotic fluid, although at lower levels than in maternal serum.[19] Peroxidase is present in amniotic fluid in increasing amounts with advancing gestational age;[20] this substance also has antibacterial activity.

In addition to these named identifiable substances, there is a separate zinc-protein complex in amniotic fluid that has an antibacterial effect.[21–23] The antibacterial effect varies with the test organism used and the pregnancy population studied and is enhanced by elevated temperature.[24] Antibacterial activity may be absent in the amniotic fluid of Ethiopian women, which has little of this complex present, and there is a high rate of maternal and newborn infection in this population.[25] All these substances, separately or in concert (lysozymes, bactericidin, transferrin, immunoglobulins, complement, peroxidase, and zinc-protein complex), have an impact that can be measured clinically. For example, prolonged rupture of membranes increases the risk of a maternal uterine infection. Despite this, fewer than 10% of women who deliver vaginally after prolonged rupture of membranes will develop a clinical infection post partum.[26]

To date, testing of the amniotic fluid for antibacterial substances has not become a standard of clinical practice. There is no agreement on the importance of the various substances that can be measured; and the correlation between laboratory and clinical results has not been uniform. For example, one recent study utilizing *Escherichia coli* as the test organism found amniotic fluid from infected patients to be noninhibitory in 70%, whereas only 32% of control samples from asymptomatic women were noninhibitory.[27] Although the differences in the populations were statistically significant, the high rate of noninhibitory fluid in the control population does not inspire clinical confidence in this laboratory test as a screen for women at high risk for infection.

THE IMMUNE SYSTEM

The host response to an invasive organism can be categorized into two large components: There is the bone marrow-derived or *B* cell system that provides the humoral response, and the thymus-derived or *T* cell system that provides cell-mediated immunity.

Humoral immunity in the host is characterized by the production of immunoglobulins. There are five major classes of immunoglobulins: IgA, IgD, IgE, IgG, and IgM. These immunoglobulins have varied roles in host defense and have a wide range of significance for the clinician. IgE is associated with the host development of allergy to antibiotics. This immunoglobulin does not cross the placenta, which is why penicillin can usually be given safely for the treatment of neonatal syphilis in the newborn of a penicillin-allergic mother. IgA, IgM, and

IgG have the most functional activity against microorganisms. There are two types of IgA, serum IgA and secretory IgA. The latter is an important component of the surface immune system of mucous membranes. IgM and IgG are important markers of the host response to infection. In response to a specific antigen, a rise in IgM occurs early and then disappears in a matter of months. The IgG response lasts for a much longer period of time. IgG crosses the placenta while IgM does not. In the evaluation of mothers or neonates for the possibility of infection acquired during pregnancy, the assessment of these two classes of immunoglobulins will usually establish the diagnosis of a recent infection in the mother.

Figure 5–1 shows the schema of the immune response of the adult host to rubella.[28] The hemagglutination-inhibition (HI) test measures antibody activity against viral surface antigen and is similar to the IgG response to rubella, for this antibody usually persists throughout the life of the host. The presence of IgM against rubella connotes recent infection. Many laboratories that are not equipped to perform IgM evaluations for rubella are able to do complement fixation (CF) tests. These tests utilize antigens from infected cell cultures, and this response appears later and disappears more rapidly than the HI response. A persistently positive HI test and absent CF antibody after a 2 to 4 week interval would indicate an old infection. Confirmation of a recent rubella infection in a pregnant woman markedly changes the prognosis for that pregnancy. This IgM testing for specific antigens can be very helpful in the newborn. Since IgM does not cross the placenta, its presence in cord blood demonstrates fetal response to an antigen. Laboratory testing for IgM depends upon the specificity and the reproducibility of the IgM to be evaluated. To date, IgM testing for rubella is quite specific and accurate.

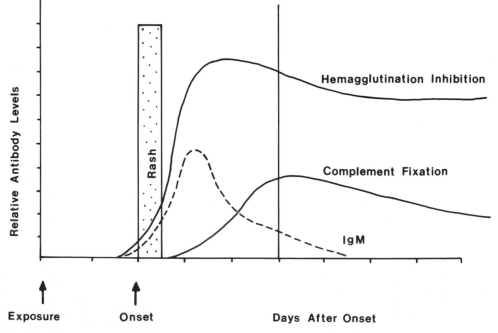

Fig. 5–1. The immune response of the human host to rubella.
(From Mann, J.M., Preblud, S.R., Hoffman, R.E., Brandling-Bennett, A.D., Hinman, A.R., and Herrmann, K.L.: Assessing risks of rubella infection during pregnancy. J.A.M.A., *245*:1647, 1981. Copyright 1981; American Medical Association.)

There still are problems in the evaluation of the IgM response to toxoplasmosis, and the test is not reliable in all clinical laboratories. It is important that the laboratory screen for the presence of rheumatoid factor, for if it is present, it can result in a positive IgM test.[29]

In addition to these laboratory evaluations that can influence patient management, there are a number of examples of the importance of these humoral factors in the etiology of disease. There are many situations in which humoral immunodeficiency can be detected with a resultant clinical impact. The majority of patients with chronic lymphocytic leukemia have bone marrows that produce immature B cells that are incapable of secreting immunoglobulins, and the result is hypogammaglobulinemia.[30] Patients with multiple myeloma produce large volumes of immunoglobulins with no activity, so although these people have normal blood levels of immunoglobulins, they react to foreign antigens as a person with agammaglobulinemia would.[31] Burn victims, so prone to serious infections, exude large amounts of serum and IgG into the damaged tissue and subsequently develop hypogammaglobulinemia.[32] Patients with the nephrotic syndrome lose large amounts of IgG in their urine and become functional hypogammaglobulinemics.[33] These types of patients are rarely part of the practice of the obstetrician-gynecologist. On oncology services, patients receiving antimetabolites and alkylating agents for the treatment of pelvic malignancies can have reduced immunoglobulin levels.[10] All of these individual syndromes or treatment responses result in a pool of patients with isolated defects of humoral immunity. These women can present with frequent infections caused by the extracellular pathogens such as pneumococci, *Hemophilus influenzae,* and *Pseudomonas aeruginosa* as well as with life-threatening infections with the viruses that cause hepatitis and poliomyelitis.[10] To date, measurement of immunoglobulin levels in women with pelvic malignancies has usually not been a significant laboratory evaluation of a failure of response to antibiotics.

In addition to the humoral immunity of the B cells, cell-mediated immunity is provided by the T cells. This cell-mediated response is complex and interrelated with other immune mechanisms. When activated by a specific antigen, these T lymphocytes undergo blast transformation with a subsequent wide variety of responses. (1) Helper T cells act on B cells to aid in the production of the humoral factors, the immunoglobulins. (2) In contrast to this helper role, suppressor T cells produce a substance that suppresses antibody formation. This function of T cells can have clinical significance. Some patients with systemic fungal infections have been observed to have increased T cell suppressor activity.[34] We have also observed increased suppressor activity in women with recurrent *Candida* vaginal infections.[35] In addition, there is increased suppressor cell activity in patients with cytomegalovirus and Epstein-Barr virus infections. (3) T cells also produce and secrete a variety of soluble factors, called lymphokines, which influence the white blood cell response to antigens. There are a range of factors from a migration inhibitory factor (MIF) to a chemotactic factor, as well as products that activate macrophages to great microbicidal activity. Recent observations of AIDS patients show the importance of this defense mechanism. In these patients, the T lymphocytes did not secrete lymphokines (rich in immune gamma-interferon) to stimulate monocyte phagocytosis.[36] This is one explanation for the high rate of infection in these patients from such intracellular organisms as protozoa *(Pneumocystis carinii* and *Toxoplasma gondii),* mycobacteria, viruses, and fungi, which are normally cleared by activated monocytes. (4) Finally, cytolytic T cells are produced that are necessary for cell-mediated immunity. When these cells are activated, they can eliminate viral-infected cells from the host. This obviously is a major component of the human control of viral infections. This T cell activity is apparent in the atypical T lymphocytes seen on peripheral blood smears of patients with mononucleosis, caused by Epstein-Barr virus.

There are a number of situations that result in impairment of cell-mediated immunity. The most dramatic for the obstetrician-gynecologist is in the patient on long-term corticosteroid therapy.[37] Recently, in evaluation of human crypto-sporidiosis infections, a moderate self-limited disease was seen in immunocompetent persons in contrast to the prolonged severe diarrhea in patients with AIDS.[38] Table 5–1 lists a variety of infections that may be seen clinically in patients with primary or acquired T cell dysfunction.[10] It is interesting to note that many of these systemic infections are seen in immunosuppressed adults undergoing renal transplant, for example, pneumonias due to cytomegalovirus, tuberculosis, and *Pneumocystis carinii.* Herpes-virus, cytomegalovirus, and *Toxoplasma* are all capable of causing serious infection in the newborn, particularly the premature infant, who is burdened by a premature immunologic system as well. Tests of T cell function are usually not available in clinical laboratories. To date, most of the evaluations have been performed as part of a research protocol in a pool of patients under investigation.

In addition to the B and T cell system, the complement system plays an important role in human host defense. This highly complex and integrated network of 11 serum proteins mediates inflammation and tissue damage and helps in the ingestion of various types of microorganisms by phagocytic cells. There are two pathways of complement activity (Figure 5–2).[39] The classic pathway is activated by cellular antigens. The alternate pathway requires only endotoxin to begin the

Table 5–1.   Infections Associated with Primary or Acquired T-Cell Dysfunction

Viral Infections
  Vaccinia
  Varicella-zoster
  Herpes simplex
  Cytomegalovirus
  Measles

Fungal Infections
  Mucocutaneous candidiasis
  Systemic candidiasis
  Cryptococcosis
  Aspergillosis

Bacterial and Mycobacterial Infections
  Tuberculosis
  Leprosy
  Bacillus Calmette-Guerin
  Listeriosis

Other Infections
  Toxoplasmosis
  Pneumocystis carinii
  Strongyloidiasis (disseminated)

(From Fauci, A.S.: Host-Defense Mechanisms Against Infections. Current Concepts. Kalamazoo, Michigan, The Upjohn Company, 1978.)

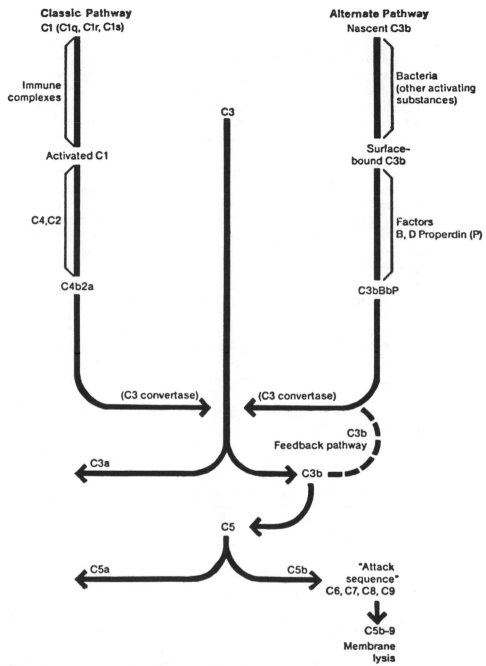

Fig. 5–2. Pathways of complement activation.
(From Goldstein, I.M.: Complement In Infectious Diseases. Current Concepts. Kalamazoo, Michigan, The Upjohn Company, 1980.)

progression of activity. The final common pathway of these two components of the complement system has a variety of important host defense functions. It helps the body kill bacteria as well as participating in the neutralization of viruses. For bactericidal activity, it produces factors that promote leukocyte chemotaxis, immune adherence, and opsonization. These complement factors also work with immunoglobulins to attack bacteria. In addition, complement increases vascular permeability.

Abnormalities of the complement system have varying degrees of import for the clinician. To date, deficiencies of the classic pathway have not been translated into recognizable human disease.[40] This is in distinction to defects in the alternative pathway of complement, which result in an increased rate of infection,[41] and to deficiencies in the final common pathway, which are also associated with clinical disease.[42] The action of complement is not always beneficial. The complement–fixing immune complex of the kidney in patients with glomerulonephritis results in the clinical syndrome of that disease.

Currently, there are few situations in which the clinician will evaluate complement in the care of patients. However, there is a correlation between low complement levels and active nephritis caused by the deposition of complement and immunoglobulins in the glomeruli of women with lupus erythematosus.[43] The measurement of complement assumes great importance in the care of the pregnant woman with lupus because low levels can be an indication of progression of renal disease.

There are other measures of complement and immunoglobulins that will have some significance for obstetrician-gynecologists in future years. Immune complexes are important markers of the interaction of the complement and humoral systems. Table 5–2 details the dynamics of immune complex formation, clearance, and deposition in tissue.[44] There are a wide variety of local and systemic factors that can influence this response, but it is already apparent that this is a measurable event in the progression of such systemic diseases as lupus erythematosus and rheumatoid arthritis as well as in malignancy. The wide variety of techniques used to measure serum immunocomplexes may account for the disparity of some of the results reported thus far. The obstetrician-gynecologist should be aware that these complexes have been reported to be present in normal pregnant women as well as in women with clinical evidence of salpingitis, condyloma acuminatum,

Table 5–2. Immune Complex Dynamics

Event	Variables
I. Encounter with antigen	1. Single event versus sustained exposure 2. Route of acquisition 3. Nature of antigen
II. Antibody synthesis	1. Genetically determined host immune response system 2. Prior encounter with antigen
III. Immune complex formation	1. In situ versus circulating
IV. Fate of immune complexes clearance by reticuloendothelial system	1. Reticuloendothelial system capacity 2. Reticuloendothelial system alteration by drugs 3. C_3b or Fc receptor
V. Deposition in tissues	1. Blood flow 2. Permeability changes 3. Antigen affinity for tissue 4. Cellular receptors (C_3b, Fc) 5. Prior tissue damage 6. Pharmacologic effects

(From Inman, R.D., and Day, N.K.: Immunologic and clinical aspects of immune complex disease. Am. J. Med., *70*:1097, 1981.)

and pelvic malignancies.[45] Their significance as a measure of progression of clinical disease will be the subject of many investigations in the next decade.

PHAGOCYTIC CELLS

In the past century, physicians and laymen have been aware of the importance of phagocytic cells in host defense. In 1887, Metchnikoff published a pioneering study on the importance of white cells in the protection against bacteria.[46] In "The Doctor's Dilemma," published in 1906, George Bernard Shaw had one of his characters intone: "Drugs are a delusion, stimulate the phagocyte."[47]

The neutrophil is the most important cell involved in primary defense against invading bacterial and viral agents. One of the most frequently ordered laboratory tests by clinicians is the total white blood cell count, with a differential count to show the total number of neutrophils as well as the number of immature forms (i.e., shift to the left). These tests have limited value because they measure only that small portion of the total number of neutrophils in circulating blood, while the bone marrow compartment contains far more neutrophils and is not measured by this exam. In addition these intravascular neutrophils have a rapid turnover, with a half-life of 6 to 7 hours.

The neutrophil has a rapid response to the invasion of bacteria into soft tissue sites. There are a number of chemotaxic factors released from tissue injury sites as well as factors in the serum that stimulate the migration of those white blood cells from the bloodstream to the site of injury. When the foreign agents are reached, phagocytosis is enhanced by various factors called opsonins, which include antibodies, complement, and other factors such as lysozymes. These opsonins render substances susceptible to phagocytosis. Phagocytosis proceeds with the ingestion of foreign substances. This is followed by intracellular killing and digestion of the microbiologic invaders. One of the laboratory evaluations of the neutrophils' ability to kill bacteria is the nitroblue tetrazolium test (NBT), which evaluates the ability of white blood cells to reduce nitroblue tetrazolium dye. In addition to this, there is a nonoxidase pathway of bacterial killing.

Any variation from normal in this scheme of white blood cell response may place the patient at increased risk for infection—either an increased rate or increased severity. For example, patients with too few white blood cells (neutropenia) are at risk for infection problems. They may have serious bacterial infections caused by *Staphylococcus, Serratia,* and *Pseudomonas* organisms. There are a number of clinical conditions associated with significant neutropenia (Table 5–3).[10] In contrast to this, normal numbers of neutrophils may be ineffective because of their inability to either engulf or destroy bacteria. Table 5–4[10] lists some of the clinical situations in which this may occur. Item six, the ineffective white blood cells of premature infants, is a major factor in the increased susceptibility of the newborn to bacterial infections.

Other types of peripheral white blood cells participate in the human host response to infection. In addition to the complex role eosinophils play in allergy, they are important in parasitic infections, particularly those due to *Schistosoma mansoni*.[48] The monocytes have a more prolonged response to infection and are involved in granuloma formation in certain types of infections such as tuberculosis and some fungal diseases.

There are a number of situations in obstetrics-gynecology in which white blood cell response can vary from normal. These should be acknowledged by the clinician in his evaluation of the patient with a suspected or proven bacterial infection.

Table 5–3. Clinical Conditions Associated wth Neutropenia

Major Categories	Individual Syndromes
I. Primary hematologic disorders	1. Aplastic anemia 2. Leukemias
II. Drug-induced	1. Suppressed production—chloramphenicol 2. Myelotoxic agents—alkylating agents, antimetabolites
III. Infections	1. Bacterial—typhoid fever, overwhelming sepsis 2. Viral—infectious mononucleosis, hepatitis
IV. Nutritional deficiencies	1. Folate (megaloblastic anemia of pregnancy) 2. B_{12} (pernicious anemia)
V. Associated with other diseases	1. Cirrhosis 2. Sarcoidosis 3. Systemic lupus erythematosus

(From Fauci, A.S.: Host-Defense Mechanisms Against Infections. Current Concepts. Kalamazoo, Michigan, The Upjohn Company, 1978.)

During pregnancy, there is a relative leukocytosis, which is more significant during labor and in the immediate postpartum period (Figure 5–3).[49] This leukocytosis is also associated with an increase in the number of immature white blood cell forms, and this also diminishes the diagnostic specificity of the white blood cell count during pregnancy. In general, the white blood cell test is used too frequently to evaluate patients without a firm clinical base. For example, the white blood cell count has been used often in patients with prolonged rupture of the membranes to detect incipient infection. I have been impressed that the elevated white count with a shift to the left is more often a marker of incipient labor than of infection.[50] There is no scientific justification for the frequently employed ritual of daily white blood cell counts in postoperative gynecologic patients as a screen for bacterial infections. There is no data to support this testing, and the patients' temperature response is a much more sensitive measure of bacterial infection. These white blood cell tests should be performed as part of the workup of patients with clinical symptoms and not as screening measures. I am distressed when an elevated white count becomes *prima facie* evidence for physician negligence in the care of a patient with postpartum infection when the laboratory result usually represented a variant of normal (Figure 5–3).[49]

Another laboratory test frequently ordered by clinicians is the sedimentation rate. Results can show elevation in women with bacterial infections, and it has

Table 5–4. Clinical Conditions with Defective Opsonic Activity

1. Agammaglobulinemia or hypogammaglobulinemia
2. Complement deficiency
3. Sickle cell anemia
4. Systemic lupus erythematosus
5. Cirrhosis
6. Premature infants

(From Fauci, A.S.: Host-Defense Mechanisms Against Infections. Current Concepts. Kalamazoo, Michigan, The Upjohn Company, 1978.)

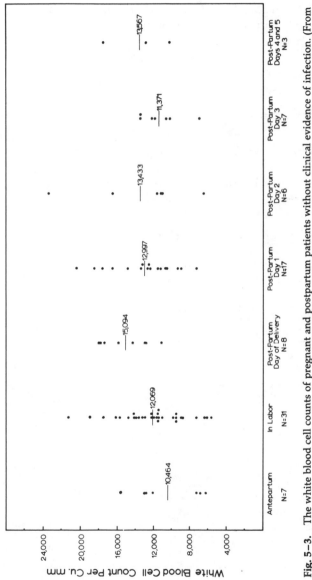

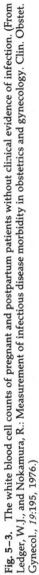

Fig. 5-3. The white blood cell counts of pregnant and postpartum patients without clinical evidence of infection. (From Ledger, W.J., and Nokamura, R.: Measurement of infectious disease morbidity in obstetrics and gynecology. Clin. Obstet. Gynecol., *19*:195, 1976.)

been touted by some experts as a valuable test to detect the presence of infection, e.g., as a screening test prior to a hysterosalpingogram or as a marker of the response of the patient with salpingitis to systemic antibiotics. There has not been uniform enthusiasm about reliance upon the sedimentation rate for a number of reasons. There are a number of physiologic changes that influence this test result. The sedimentation rate is usually higher in women than in men, and it is also uniformly elevated during pregnancy, particularly during the third trimester, labor, and the postpartum period. In addition, one study of infections following hysterosalpingogram showed no correlation between preprocedure elevated sedimentation rates and subsequent morbidity, while Eschenbach[51] could not show a parallel between the sedimentation rate and the patient's response to antibiotic treatment of salpingitis.

FEBRILE RESPONSE

Temperature elevation is a nonspecific response of the human host to most infections. The mechanisms of the production of fever have been studied in detail. Endogenous pyrogens are synthesized by the phagocytic cells of the host and act on the anterior hypothalamus-preoptic regions of the brain to produce fever.[52] These endogenous pyrogens may be stimulated by a number of exogenous pyrogens. These are noted in Table 5–5.[52]

The weight of evidence suggests that elevated temperatures are helpful in host response to infection. In animal studies in teleost fish, amphibia, reptiles, birds, and mammals, fever conferred a clear survival advantage over invading pathogens.[53] Blunting the febrile responses with antipyretics in many different animal

Table 5–5. Exogenous Pyrogens for Humans

Exogenous Pyrogens	Pyrogenic Substance
I. Viruses	1. Whole virus 2. Hemagglutinin
II. Gram-positive organisms	1. Whole organism 2. Peptidoglycans 3. Teichoic acids 4. Exotoxins 5. Enterotoxins 6. Proteins
III. Gram-negative organisms	1. Whole organism 2. Peptidoglycans 3. Lipid A
IV. Mycobacteria	1. Whole organism 2. Peptidoglycans 3. Polysaccharides 4. Protein
V. Fungi	1. Whole yeast 2. Capsular polysaccharide 3. Protein
VI. Steroids	1. Etiocholanolone
VII. Drugs	1. Penicillin 2. Prostaglandin 3. Bleomycin

(From Dinarello, C.A., and Wolff, S.M.: Fever. Current Concepts. Kalamazoo, Michigan, The Upjohn Company, 1980.)

models leads to increased mortality.[54] In the laboratory, elevated temperatures result in increased mobility,[55] increased intracellular killing of bacteria by polymorphonuclear leukocytes,[56] and greater susceptibility of antimicrobials.[57] Fever also increases the iron dependency of many bacteria.[58] In addition, it enhances the host production of antibody[59] and the antibacterial activity of amniotic fluid.[24] Clinically, those groups of patients who fail to have a good febrile response, i.e., the newborn, the aged, and the debilitated, have the worst prognosis in infectious disease. In contrast to all of these favorable outcomes, there is one study demonstrating that fever can augment mortality from endotoxin.[60]

Since the overwhelming weight of evidence supports a beneficial effect of fever in most instances of infection, the routine use of antipyretics for every febrile patient does not make therapeutic sense. If clinicians are concerned about the patient's comfort, they should be aware that the discomfort is related to both sudden elevations and drops in temperature. Giving antipyretics such as aspirin at four-hour intervals when their half-life is much shorter will result in more swings in temperature and more discomfort than if the antipyretics had not been given. Clearly, there are situations in which elevated temperatures should be reduced. If the physician is concerned about convulsions from hyperthermia or about a patient with a borderline cardiac reserve in whom the hypermetabolism may result in cardiac failure, a standard dose of antipyretics should be given initially, to be followed by a half-dose every two hours.

Febrile Response in Diagnosis

Our specialty, obstetrics-gynecology, has always been fascinated by a patient's febrile response to a bacterial infection. In the preantibiotic era, obstetrician-gynecologists established a standard of febrile morbidity, that is, a postpartum patient with an oral temperature of 100.4° F or higher on any two of the first 10 postpartum days, excluding the first 24 hours after delivery. Patients meeting this criterion were thought to have a bacterial infection and were coded as such in service statistics, and individual patients meeting this criterion were isolated from the afebrile noninfected patients.

The introduction of antibiotics into clinical practice had an impact on both morbidity and mortality figures. Unfortunately, too many obstetric services have continued to cling to the old preantibiotic definition of febrile morbidity. The patient with an incubating uterine bacterial infection given systemic antibiotics with the first rise in temperature may not satisfy this temperature definition during her hospitalization, and these patients subsequently are lost from the statistical analysis of the service. Modern obstetric services utilizing this definition must also include information on the number of women who have received systemic antibiotics, so that an accurate judgment of the number of patients with infections can be made.

There have been attempts to modify the preantibiotic obstetric definition of febrile morbidity to fit gynecologic patients.[61, 62]

1. A temperature of 101°F on two measurements at least six hours apart, excluding the first 48 postoperative hours.[61]
2. Rises in temperature up to 101°F during the first three postoperative days were usually without consequence. Those patients whose temperatures rose above this level or remained elevated after the first three days were classified as morbid.[62]

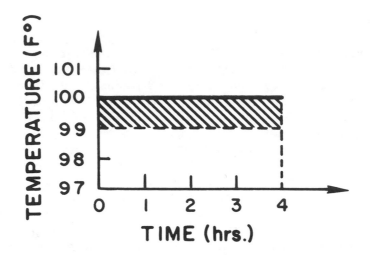

Fig. 5–4. The fever index, a quantitative indirect measure of infection in obstetric and gynecologic patients. The baseline used is 99° F, and two consecutive readings of 100° F at a four-hour interval yield four degree-hours of fever. (From Ledger, W.J., and Kriewall, R.J.: The fever index: A quantitative indirect measurement of hospital-acquired infections in obstetrics and gynecology. Am. J. Obstet. Gynecol., *115*:514, 1973.)

These investigators modified the obstetric definition of febrile morbidity in gynecologic patients in the hope that rises in temperature from atelectasis would not be included in any study of postoperative gynecologic morbidity. In this way, those patients with infections of the urinary tract, of abdominal wounds, or of the pelvis would be measured by these new standards. Evaluation of the accuracy of these defintions requires prospective studies in which there are strict controls on the use of antibiotics. Such studies have not been done. The advantage of any temperature definition is that the taking and recording of temperature are simple and reproducible measures. The disadvantage is that the significance of these febrile changes is really not known. Evaluation of rises in temperature during any treatment regimen that depends solely on these definitions of morbidity is senseless because this is an indirect measure. I am certain that reference to a temperature definition will continue to appear in the literature, but the investigators should be required to include other criteria for the evaluation of the therapeutic response, and especially for antibiotic usage.

FEVER INDEX

Another attempt to apply a measure of temperature elevation in patients with infection is the fever index, a quantitative indirect measure. Figure 5–4 demonstrates the basis for the measurement in degree-hours, utilizing a Fortran computer program for calculation.[63] This measure can be used to evaluate the temperature response of patients in many different clinical situations, including hospitalized gynecological patients with or without clinical evidence of infection (Figure 5–5).[64] Although there is some overlap between the upper and lower range of normal in patients with clinical evidence of infection, this measure does establish two distinct clinical groups. It can be used to compare gynecologic patients undergoing vaginal hysterectomy who have received either placebo or prophylactic antibiotics on the day of operation (Figure 5–6).[65] Although an indirect measure,

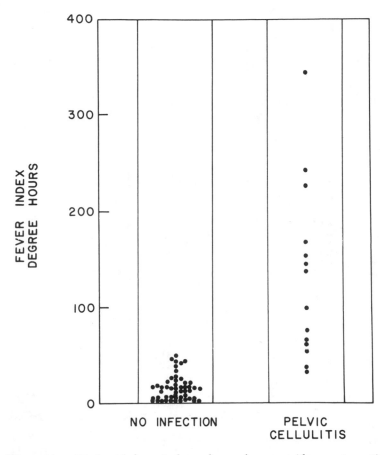

Fig. 5–5. The postoperative fever indexes, in degree-hours of women with no postoperative infection and those with a diagnosis of pelvic cellulitis who received systemic antibiotics. Although there is an overlap, this evaluation identifies two separate types of response to the operation. (From Ledger, W.J.: Infectious disease. *In* Gynecology and Obstetrics. Edited by S.L. Romney, M.J. Gray, A.B. Little, J.A. Merrill, E.J. Quilligan, and R. Stander. New York, McGraw-Hill, 1975.)

it does give a numerical basic for the evaluation of the therapeutic response of obstetric and gynecologic patients with infections who are being subjected to a prospective study. The fever index has been employed in studies of patients with septic abortions[66] and in evaluation of morbidity following cesarean section.[67]

REFERENCES

1. Westrom, L.: Incidence, prevalence, and trends of acute pelvic inflammatory disease and its consequences in industrialized countries. Am. J. Obstet. Gynecol., *138*:880, 1980.
2. Update on Kaposi's and opportunistic infections in previously healthy persons. United States. Morbid. Mortal. Wkly. Rep., *31*:294, 1982.
3. Siegal, M.: Unresolved issues in the first five years of the rubella immunization program. Am. J. Obstet. Gynecol., *124*:327, 1976.
4. Burke, J.F., Quinby, W.C., Bondoc, C.C., Sheehy, E.M., and Moreno, H.C.: The contribution of a bacterially isolated environment to the prevention of infection in seriously burned patients. Ann. Surg., *186*:377, 1977.
5. Cruse, P.J.E., and Foord, R.: A five year prospective study of 23,649 surgical wounds. Arch. Surg., *107*:206, 1973.
6. Newhouse, M., Sanchis, J., and Bienenstock, J.: Lung defense mechanisms. N. Engl. J. Med., *295*:990, 1976.

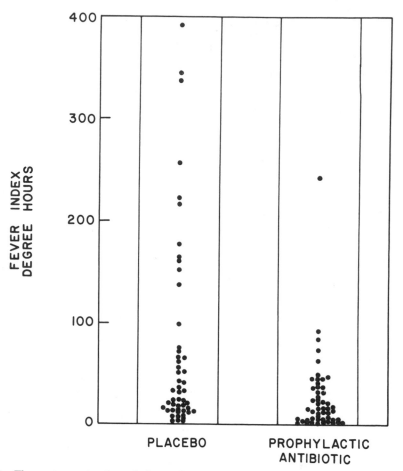

Fig. 5–6. The postoperative fever indexes of two groups of women who underwent vaginal hysterectomy; one group received placebo and the other prophylactic antibiotics. More prolonged fevers are seen in the placebo group. (From Ledger, W.J., Gassner, G., and Gee, C.: Operative care of infections in obstetrics and gynecology. J. Reprod. Med., *13*:128, 1974.)

7. Camner, P., Jarshand, C., and Philipson, K.: Tracheobronchial clearance in patients with influenza. Am. Rev. Resp. Dis., *108*:131, 1973.
8. Donaldson, R.M., Jr.: The relation of enteric bacterial populations to gastrointestinal function and disease. *In* Gastrointestinal Disease: Pathophysiocology, Diagnosis, Management. Edited by M. H. Sleisenger and J. S. Fordtran. Philadelphia, W.B. Saunders, 1973.
9. Fekety, R., and Quintiliani, R.: Current approach to the treatment of antibiotic associated diarrhea. Infect. Surg., *1*:13 (Sept.), 1982.
10. Fauci, A.S.: Host-Defense Mechanisms Against Infections. Current Concepts. Kalamazoo, Michigan, The Upjohn Company, 1978.
11. Taylor, H.A., Bradford, S.A., and Patterson, S.P.: Gonococcal arthritis in pregnancy. Obstet. Gynecol., *27*:776, 1966.
12. Draper, D.L., Donegan, E.A., James, J.F., Sweet, R.L., and Brooks, G.F.: In vitro modeling of acute salpingitis caused by *Neisseria gonorrhoeae*. Am. J. Obstet. Gynecol., *138*:996, 1980.
13. Holmes, K.K., Eschenbach, D.A., and Knapp, J.S.: Salpingitis: Overview of etiology and epidemiology. Am. J. Obstet. Gynecol., *138*:893, 1980.
14. Cherry, S.H., Filler, M., and Harvey, H.: Lysozyme content of amniotic fluid. Am. J. Obstet. Gynecol., *116*:639, 1973.
15. Larsen, B., and Galask, R.P.: Host resistance to intra-amniotic infection. Obstet. Gynecol. Surv., *30*:675, 1975.
16. Ford, L.C. Delange, R.J., and Lebherz, T.B.: Identification of a bactericidal factor (β-lysin) in amnionic fluid at 40 weeks gestation. Am. J. Obstet. Gynecol., *127*:788, 1977.

17. Gusdon, J.P.: A bactericidin for *Bacillus subtilis* in pregnancy. J. Immunol., *88*:494, 1962.
18. Larsen, B., Snyder, I.S., and Galask, R.P.: Transferrin concentration in human amniotic fluid. Am. J. Obstet. Gynecol., *117*:952, 1973.
19. Cederqvist, L.L., Ewool, L.C., Bonsnes, R.W., and Litwin, S.D.: Detectability and pattern of immunoglobulins in normal amniotic fluid throughout gestation. Am. J. Obstet. Gynecol., *130*:220, 1978.
20. Larsen, B., Galask, R.P., and Snyder, I.S.: Muramidase and peroxidase activity of human amniotic fluid. Obstet. Gynecol., *44*:219, 1974.
21. Larsen, B., Snyder, I.S., and Galask, R.P.: Bacterial growth inhibition by amniotic fluid. II. Reversal of amniotic fluid bacterial growth inhibition by addition of a chemically defined medium. Am. J. Obstet. Gynecol., *119*:497, 1974.
22. Schlievert, P., Johnson, W., and Galask, R.P.: Bacterial growth inhibition by amniotic fluid. Am. J. Obstet. Gynecol., *125*:899, 1976.
23. Applebaum, P.C., Shulman, G., Chambers, N.L., Simon, N.V., Granados, J.L. Fairbrother, P.F., and Naeye, R.L.: Studies on the growth inhibiting property of amniotic fluid from two United States population groups. Am. J. Obstet. Gynecol., *137*:579, 1980.
24. Larsen, B., and Davis, B.: Enhancement of the antibacterial property of amniotic fluid by hyperthermia. Obstet. Gynecol., *63*:425, 1984.
25. Tafari, N., Ross, S.M., Naeye, R.L., Galask, R.P., and Zaar B.: Failure of bacterial growth inhibition by amniotic fluid. Am. J. Obstet. Gynecol., *128*:187, 1977.
26. Lebherz, T.B., Hellman, L.P., Madding, R. Anctil, A., and Arje, S.L.: Double blind study of premature rupture of the membranes. Am. J. Obstet. Gynecol., *87*:218, 1963.
27. Blanco, J.D., Gibbs, R.S., Krebs, L.F., and Castaneda, Y.S.: The association between the absence of amniotic fluid bacterial inhibitory activity and intra-amniotic infection. Am. J. Gynecol., *143*:749, 1982.
28. Mann, J.M., Preblud, S.R., Hoffman, R.E., Brandling-Bennett, A.D., Hinman, A.R., and Herrmann, K.L.: Assessing risks of rubella infection during pregnancy. J.A.M.A., *245*:1647, American Medical Association.
29. Welch, P.C., Masur, H., Jones, T.C., and Remington, J.S.: Serologic diagnosis of acute lymphadenopathic toxoplasmosis. J. Infect. Dis., *142*:256, 1980.
30. Dionigi, R., Dominioni, L., and Campani, M.: Infections in cancer patients. Surg. Clin. North Am., *60*:145, 1980.
31. Frangione, B., and Franklin, E.C.: Heavy chain diseases: Clinical features and molecular significance of the disordered immunoglobulin structure. Semin. Hematol., *10*:53, 1973.
32. Munster, A.M., Hoagland, H.C., and Pruitt, B.A., Jr.: The effect of thermal injury on serum immunoglobulins. Ann. Surg., *172*:965, 1970.
33. Brenner, B.M., Hostetter, T.H., and Humes, H.D.: Molecular basis of proteinuria of glomerular origin. N. Engl. J. Med., *298*:826, 1978.
34. Stobo, J.D., Paul, S., Van Scoy, R.E., and Hermans, P.E.: Suppressor thymus-derived lymphocytes in fungal infection. J. Clin. Invest., *57*:319, 1976.
35. Witkin, S.S., Yu, I.R., and Ledger, W.J.: Inhibition of *Candida albicans*-induced lymphocyte proliferation by lymphocytes and sera from women with recurrent vaginitis. Am. J. Obstet. Gynecol., *147*:809, 1983.
36. Murray, H.W., Rubin, B.Y., Masur, H., and Roberts, R.B.: Impaired production of lymphokines and immune (gamma) interferon in the acquired immunodeficiency syndrome. N. Engl. J. Med., *310*:883, 1984.
37. Saxon, A., Stevens, R.H., Ramer, S.J., Clements, P.J., and Yu, D.T.Y.: Glucocorticoids administered in vivo inhibit human suppressor T lymphocyte function and diminish B lymphocyte responsiveness in *in vitro* immunoglobulin synthesis, J. Clin. Invest., *61*:922, 1978.
38. Current, W.L., Reese, N.C., Ernst, J.V., Bailey, W.S., Heyman, M.B., and Weinstein, W.M.: Human cryptosporidiosis in immunocompetent and immunodeficient persons. N. Engl. J. Med., *308*:1252, 1983.
39. Goldstein, I.M.: Complement in Infectious Diseases. Current Concepts. Kalamazoo, Michigan, The Upjohn Company, 1980.
40. Fearon, D.T., and Austen, K.F.: The alternative pathway of complement. A system for host resistance of microbial infection. N. Engl. J. Med., *303*:259, 1980.
41. Alper, C.A., Abramson, N., Johnston, R.B., Jr., Jandl, J.H., and Rosen, F.S.: Increased susceptibility to infection associated with abnormalities of complement-mediated functions and of the third component of complement (C_3). N. Engl. J. Med., *282*:349, 1970.
42. Miller, M.E., and Nilsson, U.R.: A familial deficiency of the phagocytosis enhancing activity of serum related to a dysfunction of the fifth component of complement (C_5). N. Engl. J. Med., *282*:354, 1970.
43. Hecht, B., Siegel, N., Adler, M., Kashgarian, M., and Hayslett, J.P.: Prognostic indices in lupus nephritis. Medicine, *55*:163, 1976.

44. Inman, R.D., and Day, N.K.: Immunologic and clinical aspects of immune complex disease. Am. J. Med., *70*:1097, 1981.
45. Witkin, S.S., and Ledger, W.J.: Circulating immune complexes in sera of patients with gynecologic disorders. Surg. Gynecol. Obstet. *159*:413, 1984.
46. Metchnikoff, E.: Sur la culte des cellules de l'organisme contre l'invasion des microbes. Ann Inst. Pasteur, *1*:321, 1887.
47. Shaw, G.B.: The Doctor's Dilemma. London, Constable, 1906.
48. Butterworth, A.E., David, J.R., Franks, D., Mahmood, A.A.F., David, P.H., Sturrock, R.F. and Houba, V.: Antibody-dependent eosinophil-mediated damage to 51 Cr-labeled schistosomula of *Schistosoma mansoni:* Damage by purified eosinophils. J. Exp. Med., *145*:136, 1977.
49. Ledger, W.J., and Nakamara, R.: Measurement of infectious disease morbidity in obstetrics and gynecology. Clin. Obstet. Gynecol., *19*:195, 1976.
50. Schreiber, J., and Benedetti, T.: Conservative management of pre-term premature rupture of the fetal membranes, in a low socioeconomic population. Am. J. Obstet. Gynecol., *136*:92, 1980.
51. Eschenbach, D.: Diagnosis and treatment of salpingo-oophoritis. *In* Antibiotics in Obstetrics and Gynecology. Edited by W.J. Ledger, The Hague, Martinus Nijhoff, 1982.
52. Dinarello, C.A., and Wolff, S.M.: Fever. Current Concepts. Kalamazoo, Michigan, The Upjohn Company, 1980.
53. Donaldson, J.F.: Therapy of acute fever: A comparative approach. Hosp., Prac. *16*:125, (Sept) 1981.
54. Vaughn, L.K., Veale, W.L., and Cooper, K.E.: Antipyresis: its effect on mortality rate of bacterially infected rabbits. Brain Res. Bull., *5*:69, 1980.
55. Nahas, G.G., Tanieres, M.L., and Lennon, J.F.: Direct measurement of leukolytic motility: Effects of pH and temperature. Soc. Exp. Biol. Med. Proc., *138*:350, 1971.
56. Sebag, J., Reed, W.P., and Williams, R.C., Jr.: Effect of temperature on bacterial killing by serum and polymorphnuclear leukocytes. Infect. Immun., *16*:947, 1977.
57. Mackowiak, P.A., Marling-Cason, M., and Cohen, R.L.: Effects of temperature on antimicrobial susceptibility of bacteria. J. Infect. Dis., *145*:550, 1982.
58. Grieger, T.A., and Kluger, M.J.: Fever and survival: The role of serum iron. J. Physiol., *279*:187, 1978.
59. Carmichael, L.E., Barnes, F.D., and Percy, D.H.: Temperature as a factor in resistance of young puppies to canine herpes virus. J. Infect. Dis., *120*:669, 1969.
60. Klastersky, J., and Kass, E.H.: Is suppression of fever or hypothermia useful in experimental and clinical infectious diseases? J. Infect. Dis., *121*:81, 1970.
61. Allen, J.L., Rampone, J.F., and Wheeless, C.R.: Use of a prophylactic antibiotic in elective major gynecologic operations. Obstet. Gynecol., *39*:218, 1970.
62. Porges, R.F.: Vaginal Hysterectomy at Bellevue Hospital: an experience in teaching residents, 1963–1967. Obstet. Gynecol., *35*:300, 1970.
63. Ledger, W.J., and Kriewall, T.J.: The fever index. A quantitative indirect measure of hospital acquired infections in obsteterics and gynecology. Am. J. Obstet. Gynecol., *115*:514, 1973.
64. Ledger, W.J.: Infectious disease. *In* Health Care of Women. Edited by S.H. Romney, M.J. Gray, A.B. Little, J.A. Marrill, E.J. Quilligan, and R. Stander. New York, McGraw-Hill Book Co., 1975.
65. Ledger, W.J., Gassner, C., and Gee, C.: Operative care of infections in obstetrics and gynecology. J. Reprod. Med., *13*:128, 1974.
66. Chow, A.W., Marshall, J.R., and Guze, L.B.: A double-blind comparison of clindamycin with penicillin plus chloramphenicol in treatment of septic abortion. J. Infect. Dis., *135*:S35, 1977.
67. Di Zerega, G.S., Yonekura, M.L., Roy, S., Nakamura, R.M., and Ledger, W.J.: A comparison of clindamycin-gentamicin and penicillin-gentamicin in the treatment of post cesarean section endomyometritis. Am. J. Obstet. Gynecol., *134*:238, 1979.

Chapter 6

A CLINICAL OVERVIEW OF INFECTIONS IN OBSTETRIC AND GYNECOLOGIC PATIENTS

CLASSIFICATION

The framework for any discussion of infections in women is a system of classification. One of the simplest and most meaningful classifications is the differentiation of infections as community-acquired or hospital-acquired (nosocomial). Community-acquired infections in women, including pharyngitis, vaginitis, urinary tract infections, and salpingitis, are those most frequently seen by an obstetrician-gynecologist, with the vast majority of these patients being treated as outpatients. In hospitalized patients with infections, the emphasis has changed in the past decade. In the 1950s, 1960s, and the early 1970s, the focus was upon serious community-acquired infections such as infection and death in patients with septic abortions from *Clostridium perfringens*[1] abortion sepsis, and death with an intrauterine contraceptive device in situ,[2] or sepsis and death in women with ruptured tubo-ovarian abscesses.[3] Recently, the emphasis on infections in hospitalized patients has switched from community to hospital-acquired infections. Surveillance studies of an obstetric[4] and gynecologic[5] service showed that the majority of infections in hospitalized patients were hospital-acquired. Bacteremia surveys of large urban obstetric-gynecologic services in Los Angeles[6] and San Antonio[7] demonstrated that the majority of such incidents were secondary to hospital-acquired infections. Increasingly, physicians must evaluate patients for postpartum and postoperative infections of the respiratory tract, the urinary tract, abdominal and vaginal incisions, or pelvic structures.

Another classification of infections in women is based upon the source of the bacterial pathogens, either exogenous (from outside sources) or endogenous (from the patients' own flora). This assessment of bacteria is detailed in Chapter 2. These two classifications can help the clinician in the initial assessment of the patient with an infection. In general, the organisms recovered from hospital-acquired infections have a greater possibility of being more resistant to antibiotics. Hospital infections frequently result after colonization of the patient by gram-negative aerobic bacteria,[8] are acquired from other patients as in epidemic diarrhea and pseudomembranous enterocolitis with patient to patient spread of *Clostridium difficile*,[9] or are carried by exogenous sources in the environment, such as transducers on the obstetric services colonized by group B beta-hemolytic streptococci.[10] Some serious gram-negative aerobic infections with organisms that are difficult to treat have been seen in the hospital. Examples of infections due to *Serratia marcescens* have been seen in the neonatal intensive care nursery[11] and of *Erwinia, Enterobacter cloacae,* and *Pseudomonas stutzeri* sepsis resulting from contaminated caps on intravenous bottles.[12] If a new organism appears with frequency in patients with hospital-acquired infection, all invasive equipment and instruments should be evaluated to see if they are serving as vehicles for the infections.

SURVEILLANCE METHODS

Most physicians who do either elective surgery or other invasive procedures tend to underestimate the incidence of hospital-acquired infections. There are many good examples of less than accurate evaluations by individual physicians. Finland found a large discrepancy between the incidence of infections reported from a hospital and the much larger number actually present when a close survey of patients was carried out.[13] In a gynecologic evaluation of over 12,000 women undergoing hysterectomy in the preprophylaxis era, Ledger and Child demonstrated a wide gap between the number of women receiving systemic antibiotics during their hospitalization and a much smaller number of women in whom a postoperative infection was coded as a final diagnosis.[14] Systemic antibiotics were given to nearly 50% of the patients, while a coded site of infection was acknowledged in less than 10%. In obstetrics, the highest incidence of fetal scalp infection following the use of fetal electrodes, many times greater than found in a number of other studies, was reported when an independent investigator, not directly involved in the care of the mother or baby, saw and evaluated these newborns each day.[15]

This underestimation of the frequency of infection should not come as a surprise to any clinician. Physicians who perform invasive diagnostic or therapeutic procedures need to have high levels of self-confidence and self-esteem. These can be undermined by too frequent recalls of individual patients who acquired infections after elective operations or invasive diagnostic procedures. One effective psychological defense mechanism is denial. This takes many forms, and this physician behavior can be recognized by direct observation during postpartum or postoperative rounds. The febrile patient whose vaginal or abdominal wound requires drainage is said to have a "seroma" or a "hematoma," not an infection. The patient with a postoperative pelvic infection who requires systemic antibiotics for cure is not coded as having an infection, and this is justified because no pelvic examination was done prior to therapy. The site of infection remains unknown, no cultures are done, and the infection is not coded. All of these frequently observed responses lead to the underestimation of the frequency of infection in postoperative and postpartum patients.

These individual shortcomings are not irreversible, for there are a number of things each practitioner can do to upgrade his diagnostic acumen and with this the quality of medical care. There is no substitute for the hands-on evaluation of the febrile postoperative or postpartum patient. Temperature elevation is the early warning system. The white blood cell count does not confirm or deny the presence of infection, and this is true for the microbiology reports as well; therefore the patient must be examined. The necessity of this physical and pelvic examination in making the diagnosis must be acknowledged by the physician, who also must have an awareness of the ability of administered antibiotics to modify the clinical picture to the point that a diagnosis of the exact site of infection cannot be made.[16] This requires adherence to guidelines of proper medical care in the approach to these patients. Antibiotics should not be prescribed for any febrile postoperative or postpartum patient without a prior examination, and the too-common practice of prolonging the postoperative use of prophylactic antibiotics[17] has to be avoided. If after examination, clinicians are unwilling to commit themselves on the chart to the site of infection, antibiotics should not be prescribed. If a urinary tract infection is suspected clinically, then antimicrobials that include the sulfas or nitrofurans, which have limited activity outside the urinary tract, should be prescribed.

If patients remain febrile after these initial evaluations, they should be reexamined. I have always been impressed at how frequently on reexamination an obvious entity like an abdominal wound infection will be discovered that either was not present or was not apparent to me on the first examination. Every clinician becomes an observant sleuth looking for the site of infection. During each abdominal and pelvic examination, one should look for induration or the purulent exudate from an infected collection or abscess. This thorough repeat examination is also important in women who remain febrile after antibiotics have been instituted. In some cases, ultrasonography may have pinpointed the location of a deep abscess that was not obvious on repeat pelvic examinations of patients who remained febrile despite the administration of antibiotics. This combination of a repeat examination and a restrictive policy of antibiotic use will improve the diagnostic accuracy of the individual physician and upgrade the medical care of individual patients. In addition to these guidelines for individual patient care, each service should have an idea of the incidence of infection.

The physician who is called upon to evaluate the febrile patient should be aware of the possibility of factitious fever. Murray has emphasized a number of clues that can suggest this diagnosis.[18] If they are present, particularly in a patient who has had paramedical training, consider the diagnosis.

1. Unexpected physical findings, i.e., a slow pulse and cool skin despite the fever.
2. Unusual laboratory findings: a normal erythrocyte sedimentation rate (ESR) and blood count and polymicrobial bacteremia.
3. Strange fever patterns.
4. Bizarre patient patterns of response, i.e., failure to cooperate with standard temperature-taking.

There are three principal means of altering the temperature reading: thermometer manipulations, falsification of the temperature chart, and self-injection of pyrogens. One recent ob-gyn report contained the record of a woman who injected herself with feces.[19] Confirmation of the diagnosis of factitious fever requires temperature-taking by the physician or obtaining a temperature reading of freshly voided urine, which will be proportionally lower than recorded oral or rectal temperature.[20] Part of the workup requires a search of the patient's room. Fortunately, these patients are rarely seen, but awareness of these warning signs may avoid a situation of prolonged patient exposure to potentially toxic antibiotics or a laparotomy for a pelvic abscess that is not present.

One way to accurately assess the frequency of infections on obstetric-gynecologic services is to establish a system of surveillance. Many hospital administrators have made the commitment to a nurse-epidemiologist, who makes rounds of the clinical microbiology laboratory and the in-patient services to survey results. The microbiology laboratory has the capability to compile antibiotic susceptibility patterns for frequently isolated organisms. This is important, for over the years I have been impressed by how gram-negative aerobic isolates, for example, *Escherichia coli,* can have susceptibility patterns that vary widely from hospital to hospital or from one city to another. An appropriate antibiotic selection in Los Angeles can be inappropriate in New York City. Even within a city, there may be differences: the gram-negative bacteria isolated from a hospital in the Bronx (New York) can be different from those recovered from patients on the other side of the city in a Manhattan hospital. Finally, the crucial ingredient in any surveillance system is a commitment by clinicians to make it work. This requires the clinicians' willingness to examine the patient and obtain cultures from suspected sites of infection prior to the initiation of antibiotic therapy.

A number of ground rules need to be established and followed in order for any surveillance system to provide meaningful and reproducible data. Firm guidelines must be established for uniform documentation of infection. If systemic antibiotics are given to the postoperative patient, she should be coded as having an infection whether or not she meets any temperature criteria of morbidity and despite the individual clinician's personal lack of acknowledgment of his patient's infection. The only difficulty with this arbitrary decision equating the use of antibiotics with postoperative infections is on services where prophylactic antibiotics are given for prolonged periods postoperatively.[17] This problem does not exist if the administration of prophylactic antibiotics is limited to the day of operation.

Another arbitrary decision is that any abdominal wound requiring drainage in the postoperative period should be coded as infected whether or not there is gross evidence of purulent material. This criterion differs from more rigid ones by general surgeons.[21] It probably overestimates the number of difficulties with wounds, but it prevents the underreporting of infections on a clinical service.

With the exception of significant bacterial colony counts from properly collected urine samples, the diagnosis of postoperative infection is not based on the microbiologic recovery of "pathogens." A number of careful microbiologic studies of the vaginal bacterial flora of sexually active women who have no clinical evidence of infection reveal the recovery of a number of "pathogenic" organisms. These findings do not lend support to any concept of the diagnosis of soft tissue infection on microbiologic grounds. The physician cannot deny the presence of infections because "pathogens" have not been isolated on bacterial culture. For example, the lack of isolation of anaerobes may be due to the clinician's poor collection of specimens. Soft tissue infection is a clinical diagnosis made by the physician in charge of the care of the patient, and it should be the basis for the prescription of systemic antibiotics. If all of these ground rules are followed, the surveillance team can provide meaningful data on the extent of infection on an obstetric-gynecologic service.

The efforts and expense of a surveillance system can pay handsome dividends for any clinical service committed to its utilization. Surveillance data will increase the clinical staff's awareness of the frequency of infections on a service and provide a stimulus for preventive efforts to decrease this incidence.

The surveillance team may be the first to recognize an epidemic of hospital-acquired infections caused by a common microorganism and should be the source of suggestions necessary for its control. If no epidemic is present, the team can prevent the ill-advised efforts of individual physicians to control the spread. This is extremely important. The appearance in a circumscribed time of a concentration of untoward events, such as wound infections, often leads to irrational behavior by clinicians. Many physicians performing surgical procedures have their own theories about the source of the outbreak and may institute such measures as prolonged preoperative hand-scrubbing, mandatory hand-dipping into caustic solutions, or the use of extra face masks. Such proposed techniques are not based on scientific data, particularly if the surveillance team demonstrates that the bacteria involved in the infectious outbreak are probably endogenous to the patient and are not transmitted by physicians or found in the environment.

The discovery of a series of infections caused by *Staphylococcus aureus* of identical antibiotic susceptibility whose common source is identified by phage type or by a group A beta-hemolytic *Streptococcus* should lead to efforts to identify the hospital personnel responsible for the epidemic of exogenous bacterial infection. In the past, such epidemiologic and microbiologic sleuthing exposed the improperly covered long hair of a house staff officer,[22] the rectal carriage of a bacterial pathogen by an anesthesiologist,[23] and the contamination of an air intake system for air conditioning.[24] In addition, new hospital construction in Los Angeles resulted in an epidemic of *Legionella pneumophilia* pneumonia because of the presence of this organism in soil at the hospital site and subsequent contamination of potable water within the institution.[25] Clearly, epidemics of infectious disease need expert investigation. Frequently one case of a *Staphylococcus* wound infection will result in other cases being seen because of contamination of the hospital environment. The surveillance team can provide guidelines for the isolation of patients with potentially dangerous infections.

In addition to these benefits, through periodic reports of antibiotic susceptibility of bacteria the surveillance team can provide a basis for the initial antibiotic prescription for patients who have clinical evidence of infection before microbiology laboratory reports are available. The limited appropriate use of antibiotics for patients should decrease the cost of hospital care. All the benefits of an active surveillance system should increase the quality of patient care on a clinical service.

A GUIDE TO STUDIES OF INFECTION IN THE OBSTETRIC-GYNECOLOGIC LITERATURE

The practicing physician needs the same discipline when reading medical literature on problems of infection that is required for the appropriate evaluation of individual patients with suspected infections. The dominant social ethic in the United States has always been success, and this theme is obvious in the perusal of our literature. We are constantly bombarded by reports of new techniques, new laboratory tests, and new drugs, all of which will improve the physician's ability to care for obstetric-gynecologic patients. Just as "all that glitters is not gold,"[26] not every initial enthusiastic report has been confirmed by subsequent evaluation.

There are a number of key points to be assessed by the discriminating reader of infectious disease literature. These points can be highlighted by the realities of clinical investigation. No one does a clinical study of a new technique or a new therapeutic approach or treats recognized clinical infections with new anti-biotic agents without a bias. If you don't believe a new treatment will be better than regimens used in the past or are suspicious that the initial report was too enthusiastic, you do not do the study. This bias is important, for it provides the impetus for initiating the study and collecting the data. However, it can be detrimental if it influences the collection of information or the analysis of the data obtained.

The first clinical studies with a new antibiotic are efficacy studies. In these, the antibiotic is employed in patients with a variety of soft tissue pelvic infections. An investigator experienced with this type of study may tend to employ these new agents in patients with early infections that are not serious. This clearly was the direction taken with the early clinical studies with metronidazole[27] and ce-foxitin.[28] After these studies have indicated effectiveness, the next step is to compare the drug with a placebo or with other antibiotics in the area of prophylaxis so the new drug can be comparatively evaluated in the treatment of infection. There are two critical points of evaluation of these clinical studies to determine whether or not the investigator bias has been dealt with in a proper way. One good method is the double-blind study, in which neither the investigator nor the patient knows which of the drugs under evaluation has been employed. Main-taining the integrity of the double-blind format is difficult. I am not aware of any other situation in clinical medicine in which everyone involved in patient care, including the nursing and house staff, is so eager to break the code. It is important in every double-blind study that the code not be broken on an individual patient until the time period of evaluation and the assessment have been com-pleted. Gibbs has emphasized the importance of the double-blind method in postcesarean endomyometritis. In a comparative trial of cefamandole versus clin-damycin and gentamicin,[29] he stressed that when the study began his house officers were convinced that clindamycin and gentamicin were superior because of pre-viously reported trials with this regimen.[30] The double-blind method was the only way to ensure that cefamandole would get a fair trial, and it was found that the two regimens had equivalent results if side-effects were included in the compar-ison.[29]

Another study illustrates the problems when investigators are not strict in their enforcement of the double-blind protocol. In a recent study purporting to show the superiority of three days of ampicillin prophylaxis over a one-day course in cesarean section patients, the code was broken in every patient requiring additional antibiotic therapy.[31] This meant that the observers, with their bias, knew which course of the prophylactic drug the patients who required additional treatment had received, and this obviously influenced their observations. When the code has been broken, a major concern is that the investigator will become more selective about the patients included in the final published analysis. For example, if the patient who received the drug regimen favored by the investigator did not respond to treatment and developed a pelvic abscess, he might drop her from the study on the pretext that the protocol was not observed because the second dose of antibiotic was given a few minutes late. This unwise after-the-fact decision-making can be avoided if the double-blind method is scrupulously maintained.

The next crucial point is the method by which patients are enrolled in a study. Before the first patient is enrolled, the investigators have to make a decision to ensure an unselected or random group of patients for every aspect of the study. One excellent method to achieve this is a random table of numbers maintained separately in the pharmacy so that the investigators do not know which regimen is next on the list when a woman is enrolled in the study. Alternatively, patients can be assigned on the basis of the last number of the hospital record. If a random table of numbers is used or hospital numbers have been employed, it is important that the study groups are equivalent when the elevation is reported. Deviation in size should make the study design suspect. For example, a study of doxycycline prophylaxis in hysterectomy patients included 46 women who received placebo and 96 women who received doxycycline.[32] These differences in sample size imply investigator selection of the patients in the study groups and make it difficult to believe any judgments of the efficacy of the prophylactic regimen. There obviously had to be preselection of the two study populations to come up with such a large discrepancy in patient numbers. Similarly, a recent study of the best length of time of ampicillin prophylaxis in cesarean section patients had dissimilar numbers in the treatment groups—46 versus 37—and no explanation of the group distribution of the eight patients dropped from the study.[31] In contrast, a study of Gibbs and colleagues had 92 patients in the cefamandole group and 106 patients in the clindamycin-gentamicin treatment group, but they noted that this difference was attributable to a number of patients in the cefamandole population whose study drug was outdated when they were enrolled for the study.[29]

In addition, the reader should closely evaluate the comparability of the study populations. In addition to equivalent numbers, the investigators should note risk factors such as the age, race, and weight of the patient and any other factors that might influence the results. For example, in patients with salpingitis, how many had an early infection and how many had one that was well established?[33] In hysterectomy patients, how long did the operation take?[34] And in cesarean section patients, how many had been in labor when the operation was performed?[35] The comparability of the study groups is in doubt when patients with highly different degrees of risk are evaluated. For example, in one prospective study evaluating mezlocillin versus ampicillin in the initial treatment of postpartum endomyometritis,[36] there were differences in the risk factors. Eight of 33 (24.2%) of the group receiving mezlocillin had delivered vaginally as compared with 16 of 37 (43.2%) of the ampicillin group. Although the treatment results were equivalent, the study groups were not, for the risk of serious postpartum infection is much lower in women delivering vaginally. This makes the interpretation of the results difficult. Every reader should feel more secure about the evaluation of treatment results when the study populations at the time of treatment closely resemble each other.

Finally, in the evaluation of studies, maintain some skepticism about the multicenter evaluation. This type of study usually permits the use of a larger study group than is possible in one institution, but sometimes the variances among institutions are greater than those attributable to any treatment regimen. This was true in the multicenter evaluation of ultraviolet light in operating rooms.[37] If multicenter evaluations are published, as they have been for neomycin, erythromycin base bowel preparation in gastrointestinal surgery,[38] and the comparison of cefoxitin and cefazolin as prophylaxis in nonelective cesarean section,[39] the reader should note whether or not the results have been documented at each individual institution. If not, then there should be hesitation about accepting the conclusions of the study, because differences noted could have been achieved by chance in a small number of subjects at one or two hospitals while no differences occurred in the majority of the study sites. This information is necessary to make an informed judgment as to the validity of the study.

The next area of critical evaluation is the analysis of the results. Any study of infection in obstetrics-gynecology should include direct and indirect measures of infection. The clinician is most interested in the direct measures, although indirect measures may reinforce a trend. The direct measures include the clinical assessment of the patient's response to treatment and whether it is preventive, as with prophylactic antibiotics, or is the care of patients with an established infection. The results should always include the number of patients with an immediate clinical cure and those who failed to respond to therapy. The immediate response to therapeutic intervention is important, but it is often an incomplete evaluation of the efficacy of a specific treatment regimen. For example, one study of the use of adrenocortical steroids in the treatment of salpingitis showed a better immediate response in those patients receiving steroids, but on laparoscopic evaluation of the pelvis several months after treatment, there were no fewer patients with blocked tubes or adhesion formation among the group that had received the steroids than among the women who were treated with antibiotics alone.[40] Similarly, one of the arguments against the uniform use of prophylactic antibiotics in patients undergoing elective termination of pregnancy has been the low incidence of postprocedure pelvic infection in women who have not received antibiotics.[41] A critical unanswered question of therapy in this population is the long-term effect of infection upon the future fertility of the groups with immediate morbidity. If future fertility is lowered by infection, a much stronger justification could be made for antibiotic prophylaxis. The clinical course of the immediate failures of response to treatment should be detailed. Failures include those women who require either additional or alternative antibiotics for a cure, those in whom a clinical diagnosis of septic pelvic thrombophlebitis is made and heparin therapy is needed, and finally those who require operative intervention for drainage of an abdominal wound or pelvic abscess or laparotomy for the removal of a pelvic abscess. The investigator must note whether the study population had early or well-established infections, because the prognosis in the two groups is so different, with a higher immediate cure rate in those with early infection and a greater number of women with well-established infections who will require operative intervention for cure.[33] In addition, it is extremely important that a minimal follow-up period of at least six weeks is used in these studies. In one evaluation of hysterectomy prophylaxis, 19% of the infections were not noted until the patients had been discharged from the hospital.[42] The indirect measures of morbidity are attempts by investigators to more completely assess the impact of the therapeutic regimens. In evaluations of prophylaxis, some studies have detailed the number of women who are febrile enough to meet the obstetric definition of temperature morbidity, the number of degree-hours of fever in the study groups, and the days of posttreatment hospitalization.[43] Each of these measures individually can suggest a therapeutic trend, for example one recent comparison of prophylactic cefoxitin versus cefazolin in women undergoing cesarean section showed significantly lower numbers of degree-hours in febrile patients in the cefoxitin population.[39] This shows a therapeutic trend but should not be accepted as the sole reason for a physician to select a particular drug, in this case cefoxitin.

Another widely employed study method is the case control method. This is a retrospective method of analysis that compares a patient population with a specific problem to a group of controls to see if there are identifiable differences in the populations. If differences are noted, these may suggest cause-and-effect relationships. This is a popular method of analysis, for it can be done retrospectively. It is the study method that supports the concepts that exogenous estrogens are a factor in endometrial carcinoma,[44] that the intrauterine device carries with it an increased risk of pelvic infections,[45] and that oral contraceptives protect women against the subsequent development of ovarian cancer.[46] One critical factor in these studies is the appropriateness of the selection of the controls. For example, in studies evaluating a possible association between reserpine and breast cancer, patients with thyrotoxicosis, renal disease, or cardiovascular disease were excluded from the control nonbreast–cancer population. Since these women would be particularly likely to be receiving reserpine, their exclusion decreases the exposure rate to reserpine among the remaining controls and falsely elevates the apparent carcinogenic risk of reserpine exposure.[47] It is very important for the reader to evaluate the control group closely to be certain that exclusions have not biased the results. Another possible source of error in the case control method is a focus upon a possible etiologic agent. Suppose, for example, that an abnormal embryo can cause maternal genital bleeding, and this bleeding results in the administration of hormonal therapy. If these pregnancies continue to term, an association may be noted between hormonal exposure and birth defects.[48] The criteria for diagnosis of the point in question are another point of contention in these case control studies. In one case control study showing a higher incidence of salpingitis among women using intrauterine contraceptive devices, a significantly higher percentage of the women with this diagnosis were afebrile.[49] Was this variance due to different criteria of diagnosis, a higher incidence of nongonococcal salpingitis among IUCD users, or an error in diagnosis? These questions need to be addressed by prospective studies. They are not answerable by the case control method. Since these case control studies can be constructed retrospectively, there is a great temptation for their widespread use in the analysis of clinical problems. Read each of these studies with careful attention to detail to be sure these or other methodologic errors have been avoided. Careful reading permits an intelligent decision about the significance of the findings.

REFERENCES

1. Decker, W.H., and Hall, W.: Treatment of abortions infected with *Clostridium welchii.* Am. J. Obstet, Gynecol., *95*:394, 1966.
2. Christian, C.D.: Maternal deaths associated with an intrauterine device. Am. J. Obstet, Gynecol., *119*:441, 1974.
3. Collins, G.G., Nix, F.G., and Cerha, H.T.: Ruptured tubo-ovarian abscess. Am. J. Obstet, Gynecol., *72*:820, 1956.
4. Ledger, W.J., Reite, A.M., and Headington, J.T.: A system for infectious surveillance on an obstetric service. Obstet. Gynecol., *37*:769, 1971.
5. Ledger, W.J., Reite, A.M., and Headington, J.T.: The surveillance of infection of an inpatient gynecology service. Am. J. Obstet, Gynecol., *113*:662, 1972.
6. Ledger, W.J., Norman, M., Gee, C., and Lewis W.: Bacteremia on an obstetric gynecologic service. Am. J. Obstet. Gynecol., *121*:205, 1975.
7. Blanco, J.D., Gibbs, R.S., and Castaneda, Y.S.: Bacteremia in obstetrics: Clinical course. Obstet. Gynecol., *58*:621, 1981.
8. Tillotson, J.R., and Finland, M.: Bacterial colonization and clinical superinfection of the respiratory tract complicating antibiotic treatment of pneumonia. J. Infect. Dis., *119*:597, 1969.

9. Fekety, R., Kim, K.H., Brown, D., Batts, D.H., Cudmore, M., and Silva, J., Jr.: Epidemiology of antibiotic associated colitis. Isolation of *Clostridium difficile* from the hospital environment. Am. J. Med., *70*:906, 1981.

10. Davis, J.P., Moggio, M.V., Klein, D., Tiosejo, L.L., Welt, S.I., and Wilfert, C.M.: Vertical transmission of group B streptococcus: Relation to intrauterine fetal monitoring. J.A.M.A., *242*:42, 1979.

11. Christensen, G.D., Korones, S.B., Reed, L., Bulley, R., McLaughlin, B., and Bisno, A.L.: Epidemic *Serratia marcescens* in a neonatal intensive care unit: Importance of the gastrointestinal tract as a reservoir. Infect. Control *3*:127, 1982.

12. Felts, S.K., Schaffner, W., Melly, M.A., and Koenig, M.G.: Sepsis caused by contaminated intraveous fluids. Ann. Intern. Med., *77*:881, 1972.

13. Finland, M.: Excursions into epidemiology: Selected studies during the past four decades at Boston City Hospital. J. Infect. Dis., *128*:76, 1973.

14. Ledger, W.J., and Child, M.: The hospital care of patients undergoing hysterectomy. An analysis of 12,026 patients from the Professional Activity Study. Am. J. Obstet. Gynecol., *117*:423, 1973.

15. Okada, D.M., Chow, A.W., and Bruce, V.T.: Neonatal scalp abscess and fetal monitoring: Factors associated with infection. Am. J. Obstet. Gynecol., *129*:185, 1977.

16. Ohm, M.J., and Galask, R.P.: The effect of antibiotic prophylaxis on patients undergoing abdominal hysterectomy. I. Effect on morbidity. Am. J. Obstet. Gynecol., *125*:442, 1976.

17. Shapiro, M., Townsend, T.R., Rosner, B., and Kass, E.H.: Use of antimicrobial drugs in general hospitals: Patterns of prophylaxis. N. Engl. J. Med., *301*:351, 1979.

18. Murray, H.W.: Factitious fever updated. Arch. Int. Med., *139*:739, 1979.

19. Hustead, R.M., Lee, R.A., and Maruta, T.: Factitious illness in gynecology. Obstet. Gynecol., *59*:214, 1982.

20. Murray, H.W., Tuazon, C.U., Guerrero, I.C., Claudio, M.S., Alling, D.W., and Sheagren, J.N.: Urinary temperature: A clue to early diagnosis of factitious fever. N. Engl. J. Med., *296*:23, 1977.

21. Cruse, P.J.E., and Foord, R.: A five year prospective study of 23,649 surgical wounds. Arch. Surg., *107*:206, 1973.

22. Dineen, P., and Drusin, L.: Epidemics of postoperative wound infections associated with hair carriers. Lancet, *2*:1157, 1973.

23. McIntyre, D.M.: An epidemic of *Streptococcus pyogenes* puerperal and postoperative sepsis with an unusual carrier site—the anus. Am. J. Obstet. Gynecol., *101*:308, 1968.

24. Dondero, T.J., Jr., Rendtorff, R.C., Mallison, G.F., Weeks, R.M., Levy, J.S., Wong, E.W., and Schaffner, W.: An outbreak of Legionnaires' disease associated with a contaminated airconditioning cooling tower. N. Engl. J. Med., *302*:365, 1980.

25. Haley, C.E., Cohen, M.L., Halter, J., and Meyer, R.D.: Nosocomial Legionnaires' disease: A continuing common source epidemic at Wadsworth Medical Center. Ann. Intern. Med., *90*:583, 1979.

26. Shakespeare, W.: Merchant of Venice, Act II, Scene VII, Line 65.

27. Ledger, W.J., Gee, C.L., Pollin, P., Lewis, W.P., Sutter, V.L., and Finegold, S.M.: A new approach to patients with suspected anaerobic post-partum pelvic infection. Transabdominal uterine aspiration for culture and metronidazole for treatment. Am. J. Obstet. Gynecol., *126*:1, 1976.

28. Ledger, W.J., and Smith, D.: Cefoxitin in obstetric and gynecologic infections. Rev. Infect. Dis., *1*:199, 1979.

29. Gibbs, R.S., Blanco, J.D., Castaneda, Y.S., and St. Clair, P.J.: A double-blind randomized comparison of clindamycin-gentamicin versus cefamandole for treatment of post-cesarean section endomyometritis. Am. J. Obstet. Gynecol., *144*:261, 1982.

30. DiZerega, G., Yonekura, L., Roy, S., Nakamura, R.M., and Ledger, W.J.: A comparison of clindamycin gentamicin and penicillin gentamicin in the treatment of post cesarean endomyometritis. Am. J. Obstet. Gynecol., *134*:238, 1979.

31. Elliott, J.P., Freeman, R.K., and Dorchester, W.: Short versus long course of prophylactic antibiotics in cesarean section. Am. J. Obstet, Gynecol., *143*:740, 1982.

32. Wheeless, C.R., Jr., Dorsey, J.H., and Wharton, L.R., Jr.: An evaluation of prophylactic doxycycline in hysterectomy patients. J. Reprod. Med., *21*:146, 1978.

33. Ledger, W.J.: Selection of antimicrobial agents for treatment of infections of the female genital tract. Rev. Infect. Dis., *5*:S98, 1983.

34. Shapiro, M., Munoz, A., Tager, I.B., Schoenbaum, S.C., and Polk, B.F.: Risk factors for infection at the operative site after abdominal or vaginal hysterectomy. N. Engl. J. Med., *307*:1661, 1982.

35. Gibbs, R.S., Jones, P.M., and Wilder, C.J.Y.: Internal fetal monitoring and maternal infection following cesarean section. Obstet. Gynecol., *52*:193, 1978.

36. Sorrell, T.C., Marshall, J.R., Yoshimori, R., and Chow, A.W.: Antimicrobial therapy of postpartum endomyometritis. II. Prospective randomized trial of mezlocillin versus ampicillin. Am. J. Obstet. Gynecol., *141*:246, 1981.

37. Committee on Trauma, Division of Medical Sciences-National Research Council: Postoperative wound infections: The influence of ultraviolet irradiation of the operating room and of various other factors. Ann. Surg., *160*:(Supp. 1), 1964.

38. Clarke, J.S., Condon, R.E., Bartlett, J.G., Gorbach, S.L., Nichols, R.L., and Ochi, S.: Pre-operative oral antibiotics reduce septic complications of colorectal operations: Results of prospective, randomized, double-blind clinical study. Ann. Surg., *186*:251, 1977.
39. Stiver, H.G., Forward, K.R., Livingstone, R.A., Fugere, P., Le May, M., Verschelden, G., Hunter, J.D.W., Carson, G.D., Beresford, P., and Tyrrell, D.L.: Multicenter comparison of cefoxitin versus cefazolin for prevention of infectious morbidity after nonelective cesarean section. Am. J. Obstet. Gynecol., *145*:158, 1983.
40. Falk, V.: Treatment of acute non-tuberculous salpingitis with antibiotics alone and in combination with glucocorticoids. Acta Obstet. Gynecol. Scand., *44*, Suppl. 6, 1965.
41. Hodgson, J.E., Major, B., Portmann, K., and Quattlebuum, F.W.: Prophylactic use of tetracycline for first trimester abortions. Obstet. Gynecol., *45*:574, 1975.
42. Polk, B.F., Tager, I.B., Shapiro, M., Goren-White, B., Goldstein, P., and Schoenbaum, S.C.: Randomized clinical trial of perioperative cefazolin in preventing infection after hysterectomy. Lancet, *1*:437, 1980.
43. Young, R., Platt, L., and Ledger, W.J.: Prophylactic cefoxitin in cesarean section. Surg. Gynec. Obstet., *157*:11, 1983.
44. Horwitz, R.I., and Feinstein, A.R.: Alternative analytic methods for case control studies of estrogens and endometrial cancer. N. Engl. J. Med., *299*:1089, 1978.
45. Westrom, L., Bengtsson, L., and Mardh, P.: The risk of developing pelvic inflammatory disease in women using intrauterine devices as compared to non-users. Lancet, *2*:221, 1976.
46. Cramer, D.W., Hutchison, G.B., Welch, W.R., Scully, R.E., and Knapp, R.C.: Factors affecting the association of oral contraceptives and ovarian cancer. N. Engl. J. Med., *307*:1047, 1982.
47. Armstrong, B., Stevens, N., and Doll, R.: Retrospective study of the association between use of rauwolfia derivatives and breast cancer in English women. Lancet, *2*:672, 1974.
48. Hayden, G.F., Kramer, M.S., and Horwitz, R.I.: The case control study. J.A.M.A., *247*:326, 1982.
49. Eschenbach, D.A., Harnisch, J.P., and Holmes, K.K.: Pathogenesis of acute pelvic inflammatory disease: Role of contraception and other risk factors. Am. J. Obstet. Gynecol., *128*:838, 1977.

Chapter 7
ANTIMICROBIAL AGENTS

One of the cornerstones of obstetric and gynecologic practice is the utilization of chemotherapeutic agents for the treatment of infection. This occurs frequently. For the busy practitioner, there are few days in which prescriptions for chemotherapeutic agents are not written, both for hospitalized patients and outpatients. A wide variety of products is available. With antibiotics, they range from high dose intravenous antibiotics with a high potential for toxicity when given to seriously ill patients to the more commonly employed oral antibiotics that are less often seriously toxic. In addition, clinicians have other chemotherapeutic agents that work against nonbacterial pathogens in diseases such as *Trichomonas vaginalis* vaginitis, amoebic liver abscess, systemic candidiasis, and *herpes simplex* encephalitis. Systemic drug forms are not the only choice for the obstetrician-gynecologist, as there are local antibiotic, antifungal, and antiviral agents that can be given to patients.

PHARMACOKINETICS OF ANTIBIOTICS

The physician who is prescribing antibiotics should be aware of the many factors that influence serum and tissue levels. The antibiotic selected that kills the offending organisms in the laboratory will be ineffective in the patient if the routes or timing of the administration do not permit effective levels to be attained. Precise knowledge of the pharmacokinetics of antibiotics will help avoid therapeutic misadventure.

The mode of antibiotic administration determines serum and tissue levels in individual patients. Varying concentrations can be achieved when the intravenous, intramuscular, or oral route is employed.

The highest levels can be reached by the intravenous route, especially by bolus infusion, i.e., the antibiotic is added to a small volume of diluent and administered rapidly in 30 minutes or less. By contrast, the constant intravenous infusion of antibiotic over a period of hours results in lower levels in the bloodstream than the peak levels seen with the bolus method, but the constant infusion avoids the trough stage in which the antibiotic concentration in the blood falls below therapeutic levels before the next bolus dose is given. Although there are enthusiastic proponents of each technique of intravenous antibiotic administration, there have been no comparative clinical trials of patients with pelvic infections that demonstrate the superiority of one method over another. In an animal model designed to simulate an abscess, the bolus method resulted in higher antibiotic levels in the fibrin clot.[1] This is the way I usually order intravenous antibiotics, but other characteristics of antibiotics will influence the technique of intravenous administration. For example, bolus administration is not practical with doxycycline, because this approach results in a high incidence of superficial thrombophlebitis.[2] Also, there are limits on the amount of antibiotic given. The constraint of the potential toxicity of the aminoglycosides limits the amount of these agents that can be given intravenously as opposed to the much higher doses given of penicillins and cephalosporins.

The physician should also be aware of the chemistry of these agents. When carbenicillin and gentamicin are combined in the same intravenous solution, they will chemically bind, inactivating both and resulting in a lower amount of antibiotic being given to the patient.[3] The stability of the antibiotic in the intravenous fluid can also affect levels achieved. For example, there is loss of ampicillin activity when it is either added to hyperalimentation solutions[4] or kept in 5% glucose and water solutions for more than 12 hours.[5] If at all possible, ampicillin should be administered intravenously in a saline solution, or if glucose and water is the solution of choice, the ampicillin should be added and given immediately to the patient instead of being stored on the floor for up to 24 hours.

In addition to the impact upon peak levels reached by the rapid infusion of intravenous antibiotics, the patients' intravascular volume and the volume of distribution of the antibiotic inversely influence the levels. The greater the blood volume and/or the volume of distribution, the lower the peak serum levels of drug achieved. For antibiotics, the volume of distribution refers to the volume of fluid into which the antibiotic distributes throughout the body and its uptake in tissue. The influence of these two factors upon the blood drug levels attained is illustrated by the lower blood levels recorded when intravenous antibiotics are given during pregnancy. Pregnancy is associated with an increased blood volume, and in the case of ampicillin, there is a markedly increased volume of distribution (Table 7–1).[6] In the nonpregnant state, blood volume and the volume of distribution of an antibiotic usually correlate with patient size. The bigger the patient, the larger these volumes. This is the rationale for modifying the dosage of aminoglycosides based upon the patient's weight. There are exceptions. Massively obese patients have lower than expected blood volumes and volumes of distribution. Thus, they require lower doses of aminoglycosides to avoid toxicity.[7] It is especially important for the clinician to control peak and trough levels of aminoglycosides in this population so that toxicity of the eighth cranial nerve and of the kidney caused by too high serum levels can be avoided. The peak blood sample should be obtained 30 to 60 minutes after the infusion has been started, and the trough level should be obtained just prior to the administration of the next dose. For seriously ill patients, I believe that the intravenous route of

Table 7–1. The Impact of Pregnancy Upon the Volume of Distribution and Half-Life of Ampicillin

Clinical Status	Volume of Distribution ± SD	Half-Life ± SD
Pregnant	0.55 ± 0.28	39 min ± 8.1
Nonpregnant	0.41 ± 0.20	44 min ± 6.8
	Differences are significant $p < 0.05$	$p < 0.05$

(From Philipson, A.: Pharmacokinetics of ampicillin during pregnancy. J. Infect. Dis., *136*:370, 1977.)

administration is the treatment of choice, because it provides exact dosing and there is the capability of achieving the highest serum levels. The serum levels that can be expected and the serum half-life with intravenous infusion in non-pregnant women are noted in Table 7–2.[8, 9] The serum half-life of the antibiotic is the length of time required to eliminate one-half of the dose from the body.

The intramuscular route of administration results in lower peak serum levels than those obtained intravenously, and this peak requires a longer period of time to reach than in the intravenous approach (Figure 7–1).[9] Other factors can result in lower than expected levels of antibiotics in the blood. For example, intramuscular chloramphenicol is poorly absorbed, and therefore this route of administration for prophylaxis in patients undergoing vaginal hysterectomy produced poor results.[10] The aminoglycosides are notoriously inconsistent in their absorption when given intramuscularly,[11] and for this reason I believe that only the intravenous routes should be employed when these antibiotics are prescribed. Despite these shortcomings, I favor the intramuscular administration of a cephalosporin preoperatively for the prevention of pelvic infections in gynecologic patients.[12]

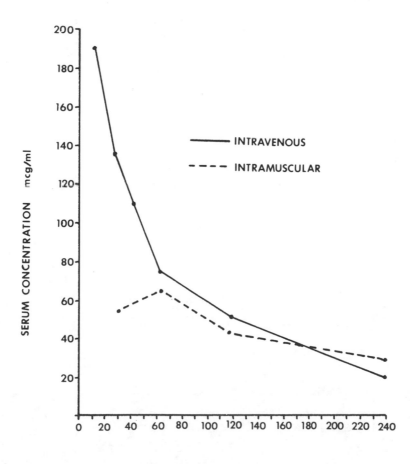

TIME AFTER INJECTION, MIN.

Fig. 7–1. The differences in serum levels of antibiotics achieved with the intramuscular or intravenous route.

Table 7-2. Intravenous Antibiotics

	Antibiotics	Dose	Serum Concentration μg/ml	Half-Life	Protein Binding (%)	Therapeutic Considerations
I.	Penicillins					
	Penicillin G	1,000,000 U	10	30 min	55	1.7 of Na$^+$ or K$^+$
	Ampicillin	1.0 gm	40	30–60 min	17	3 mEq of Na$^+$
	Carbenicillin	5.0 gm	200–300	75 min	50	Watch for bleeding, hypokalemia
	Ticarcillin	3.0 gm	150–200	60 min	50	4.7 mEq of Na$^+$ per gm
	Methicillin	1.0 gm	20–40	30–60 min	35	5.2 mEq of Na per gm
	Nafcillin	15 mg/kg	20–40	75 min	87	Interstitial nephritis
	Oxacillin	1.0 gm	40	30 min	93	
	Piperacillin	2.0 gm	300	55 min	16	2.9 mg Na per gm
	Mezlocillin	2.0 gm	150–200	60 min	26–42	
II.	Cephalosporins					
	Cephalothin	1.0 gm	40–60	30 min	65	2.5 mEq of Na$^+$ per gm
	Cefazolin	1.0 gm	90–120	90 min	85	2.0 mEq of Na$^+$ per gm
	Cefoxitin	1.0 gm	60–80	60 min	70	2.3 mEq of Na$^+$ per gm
	Cefamandole	1.0 gm	60–80	60 min	70	3.3 mEq of Na per gm
	Cefoperazone	1.0 gm	90–120	96–156 min	87–93.5	Diarrhea
	Ceftizoxime	1.0 gm	100	90 min	30%	
	Cefotaxime	1.0 gm	100	60 min	50%	
III.	Aminoglycosides					
	Gentamicin	1.5 mg/kg	5–7	120 min	low	Eighth nerve and renal toxicity
	Tobramycin	2.0 mg/kg	5–8	120 min	low	
	Amikacin	7.5 mg/kg	20–30	120 min	low	
IV.	Tetracyclines					
	Tetracycline	250 mg	3–4	6–12 hr	20–67	
	Doxycycline	100 mg	2–5	14–24 hr	25–93	
V.	Erythromycin	500 mg	5	1.5–2 hr	73	High incidence of phlebitis
VI.	Clindamycin	600 mg	25–30	2–3 hr	93%	Diarrhea
VII.	Chloramphenicol	500 mg	6–10	1.5–3.5 hr	60	Aplastic anemia
VIII.	Metronidazole	500 mg	16–20	6–8 hr	less than 20%	Alcohol intolerance

This route avoids concern that the intravenous fluid containing the antibiotic will not be infused during the procedure because of the need of the anesthesiologist to administer other fluids. In addition, intramuscular antibiotics can be employed in the treatment of sexually acquired diseases, including gonorrhea and syphilis.

Generally, the lowest drug serum levels are achieved with oral antibiotics. Table 7–3 lists the oral antibiotics most frequently employed by the obstetrician-gynecologist and documents the serum levels usually obtained, the half-life of the antibiotics, protein binding, and other therapeutic considerations.[8, 13] Oral agents are usually a more comfortable route of administration of antibiotics for the patient, although diarrhea is more common with many of the families of drugs used. The clinician should avoid the substitution of oral agents for active parenteral antibiotics that have given a good clinical response if the oral agents are not equivalent. **In the treatment of soft tissue pelvic infection there is no oral antibiotic equivalent to the aminoglycosides, the broad-spectrum penicillins (i.e., Carbenicillin, Ticarcillin, Piperacillin, Mezlocillin), or any parenteral cephalosporins.** The reasons for this vary with each family of antibiotics. The aminoglycosides are poorly absorbed from the gastrointestinal tract. With the penicillins, the high levels needed to cover gram-negative anaerobes cannot be achieved with oral medications. For the cephalosporins, the oral agents are not equivalent. This is particularly true of cefoxitin, which is the most resistant to the beta-lactamases and most active against *Bacteroides fragilis.* There is no oral cefoxitin to prescribe.

Another important consideration for the clinician when planning the dosage of antibiotics is the amount of binding of antibiotic to protein in the serum. Serum binding of antibiotics can have significant therapeutic implications[14] for the clinician. The unbound free antibiotic in the serum provides antibacterial activity. This is most important in the evaluation of serum bactericidal activity.[14] Table 7–4 lists the very large differences between broth minimum inhibitory concentration (MIC's) and serum MIC's of various penicillins. These are directly related to the protein binding of the antibiotic; the lower the percentage of protein binding, the greater the serum bactericidal activity. With the various penicillins, those with the least protein binding had more of the administered dose available for antibacterial action. In addition, the free antibiotic is all that is available for passage from the intravascular compartment to other tissue spaces (Figure 7–2).[15] This influence of drug binding to protein on movement of antibiotic to other sites is best illustrated by the blood levels of antibiotics achieved in the fetus when systemic antibiotics are given to the mother. Highly bound penicillins like dicloxacillin achieve much lower serum levels in the fetus than less protein-bound penicillins such as ampicillin.[16, 17] Even with ampicillin, which is only 17% protein bound, the binding to protein means that the peak serum level in the fetus is never as high as that in the mother (Figure 7–3).[17] The serum binding of antibiotics in the laboratory does not always correlate with laboratory measurements of passage of antibiotic to the fetus. The protein binding of cephalosporins in the bloodstream occurs slowly[18] and does not limit bactericidal activity or movement of the antibiotic from the bloodstream to other tissue sites, for these events occur before protein binding takes place. In other words, the measurement of protein binding of cephalosporins in the laboratory is a static process and does not parallel the pharmacokinetics of these antibiotics in the body as accurately as it does for the penicillins.

Table 7–3. Oral Antibiotics

	Antibiotics	Dose	Serum Concentration μg/ml	Half-Life	Protein Binding	Therapeutic Considerations
I.	Penicillins					
	Penicillin G	500 mg	2	30–60 min	55%	Poorly absorbed
	Penicillin V	250 mg	2–3	30 min	80%	Preferred to penicillin G
	Ampicillin	500 mg	4–6	45–90 min	17%	
	Amoxicillin	500 mg	7–8	1 hr	low	Better absorbed than ampicillin
	Carbenicillin	764 mg	5–10	50–60 min	50%	Urinary tract infection treatment only
	Cloxacillin	500 mg	8	45 min	94%	
	Dicloxacillin	250 mg	8	45 min	97%	Half-life unchanged in renal failure
II.	Cephalosporins					
	Cephalexin	500 mg	15–20	30–60 min	low	Limited to urinary tract infections
	Cephradine	500 mg	15–20	30–60 min	low	
	Cefadroxil	500 mg	15–20	75 min	low	
III.	Tetracyclines					
	Tetracycline	250 mg	2–3	6–12 hr	60%	Absorption diminished with use of daily products
	Doxycycline	100 mg	1–1.5	15–25 hr	80–95%	Absorption as for Tetracycline
	Minocycline	100 mg	1.5–2.0	15–20 hr	75%	Not cleared by kidneys Frequent CNS symptoms
IV.	Erythromycins					
	Base	500 mg	0.5–1.0	90 min	73%	Hepatocellular toxicity
	Estolate	250 mg	2.5–3.0	—	—	
V.	Clindamycin	300 mg	4–5	2–4 hr	95%	Diarrhea, pseudomembranous enterocolitis
VI.	Chloramphenicol	250 mg	4–8	3 hr	50–60%	Inhibits metabolism of dilantin and hypoglycemic and oral anticoagulants
VII.	Metronidazole	250 mg	4–6	6–10 hr	<10%	Antabuse effect with alcohol
VIII.	Ketoconazole	400 mg	10	8–12 hr	—	Hepatic toxicity with huge doses

Table 7–4. Minimum Inhibitory Concentrations (MIC) of Various Penicillins Diluted in 100% Human Serum or Trypticase Soy Broth Against a Penicillin-G Sensitive *Staphylococcus*

Penicillin Analogs	MIC mg/ml	
	Broth	Serum
Benzyl (G)	0.04	0.07
Phenoxymethyl (V)	0.04	0.10
Ampicillin	0.15	0.15
Methicillin	1.5	1.5
Nafcillin	0.3	2.5
Oxacillin	0.3	4.25
Cloxacillin	0.2	5.5
Dicloxacillin	0.1	5.5

Another factor in the serum and tissue levels of antibiotics in the body is the elimination of the administered antimicrobial agents. There is good evidence that the clearance of antibiotics by the kidneys is related to the amount of free antibiotic in the serum (Figure 7–4).[15] In general, poorly bound antibiotics are excreted more rapidly from the body via the urinary tract. This may be the cause of the poor record of cephalothin as a preventive antibiotic in bowel surgery.[19] This drug has a short half-life and is cleared so quickly from the body that effective serum and tissue levels may not be present when the operation begins. This is especially true if there has been any delay in the start of the operation from the time the on-call antibiotic dose has been given. The advantage of cefazolin as a prophylactic antibiotic is related to its greater binding to protein and its slower elimination from maternal serum. The rapid clearance of certain antibiotics by the kidney may have an impact upon prescription strategies. Table 7–5 lists the antibiotics that are wholly or partly cleared by the kidney.[8] Patients taking antibiotics that

INTRAVASCULAR SPACE

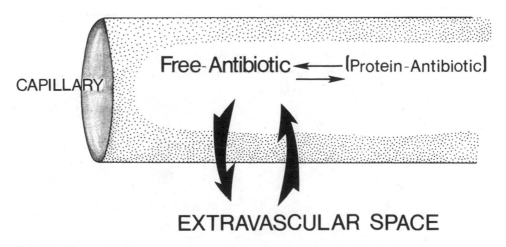

Fig. 7–2. Free antibiotic available for passage from intravascular to extravascular space.

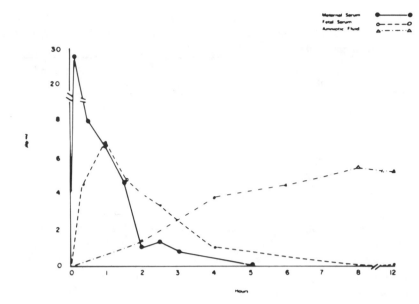

Fig. 7–3. Levels of antibiotics achieved in mother and fetus with administration to the mother. (From Bray, R. F., Boe, R. W., and Johnson, W. L.: Transfer of ampicillin into fetus and amniotic fluid from maternal plasma in late pregnancy. Am. J. Obstet. Gynecol., *96*:938, 1966.)

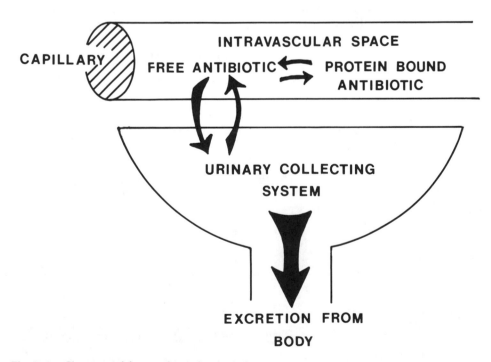

Fig. 7–4. Clearance of free antibiotic by the kidneys.

Table 7-5. Concentrations of Antibiotics in the Serum and Urine

	Antibiotics	Dose	Serum Concentration μg/ml	Urine Concentrate mg/ml
I.	Penicillins			
	Penicillin G	500 mg	2	150–300
	Penicillin V	250 mg	2–3	200–400
		1.0 gm IV	40	500–1000
	Ampicillin	500 mg po	4–6	250–500
	Amoxicillin	500 mg	7–8	500–2500
	Carbenicillin	5.0 IV	200–300	2500–5000
		764 mg	5–10	1000
II.	Cephalosporins			
	Cephalothin	1000 mg IV	40–60	1000–2000
	Cefazolin	1000 mg IV	90–120	1000–2000
	Cephalexin	500 mg	15–20	500–1000
	Cephradine	500 mg	15–20	500–1000
	Cefadroxil	500 mg	15–20	> 1000
	Cefamandole	1.0 gm IV	60–80	1000–5000
	Cefoxitin	1.0 gm IV	60–80	1000–5000
III.	Tetracyclines			
	Tetracycline	250 mg	2–3	200–300
	Doxycycline	100 mg	1–1.5	100–200
	Minocycline	100 mg	1.5–2.0	100–200
IV.	Erythromycin			
	Base	500 mg	0.5–1.0 mg	—
	Estolate	250 mg	2.5–3.0 mg	—
V.	Sulfisoxazole	1000 mg	50–100	500
VI.	Nitrofurantoin	100 mg	0.5–4.8	
VII.	Trimethoprim and sulfamethoxazole			
	Trimethoprim	160 mg	2–3	50–100
	Sulfamethoxazole	800 mg	40–60	100–500
VIII.	Aminoglycosides			
	Gentamicin	1.5 mg/kg IV	5–7	100–500
	Tobramycin	2 mg/kg IV	6–8	200–500

are largely eliminated from the body by the kidney may have lower than expected drug serum levels if they have efficient renal clearance mechanisms. This has been illustrated with aminoglycosides; low serum levels were found in postpartum patients, in whom renal clearance is increased,[20] and in young women who are in the hospital on the gynecologic service who have good renal function.[21] It is particularly important to measure peak and trough aminoglycoside levels in these women to be sure that adequate serum levels are attained for the coverage of gram-negative aerobic organisms.

THERAPEUTIC STRATEGY WITH ANTIBIOTICS

There are a number of unique clinical situations for the obstetrician-gynecologist in which antibiotics are prescribed. These include urinary tract infections, soft tissue pelvic infections, pregnancy, and prophylaxis. The goal for treatment strategies in every patient should be to utilize the least toxic antibiotic that will result in a clinical cure. To achieve this requires specific understanding of the varied problems associated with each group of patients.

Urinary Tract Infections

Urinary tract infections offer a favorable clinical situation for the obstetrician-gynecologist in that almost all of them are caused by a single species of bacteria, so that one rarely needs to prescribe more than one antibiotic for treatment. Most of the antibiotics commonly employed for urinary tract infections are cleared by the kidney and are present in higher concentrations in the urine than can be achieved in the serum (Table 7–5).[8] This higher urine concentration means that on occasion some antibiotics may be effective in vitro at higher concentrations than are found in laboratory testing showing resistance. In addition to this advantage, there are a number of other therapeutic aids for the clinician. In the case of doxycycline and minocycline, although they are adequately cleared from the body by the gastrointestinal tract so that dosage modification are not necessary in women with renal failure, these antibiotics achieve good levels in the urinary tracts of patients with normal renal function for the treatment of infections there. Erythromycin is another interesting drug for the clinician. It achieves good concentrations in the urine, and its activity against gram-negative aerobes increases manyfold if the urine is kept alkaline.[22] This can usually be achieved by the use of sodium bicarbonate or the diuretic, acetazolamide. In addition to the many antibiotics employed by the physician for the treatment of other sites of infection, the sulfas and the nitrofurantoins are sufficiently concentrated in the urine to be effective. Their prescription should be limited to patients suspected of having only urinary tract infections. They have the great advantage of not masking signs and symptoms of infections outside the urinary tract, for they do not penetrate other soft tissue sites in high enough concentrations to be effective. For the treatment of lower urinary tract infections, they work as well clinically as the oral penicillins and oral cephalosporins, which can modify the clinical presentation of soft tissue infections. The nitrofurantoins also have a unique clinical advantage because they do not alter the bacterial flora of the gastrointestinal tract. This means that long-term therapy or prophylaxis can be employed without the emergence of resistant gram-negative aerobes. The drugs trimethoprim and sulfamethoxazole are also effective against the gram-negative bacteria associated with urinary tract infections.

There are cautions to be acknowledged in the treatment of urinary tract infection. Renal function can be reduced in acute pyelonephritis of pregnancy, resulting in excessively high serum antibiotic levels if standard doses of antibiotics primarily cleared by the kidney are given to a woman with this transient change in renal function.[23] There is evidence that high serum levels of tetracycline have been obtained when used in the treatment of pyelonephritis in pregnant women.[24] This accounts in part for the syndrome of fatty liver and death noted in pregnant women with pyelonephritis who were treated with high doses of tetracycline.[25] In addition, the appropriate length of therapy for urinary tract infections has not been established. A number of recent studies offer some guidelines for therapeutic strategies. For patients with asymptomatic bacteriuria and cystitis, a single dose treatment has been studied, but most physicians use 3 to 10 day regimens.[26] Although the single dose regimen has been effective in nonpregnant women, it has been much less effective in a pregnant population and is not currently recommended.[27] For pyelonephritis, some physicians have utilized a 10 day course of therapy, while others recommend 20 days.[28] Prospective comparative studies to determine the relative effectiveness of these alternative regimens have not been done. There are other controversies in the care of pregnant women with pyelonephritis. One study in Texas showed a great benefit from continual prophylaxis with antimicrobial agents for the remainder of the pregnancy. The incidence of recurrent pyelonephritis was markedly reduced.[29] In contrast, a recent study from the University of Southern California showed no benefit from continued prophylaxis.[30] Because I am not convinced of the latter investigators' ability to assure compliance of asymptomatic patients in a population of urban poor served by a large county hospital, I still prescribe long-term nitrofurantoin prophylaxis in pregnant women after successful treatment of pyelonephritis.

Soft Tissue Pelvic Infections

The antibiotic treatment of soft tissue pelvic infections requires some knowledge of the bacteria involved in the infection. These infections are multibacterial, i.e., many organisms are involved, and there is microbiologic evidence that anaerobes are important components. Anaerobes can be recovered from the infection site in over 70% of the cases,[31] and they can be isolated from the blood cultures of patients with pelvic infections and associated bacteremia in over 25% of cases;[32] further, in the most serious cases, those patients with pelvic abscesses, anaerobes are invariably found.[33] Part of the antibiotic planning for a patient with a soft tissue pelvic infection should include antibiotic coverage of anaerobes.

There are many shortcomings of the clinical studies of antibiotic treatment of women with pelvic infections. Some obvious clinical assessments can be made. Did the patient respond to antibiotic therapy, and if she was a treatment failure with the initial selection of antibiotics, did she require additional antibiotics or heparin for a cure, or did she need operative drainage or removal of an abscess? Unfortunately, in these mixed bacterial infections, this is very superficial information. What we would really like to know is the variety of organisms present at the site of infection when treatment begins, what organisms are eliminated with treatment successes, and what organisms remain when there is a failure of response to systemic antibiotics. This would be very helpful so that recommendations for future therapies can be made. These important observations are not possible, however, because of the nature of human pelvic infections. These infections are internal, and the access sites for culture through the vagina and endocervix have an abundant surface bacterial flora. At the present time, it is impossible to differentiate surface contaminants from bacterial pathogens with available microbiologic techniques. In a few selected cases, laparoscopy before therapy enables us to sample the infection site,[34] but laparoscopy is not accepted as a routine diagnostic procedure in such women in the United States. In those women who are treatment failures, i.e., who require surgical drainage or removal of the abscess, we can get good microbiologic data from pus, but they represent a small minority of the total number of patients treated with pelvic infections. With these shortcomings, it is natural to look to an animal model of infection.

The model of infection that has had the greatest influence upon the treatment of soft tissue pelvic infections was devised and studied by Gorbach, Bartlett, and their colleagues at the University of California Los Angeles and Tufts University College of Medicine in Boston.[35-39] In order to mimic the mixed bacterial flora of intraabdominal soft tissue infections, they used rat feces as their inoculum, which contained huge quantities of many species of anaerobes and many gram-negative aerobes as well. This was mixed with barium sulfate, placed in a gelatin capsule, and inserted into the peritoneal cavity of rats. As the gelatin dissolved, a distinctive animal response was seen. In the early phases, the animals became acutely ill, developed peritonitis, and had gram-negative aerobic sepsis; approximately 40% died. The survivors would appear better for a day or two and then would get sick again; if sacrificed, they were found to have intraabdominal abscesses in which anaerobic bacteria predominated. The investigators theorized a biphasic response to infection, an early onset phase with sepsis and death in which gram-negative aerobic bacteria predominated, and a late onset phase with abscess formation in which anaerobic bacteria were important (Figure 7–5).[35] This was an effective

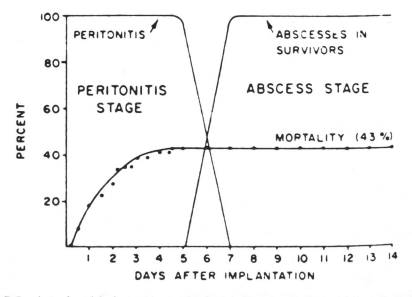

Fig. 7–5. Animal model of mixed bacterial infection. There is a biphasic response. Early onset sepsis and late onset abscess formation. (From Weinstein, W. M., Onderdonk, A. B., Bartlett, J. G., and Gorbach, S.L.: Experimental intra-abdominal abscesses in rats. Development of an experimental model. Infect. Immun., *10*:1250, 1974.)

animal model to evaluate modifications produced by therapy for the end-points, since death and abscess formation were easy to measure. The next step in the experiment was to determine the impact of systemic antibiotics upon the observed response. The results of the many different antibiotics alone or in combination are noted in Table 7–6.[36-39] In general, most of the results were as expected. Antibiotics effective against only gram-negative aerobes (e.g., gentamicin) markedly reduced the first stage of infection, while antibiotics primarily effective against anaerobes with no gram-negative aerobic action (e.g., clindamycin) had no effect on the first stage but markedly reduced the number of abscesses in the survivors. A combination of clindamycin and gentamicin had superior results over the traditional clinical regimens of a tetracycline alone or a combination of penicillin and an aminoglycoside. Second and third generation cephalosporins such as cefoxitin and cefotaxime with a broader spectrum of gram-negative anaerobic coverage produced better results than the traditional regimens or those with first generation cephalosporins. Carbenicillin in high doses in combination with gentamicin also produced better results than the traditional penicillin and aminoglycoside regimen. There were unexpected results. Metronidazole reduced the incidence of early onset mortality despite its lack of activity in vitro against gram-negative aerobes. Chloramphenicol had a poor record in preventing late onset abscess formation. The reasons for these surprising results with metronidazole and chloramphenicol are still not clear to me.

Before any of the lessons of these experimental results can be applied to the clinical experience of obstetrician-gynecologists, several important questions must

Table 7–6. Results of Treatment with Antimicrobial Agents for Rats with Intraabdominal Sepsis

	Treatment Group	Death from Sepsis	Abscess	Cured
I.	Untreated controls	108 of 295 (37%)	187 of 187 (100%)	0 of 295 (0)%
II.	Limited-spectrum antibiotics			
	Aminoglycosides (gentamicin or amikacin)	4 of 97 (5%)	81 of 93 (98%)	2 of 87 (2%)
	Clindamycin	37 of 89 (42%)	3 of 53 (6%)	49 of 89 (55%)
III.	Frequently employed regimens			
	Penicillin and aminoglycoside (amikacin)	0 of 30 (0%)	22 of 30 (73%)	80 of 30 (27%)
	Doxycycline	7 of 30 (23%)	7 of 23 (30%)	16 of 30 (54%)
IV.	Cephalosporins alone			
	Cefazolin (H)	0 of 30 (0%)	8 of 30 (27%)	22 of 30 (73%)
	Cephalothin (H)	3 of 50 (16%)	4 of 42 (10%)	38 of 50 (76%)
	Cefamandole (H)	1 of 30 (3%)	7 of 29 (24%)	22 of 30 (73%)
	Cefoxitin (L)	0 of 30 (0%)	20 of 30 (7%)	28 of 30 (93%)
	Cefotaxime (L)	1 of 29 (3%)	1 of 28 (4%)	27 of 29 (93%)
	Moxalactam			
V.	New combination therapy			
	Carbenicillin and gentamicin	2 of 60 (3%)	4 of 58 (7%)	54 of 60 (90%)
	Clindamycin and gentamicin	10 of 158 (7%)	6 of 148 (5%)	142 of 158 (90%)
VI.	Unexpected results			
	Chloramphenicol	2 of 60 (3%)	34 of 58 (59%)	24 of 60 (40%)
	Metronidazole	5 of 50 (10%)	6 of 45 (13%)	39 of 50 (78%)

H = high doses; L = low doses

be answered. Does the model of infection in the animal create infections similar to those in the human? Are there early onset infections and late onset infections in the human? Is the therapeutic situation in the human similar to that in the animal model? In the animal model, the timing of antibiotic administration is very important. In the studies shown in Table 7–6, the antibiotics were given four hours after the insertion of the capsule. If the initial dose of the antibiotics was delayed until the animals became symptomatic, the antibiotics were much less effective. In the human, we do not begin antibiotics until the patient becomes symptomatic, and this can represent a range from hours to many days.

There are many parallels between the animal model and clinical infections seen in the human. Early onset infections are seen, and *Escherichia coli* has been the most common bloodstream isolate in obstetric-gynecologic patients with bacteremia.[32, 40] There are differences, however. Gram-positive aerobes[32, 40] such as the group B beta-homolytic streptococci[32, 40, 41] and anaerobic bacteria[32, 40] are also frequently recovered in these early onset problems.[32, 40] In addition, death from sepsis is a rare event on an obstetric-gynecologic service, and the very best results with administered antibiotics in the animal model still have associated mortality (see Table 7–6). This probably reflects the enormous numbers of bacteria released in the peritoneal cavity of the rat as the gelatin of the fecal capsule dissolves in comparison to the much smaller bacterial inoculum in pelvic infections in the human. The late onset problems are very similar to the clinical picture seen in humans. Abscesses take many days or weeks to develop, and in the pelvis they are invariably caused by anaerobic bacteria, particularly gram-negative anaerobic rods such as *Bacteroides fragilis, B. bivius,* and *B. disiens.* Although the animal model infection is more severe than most pelvic infections in the human, the timing of the symptoms, the clinical picture seen, and the microorganisms involved seem to parallel human experience. The similarities are close enough to indicate that the lessons learned in the therapy of the massive mixed bacterial contamination of the peritoneal cavity in animals could have some bearing on the treatment of pelvic infections in the human.

Another important question that is too infrequently asked is the comparability of the situation for antibiotic treatment in the human and the animal model. Treatment of infection in the human does not begin until it has progressed to the point that symptoms occur in the form of fever, pain, and others. In addition, some women are first examined by physicians well after the development of a pelvic abscess. There is a big difference in the prognosis for response to antibiotic therapy, depending upon the timing of the initiation of treatment. To illustrate this, I have divided patients with infections into two categories, early and well-established infections. The early infections include patients with symptoms for four days or less and who have no discrete pelvic mass on examination. Those with well-established infections either have had symptoms for five days or more or have had an indurated pelvic mass on examination. Looking at these two groups of patients, there was a marked difference in prognosis after antibiotic therapy (Table 7–7).[42] The cure rate was much higher and the number of women needing operative intervention was much lower in the early onset group. The data in this table of clinical response should have two relevant lessons for clinicians.

The first lesson is important for the evaluation of current literature. There are many new antibiotics, primarily penicillins and cephalosporins, that are being

Table 7-7. Therapy Outcome in Early and Well-Established Infections

Stage of Infection	Total	Number (%) Cured	Surgical Intervention
Early	403	337 (83.6%)	26 (6.4%)
Well established	98	47 (48%)	50 (51%)

introduced into clinical practice. These have great appeal to the physician because they have less toxicity than some of the combinations of antibiotics that have been used in the treatment of serious pelvic infections. There is also the benefit of having to prescribe only one antibiotic.[43] But the clinician must carefully evaluate the patient populations in the study groups in which new antibiotics have been tested. If the new antibiotics have been used solely in patients with early infections, one would expect the results to be better than those obtained with standard antibiotic regimens prescribed in the treatment of well-established infections. Decisions about the best antibiotic regimen for a specific pelvic infection require carefully controlled prospective clinical trials. To date, few of these have been done. Good populations for the evaluation of the best antibiotics for patients with early infections are women who develop postpartum uterine infections following delivery by cesarean section. A number of studies in this setting have a parallel with the animal model. In one, clindamycin and gentamicin gave better clinical results than the traditional penicillin-aminoglycoside regimen,[44] while in the other, clindamycin and gentamicin have a higher percentage of clinical cures than cefamandole, although more patients receiving clindamycin developed diarrhea.[45] Similar results were seen in a comparative trial of moxalactam versus clindamycin-gentamicin.[46] All of the trials with a combination of clindamycin and an aminoglycoside or a newer cephalosporin or penicillin alone have shown much greater success in the prevention of the late developing abdominal wound or pelvic abscess following postpartum endomyometritis after cesarean section than the old combination of penicillin G and an aminoglycoside. The strategy of using ampicillin alone or penicillin and an aminoglycoside in that type of infection should be abandoned. The largest clinical experience in the treatment of postcesarean endomyometritis has been with the combination of clindamycin and an aminoglycoside. There are concerns about potential gastrointestinal toxicity of clindamycin and the need to obtain serum levels in young, healthy postpartum women receiving aminoglycosides. As a result, there is interest in alternative treatment regimens. The newer cephalosporins, particularly cefoxitin and the newer penicillins, have a broad anaerobic coverage. There is an appeal of using a single antibiotic in this treatment. Although the studies to date have looked at minimal numbers of the patients, the results have been encouraging for this initial approach. Metronidazole remains an excellent anaerobic agent. Unfortunately, there have been a limited number of comparative studies published,[47] and I am not sure what drug should be used to provide aerobic coverage. Although many people prescribe aminoglycosides, a newer cephalosporin such as cefoxitin or cefoperazone is favored. There is little information available on the treatment regimens for other early infection. In women with infections as a result of abortions, all of the studied regimens seem effective, and the curettage is the most important factor in cure.[42] In salpingitis, the newer cephalosporins give better immediate results than the regimen of a penicillin or a tetracycline alone.[42] This therapeutic evaluation does not take into account the possible significance of *Chlamydia* or the number of women who have early cures but are left with blocked tubes. In postpartum infection following vaginal delivery, the few studies that have been done suggest good results with any agent. The initial choice does not seem as important as it does following cesarean section. In postoperative pelvic infections, anaerobes seem important, but studies on the best initial therapy for these women are limited. Unless they appear seriously ill, a newer cephalosporin, with cefoxitin or cefoperazone or one of the newer penicillins, either piperacillin or mezlocillin, is preferred.

The second point of emphasis involves antibiotic strategies in the care of women with well-established infections. In the antibiotic treatment of women with pelvic infections, the failure of the patient to respond to antibiotic treatment elicits a standard response. The organisms causing the infection are resistant to the antibiotic being employed, and a switch of antibiotics is needed for cure. This is seldom the case in the care of patients with a well-established infection if appropriate initial antibiotics have been used. When antibiotic therapy is begun, antibiotics should be given with a broad spectrum of activity against gram-negative aerobes and all anaerobes, particularly the gram-negative anaerobic rods. If there

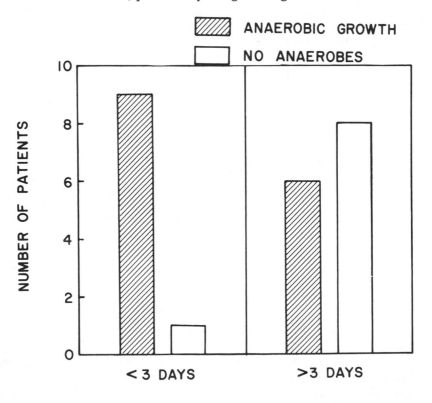

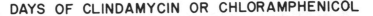

Fig. 7–6. Marked differences in elimination of anaerobes from abscess material, depending upon length of prior antibiotic therapy. (From Ledger, W. J., Gee, C. L., Pollin, P., NaKamura, R. M., and Lewis, W.: The use of pre-reduced media and portable jars for the collection of anaerobic organisms from clinical sites. Am. J. Obstet. Gynecol., *125*:677, 1976.)

Table 7–8. Resistance Rates of *Bacteroides fragilis* Group

Antimicrobial Agent	% Resistant
Metronidazole	0
Chloramphenicol	0
Clindamycin	6
Cefoxitin	8
Piperacillin	12
Moxalactam	22
Cefotaxime	54
Cefoperazone	57
Tetracycline	63

is no response to a minimum of three days of therapy, the clinician's concern should be that there is a pelvic abscess that requires drainage or removal for a cure. The emphasis upon a minimum of three days of therapy is based upon the microbiologic results from purulent material obtained from patients who failed to respond to antibiotic therapy (Figure 7–6).[48] A minimum of three days seemed necessary to eliminate anaerobes from the abscess. This strategy will avoid the long delays when various combinations of antibiotics are unsuccessfully employed because the patient needs operative intervention.

Although this discussion emphasizes the importance of operative intervention in the treatment of well-established infections, there are many women who respond to systemic antibiotics alone. There are two important therapeutic considerations for the practitioner. The first is the focus upon the antibiotic susceptibility of *Bacteroides fragilis,* an important gram-negative anaerobic rod that is so often involved in pelvic abscesses. Tally and coworkers have recently published a nationwide survey of susceptibility patterns of this organism, and the results are noted in Table 7–8.[49] It is important to note that a few strains are resistant to clindamycin. In addition to this consideration, different antibiotics have varying degrees of effectiveness against the huge bacterial inoculum found in the pelvic abscess. Table 7–9 notes the effectiveness of various antibiotics in reducing the numbers of anaerobes in a high inoculum model.[50] Based on these two separate observations in the laboratory, metronidazole and clindamycin seem the best choices for coverage of gram-negative anaerobes in well-established infections. Further confirmation awaits prospective clinical trials.

Table 7–9. Activity of Antibiotics Against *Bacteroides fragilis*

Antibiotic	Reduction in Bacterial Counts ± SEM
Metronidazole	6.7 ± 0.6
Clindamycin	5.0 ± 0.6
Moxalactam	3.8 ± 0.6
Cefoxitin	3.5 ± 0.6
Cefotaxime	1.1 ± 0.3
Carbenicillin	1.0 ± 0.3
Cephalothin	0.4 ± 0.2
Cefoperazone	0.1 ± 0.1

Pregnancy

Pregnancy is associated with a series of unique concerns for the clinician who prescribes antibiotics. The obstetrician-gynecologist is aware of the physiologic changes in the pregnant woman and should know their impact upon the choice of antibiotics and the dosing pattern for appropriate therapy. In addition, there should be awareness of the effect of any antibiotics prescribed upon the fetus and the newborn. The Physicians' Desk Reference (PDR) and the written inserts for the individual antibiotics provide little guidance for the physician. With the exception of penicillin and erythromycin, these reference sources state only that the safety of this agent during pregnancy has not been established.

There are many reasons for reservations about the safety of some antibiotics for the pregnant woman. Some antibiotics have specific actions that are dangerous for pregnant women. Tetracycline in high doses has led to fatty liver and death when given during pregnancy.[25] The combination of trimethoprim and sulfasoxizole is an antifolate. This accounts for its action against bacteria, but this can be detrimental for the pregnant woman because of the heavy demand for folic acid by the fetus during pregnancy. Theoretically this could increase the risk for folic acid deficiency during pregnancy, although this drug has been widely used by the British in pregnant women in the second and third trimesters without any reported toxicity.[51] If the pregnant woman has diminished renal function because of pyelonephritis[23] or pregnancy-associated hypertension, drugs primarily cleared by the kidney, such as the aminoglycosides or standard tetracyclines can reach toxic levels in the bloodstream. Further, many unique maternal functions during pregnancy may be modified by antibiotic administration. During pregnancy, there is a remarkable increase in estriol production and excretion in the urine. The production and clearance of this hormone are complicated interrelated mechanisms involving the mother and the fetus. Part of the metabolic pathway involves estriol bound to protein excreted in the bile, with bacteria in the gastrointestinal tract breaking this bond and permitting the reabsorption of free unconjugated estriol into the bloodstream, where it will be cleared by the kidney. Antibiotics such as ampicillin[52, 53] and erythromycin[54] decrease the number of bacteria in the bowel. The reduction in the number of bowel bacteria results in less breaking of the estriol-protein complex, with more conjugated estriol cleared unchanged by the gastrointestinal tract and less unconjugated estriol reabsorbed and subsequently cleared by the kidneys. This does not adversely affect the pregnancy in any way that we know, but it can make the laboratory determination of estriol lower than would be expected from the maternal-fetal production of the hormone. Physician intervention for fetal stress on the basis of low estriol levels caused by antibiotic administration would be ill-advised.

The clinician should be aware of the risks to the fetus and newborn when antibiotics are prescribed during pregnancy. During organogenesis in the first trimester, there is a justified fear of the use of any drug because it may interfere in some way with the normal sequence of events that results in the formation of a normal embryo. All physicians and patients know the tragic story of thalidomide and want to avoid its repetition. In general, there should be a prohibition against the use of any antibiotics in the first trimester of pregnancy, but some women do develop bacterial infections that require therapy. The patient should receive the appropriate antibiotic for cure, but if the physician has any therapeutic leeway, agents like penicillin that act on the bacterial cell wall should be selected, because there is no comparable site of activity in mammalian cells. On theoretical grounds, avoid the use of the antifolate combination trimethoprim-sulfamethoxazole because of the potential risk of malformation, although it has been used by British investigators in the first trimester without observed ill-effects.[51] Beyond the first trimester, there are defined actions of antibiotics on the fetus and newborn that should be acknowledged. However, it is important to differentiate reported dangerous side-effects from theoretical concerns. There are examples: Tetracycline has an adverse effect on tooth development in the fetus and newborn, resulting in a brownish discoloration of the teeth.[55] This is an observed clinical effect. In animals, tetracyclines inhibit long bone growth,[56] but this has not been reported in humans. There are many references to the toxicity of the sulfas and chloramphenicol for the fetus and newborn. Most practitioners prohibit the use of sulfas during the third trimester to avoid hyperbilirubinemia in the newborn and of chloramphenicol to avoid the gray baby syndrome in the newborn. In fact, however, these last two prohibitions are based on theory and not on observed clinical outcomes. The difficulties with neonatal hyperbilirubinemia were related to the use of long-acting sulfas in pregnant women.[57] Since the serum half-life of sulfisoxizole is approximately 6 hours, and there are alternative drugs for the treatment of urinary tract infections in pregnant women, I would avoid the use of this agent in the third trimester. For chloramphenicol, the gray baby syndrome has only been reported with administration of this drug to the newborn,[58] never when the drug was given only to the mother. Fortunately, the use of chloramphenicol is rarely indicated during pregnancy.

The most important antibiotic information for the physician caring for the pregnant woman is a knowledge of the lower than expected serum levels of antibiotics achieved when standard doses are given. This phenomenon has been most extensively studied by Philipson[6] and has been noted with parenteral as well as oral administration. The increased maternal blood volume during pregnancy and the increased volume of distribution, greater renal clearance, and the passage of antibiotics to the fetus are all factors in this observed phenomenon. It has been reported for all of the penicillins, cephalosporins, and aminoglycosides.[59] In cases in which high serum levels are needed for a clinical cure, either higher doses or more frequent administration of antibiotics may be necessary.

Prophylactic Antibiotics

There has been a wide shift in obstetric-gynecologic opinion about prophylactic antibiotics in the past two decades. Medical thought has switched from condemnation of this method of therapy to overenthusiasm, and expensive, potentially toxic antibiotics have been used in inappropriate cases for a prolonged length of therapy. This area of treatment gives the physician wide latitude in which to make errors of judgment. It is important to understand the principles of antibiotic prophylaxis and to be knowledgeable about the clinical studies to date so that appropriate use of this form of therapy will be possible.

The scientific cornerstone for the use of systemic antibiotic prophylaxis in women undergoing obstetric-gynecologic procedures is based upon the work by Burke.[60] The results of the attempt to modify a local response to bacterial contamination by systemic antibiotics are noted in Figure 7-7.[60] The local lesions

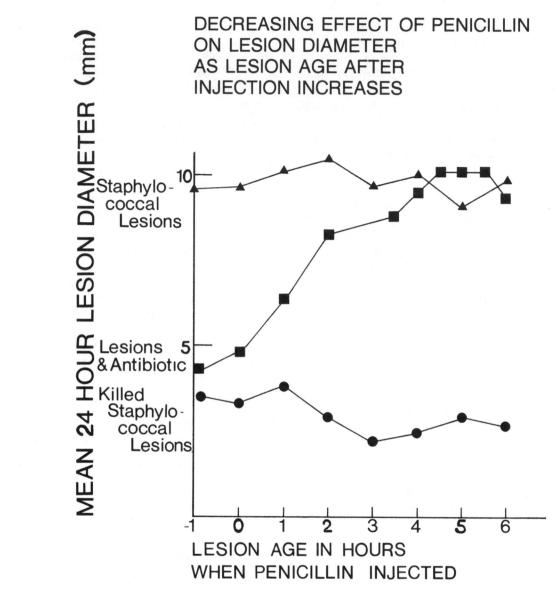

Fig. 7–7. Modification of local response to bacteria with systemic antibiotics. Those given prior to or at the time of the bacterial contamination are the most effective. (From Burke, J. F.: The effective period of preventive antibiotic action in experimental incisions and dermal lesions. Surgery, *50*:161, 1961.)

produced by live staphylococci were reduced in size when intravenous penicillin was given either before or at the time of the bacterial insult. When the penicillin was given three or more hours after the injection of bacteria, no effect was noted. This observation has been confirmed clinically. If antibiotics were given as prophylactic agents before or at the time of the surgery, they worked.[61, 62] If they were given after the operation was completed, they were ineffective.[63] In an attempt to provide a basis for rational physician judgment about prophylaxis, I have developed a series of guidelines for antibiotic prophylaxis[12] that should be applicable to obstetric-gynecologic practice for the lifetime of this edition.

Guideline One. *There should be a significant risk for the development of infection at the operative site.*

The critical word to be evaluated in this guideline is significant. Significant usually relates to frequency of postoperative infections. Postoperative infections can be frequent following vaginal hysterectomy and cesarean section in the woman in labor. Significant can also be related to severity. The rare postoperative adnexal abscess following vaginal hysterectomy is a life-threatening problem,[64] as is the serious pelvic infection following cesarean section.[65] Significant may be related to the change in desired outcome caused by the infection. Infection following reconstructive tubal surgery is rare, but when it occurs, it is a tragedy for the patient involved. The concept of significant risk is the most important question to ask when contemplating the use of antibiotic prophylaxis.

Guideline Two. *The operation should be associated with endogenous bacterial contamination.*

This guideline should be obvious to all physicians. Systemic antibiotics, to work, must be applied to operations in which there is bacterial soiling of the operative site. This is the case in vaginal hysterectomy where bacterial contamination has been noted[12] and is certainly true in the patient in labor undergoing cesarean section.[66] In vaginal hysterectomy, surface preparation of the vagina markedly reduces the number of bacteria, but contamination obviously occurs from the endocervix. One of the more interesting strategies to reduce postoperative infection by reducing bacterial contamination came with the use of hot conization of the cervix prior to hysterectomy.[67] This effort was associated with a reduced postoperative infection rate. Recently there has been enthusiasm for uterine wound antibiotic solution lavage in cesarean section prior to closure of the incision,[68] which undoubtedly reduces bacterial contamination and has resulted in a reduced rate of postoperative infection. *Chlamydia* organisms have been recovered from the pelvises of women with no clinical evidence of infection or inflammation.[69] These organisms may account for the occasional unexpected postoperative infection in that population.

Guideline Three. *The antibiotic used for prophylaxis should have laboratory evidence of effectiveness against some of the contaminating microorganisms.*

The key word in this guideline is some, and the use of this modifier reflects our lack of understanding of the nature of protection against infections with antibiotic prophylaxis. Consider vaginal hysterectomy. Equivalent rates of success in preventing infection have been reported with cephaloridine[61] and metronidazole.[70] Each of these antibiotics has a widely differing antibacterial activity, with metronidazole limited to anaerobic bacteria, while cephaloridine has much more limited anaerobic coverage but more extensive aerobic activity. This is an important point in antibiotic prophylaxis in obstetrics-gynecology. The volume of bacterial contamination is not as great as in large bowel surgery, and the choice of antibiotic for successful prophylaxis does not seem to be as critical as it is in patients with established infections. There are other possibilities. On the initiation of these mixed bacterial infections, the interaction of many strains of bacteria can produce an environment in which proliferation of organisms is enhanced, with resultant serious infection. Coverage of some of these organisms can break this synergism and permit host defense mechanisms to control those bacteria not covered by the antibiotic. In animal model studies, there is good evidence that strains of *Bacteroides fragilis* without a capsule alone or the enterococcus group alone represents little threat, but in combination they can result in a serious infection.[71] The clinician should be on guard against theoretical arguments that one antibiotic is best for prophylaxis because of better antimicrobial coverage in the laboratory. Certainly, the newer cephalosporins like cefoxitin[72] and the newer penicillins like pipera-cillin[73] and mezlocillin[74] have been effective prophylactic agents. The question that needs to be addressed by the physician is whether or not they are better than the currently used first generation cephalosporins, which are less expensive. The answer can only come from prospective comparative studies.

Guideline Four. *The antibiotic used for prophylaxis should have clinical evidence of effectiveness.*

This is the most important of all of the guidelines. If there is no clinical evidence of effectiveness in reducing the numbers and severity of postoperative infections, there really is no justification for use. There are a number of important points of evaluation. Does the antibiotic reduce the number and severity of infections? In addition, what is the long-term effect? If, for example, the incidence of infection following a first trimester termination is very low but when such infections occur they cause subsequent infertility, a stronger case for prophylaxis could be made.

There are a number of procedures in which the effectiveness of prophylactic antibiotics has been clearly demonstrated. In vaginal hysterectomy, prophylactic antibiotics work well,[12, 61, 62, 70] and there have been a multitude of other studies indicating this effectiveness. To date, there has been no conclusive evidence to suggest that one antibiotic is any more effective than any other. There is also a very large volume of studies that show a lowering of the postoperative infection rate when prophylactic antibiotics are used for cesarean section.[66, 72–75] I believe that they are indicated for the patient in labor who requires a cesarean section, but the physician should be aware that serious infections can still be seen in these women. If these patients show evidence of an infection after cesarean section, they still should be treated aggressively. There are other operations for which the reported experience is not as great but in which prophylactic antibiotics are effective. In vaginal hysterectomy preceded by conization[76] and in radical hysterectomy,[77] the antibiotics are effective. First trimester pregnancy terminations have a low rate of infection, but two studies utilizing prophylactic antibiotics showed a reduction in the resulting rate of infection.[78, 79] Finally, one recent study showed a reduction in the infection rate following hysterosalpingography, particularly in those women with hydrosalpinx.[80]

In contrast, uniform effectiveness has not been demonstrated in several procedures. The most striking example of this has been abdominal hysterectomy. Although some studies have shown effectiveness of prophylactic antibiotics,[62, 81, 82] others have shown no benefit.[83, 84] Our own experience with abdominal hysterectomy at The New York Hospital has been that systemic antibiotics have not been effective.[85] The decision about the use of prophylactic antibiotics in this operation has to be individualized, based upon the physician's own experience or the experiences of the services.

There are many other procedures in which prophylactic antibiotics are given for which a data base is not available to render a decision. These include the insertion and removal of an intrauterine device, tubal ligation, and reconstructive tubal surgery. If the physician makes a personal judgment that prophylaxis is indicated in this area, then the importance of *Chlamydia* infections in salpingitis should be acknowledged.

Guideline Five. *The antibiotic used for prophylaxis should be present in the wound some time during the operation.*

This guideline will be the most critical area of evaluation in prophylaxis in the next decade. To be effective, these agents must be present at the operative site to prevent the problems resulting from local bacterial contamination. According to Burke's experiment (Figure 7–8),[86] if antibiotics are not present within three hours of the seeding of the wound with bacteria, they will not work.

A most important influence on the prescription of prophylactic antibiotics is the pharmacokinetics of the agent to be ordered. The delivery of the antibiotic to the operative site will be influenced by the serum peak, protein binding, volume of distribution, and the half-life. Higher serum levels are achieved with intravenous as compared with intramuscular administration. With the penicillins, the higher protein binding of some forms such as dicloxacillin means there is little free antibiotic available for diffusion into the wound. Antibiotics with a large volume of distribution have greater diffusion into all tissue spaces, and particularly into the wound. I believe the most important factor in the selection of an antibiotic is the half-life of the agent, that is, the length of time required for one-half of the administered antibiotic to be cleared from the serum. In gynecology, our focus has been on the preoperative on-call dose. If the antibiotic is given by rapid intravenous infusion, and if there is a delay in the start of the operation or the procedure is prolonged, little or no antibiotic will be available at the wound site. This fact has been ignored in many clinical protocols and may account for the failure of antibiotic prophylaxis in abdominal hysterectomies that lasted more

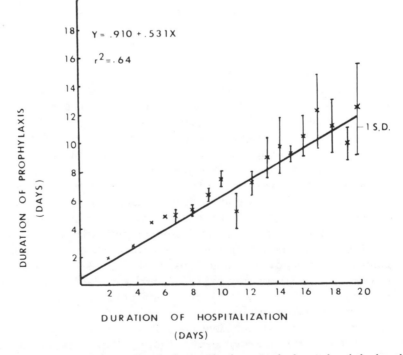

Fig. 7–8. The direct correlation between the length of stay in the hospital and the length of time of antibiotic prophylaxis. (From Shapiro, M., Townsend, T. R., Rosner, B., and Kass, E. H.: Use of antimicrobial agents in general hospitals. N. Engl. J. Med., *301*:351, 1979.)

than three hours.[82] It may also account for the lack of effectiveness of cephalothin, which has a short half-life, in bowel surgery.[19] In gynecology, there are two approaches to this on-call dose problem. One is to use an intramuscular route of administration on-call. The alternative is to select antibiotics with longer half-lives. For the cephalosporins specifically, there is great appeal to the use of cefazolin, cefoperazone, and cefotetin, all of which have long half-lives. In addition to the on-call concerns, it may be much more appropriate to give the next dose of antibiotics intraoperatively in 1 to 2 hours rather than in 4 to 6 hours, as is so widely done.

The timing of the initial dose of antibiotic prophylaxis for cesarean section is a difficult decision. In gynecologic procedures, this dose is given preoperatively. With cesarean section, preoperative administration of the antibiotic to the mother results in therapeutic levels for the fetus (see Figure 7–4).[17] As noted in the figure, the antibiotics rapidly pass to the fetus, although the peak levels are not as high as in the adult because of protein binding. For the pediatrician, this means that the newborn will have therapeutic levels of antibiotics; these can modify blood culture results and make the task of confirming newborn sepsis more difficult. In this situation, some difficult decisions have to be made by the pediatrician. On some neonatal services, all such newborns are given therapeutic antibiotics for a few days, because of the concern about potential failure to make the diagnosis. To avoid this problem, a number of obstetric investigators have given the antibiotic to the mother after the cord has been clamped.[66, 72] The result seemed equivalent to that obtained with preoperative dosing, and at least one prospective study showed clinical results equivalent to those with preoperative dosing.[87] Antibiotics given in this manner were effective. This intraoperative approach is not free of problems, however. One study reported two deaths from cardiovascular collapse when intravenous cephalothin was given to patients under general anesthesia.[88] The mechanism is not known. As an alternative, intraperitoneal lavage with an antibiotic solution has been tried, and it has been effective.[68, 89, 90] This avoids the bolus effect of a sudden intravenous infusion. Another study demonstrated peritoneal absorption with measurable serum levels that persist after the lavage has been completed.[91] This is an appealing approach, and I believe will be the method of choice for future prophylaxis. The only problem thus far has been one study in which this approach was not effective, while intravenous prophylaxis still worked.[92] Further studies will be needed.

Guideline Six. *Short-term administration of antibiotics for prophylaxis should be employed.*

This is still one of the most poorly understood areas of medical therapy in obstetrics-gynecology. Despite evidence from the experimental studies of Burke (see Figure 7–7)[60] and nearly every paper on prophylaxis in obstetrics-gynecology confirming that short-term prophylaxis works, many physicians disregard this guideline. One study of antibiotic use in the hospital showed a direct correlation between the length of stay in the hospital and the length of time of antibiotic prophylaxis[86] (see Figure 7–8). Too many physicians equate a longer course of therapy with better results.

There is accumulating evidence that short-term prophylactic therapy produces clinical results that are equivalent to those of long-term therapy. One evaluation of short-term and long-term prophylaxis in vaginal hysterectomy demonstrated no difference in the results when comparing postoperative morbidity and the fever index[12] (Table 7–10). A number of studies of vaginal hysterectomy using a single preoperative dose of cephaloridine,[93] cephradine,[94] metronidazole,[95] carbenicillin,[96] or cefoxitin[97] have all shown clinical effectiveness. With cesarean section, the picture is mixed. One study has shown a single dose of cefoxitin as effective as three,[98] while another study found three days of ampicillin prophylaxis superior to one.[99] The latter study had major problems of study design. The burden of evidence seems to support the effectiveness of short-term prophylaxis.

There are many observations that document greater potential for toxicity with long-term prophylaxis. Long-term prophylaxis has resulted in colonization of the vagina with *Pseudomonas aeruginosa*,[83] an increase in the number of infections due to gram-negative *Klebsiella aerogenes*,[100] and death due to pseudomembranous enterocolitis.[101] Such events are uncommon but they are avoidable with a short-term strategy.

Guideline Seven. *Antibiotics with an important antibacterial spectrum of activity should be reserved for treatment and not used for prophylaxis.*

This guideline is on the shakiest scientific ground. New and theoretically more effective antibiotics should be reserved for treatment, but I have not been convinced to date that short-term antibiotic prophylaxis has resulted in ecology pressures in the hospital with the emergence of resistant strains. The most detailed evaluation of this point by Grossman and coworkers could not demonstrate an increase in the percentage of organisms resistant to the antibiotics used for prophylaxis.[84]

The cutting point for decision-making in this area is clinical results. If a new agent produces clearly superior results in comparison with the other antibiotics, then a point can be made for its use. To date this has not been demonstrated in vaginal hysterectomy. Although the newer cephalosporins and penicillins have been effective as prophylactic antibiotics, they have not been noted to be superior to the first generation cephalosporins such as cephaloridine, cephalothin, and cefazolin. In cesarean section, there is one study in which cefoxitin prophylaxis resulted in a lower postoperative fever index than cefazolin,[102] although the clinical results were similar. Again, a solid data base demonstrating superiority has not been presented. Also, the newer agents can be associated with problems. Moxalactam used for prophylaxis was associated with an unexpectedly high number of postoperative enterococcal urinary tract infections.[103] Until prospective studies

Table 7–10. Postoperative Course with Short-Term vs. Long-Term Prophylactic Antibiotics

Clinical Outcome	Short Term	Long Term
No infection	41	39
Urinary tract infection	2	1
Pelvic cellulitis	5	8
Total	48	48
Indirect Measures		
Standard temperature morbidity	10	15
Mean post-operative stay	4 days	4.5 days
Mean fever index ± SD	38.5 ± 43.4	36.4 ± 34.2
Median fever index	31.1	27.3

demonstrate better results, clinicians can continue to use first generation cephalosporins for prophylaxis.

Guideline Eight. *The benefits of antibiotic prophylaxis should outweigh the risks.*

This is the final decision for every physician contemplating the use of prophylactic antibiotics. For women undergoing vaginal hysterectomy, conization and then hysterectomy, radical hysterectomy, for those in labor requiring a cesarean section and for women who need termination of a first trimester pregnancy, antibiotic prophylaxis is indicated. I do not use it routinely for abdominal hysterectomy, hysterosalpingograms, manipulation with intrauterine devices, or tubal ligations, but there are some high-risk patients in whom I do prescribe these drugs. For example, I order them for a massively obese woman who needs an abdominal hysterectomy or a woman who needs a tubal ligation but will not agree to have her intrauterine device removed preoperatively. To date, these are individual therapeutic decisions. Prospective studies may modify this approach.

Other Types of Prophylaxis

The obstetrician-gynecologist will have other situations in which antibiotic prophylaxis is indicated. The largest group of patients in whom prophylaxis is necessary are those at risk for bacterial endocarditis. Such patients have valvular heart disease, congenital heart disease, a previous history of endocarditis, prosthetic heart valves, and recently it has been noted that women with a prolapsed mitral valve are also at risk.[104] I believe that prophylactic antibiotics should be employed in these women if they undergo any minor or major operative manipulation of the lower genital tract, including D and C, conization, insertion or removal of an intrauterine device, hysterectomy, vaginal delivery, or cesarean section. The American Heart Association recommendations are noted in Table 7–11.[105] The physician and patient should be aware that despite appropriate use of antibiotics, some cases of bacterial endocarditis will still occur.[106]

Another group more frequently seen by obstetrician-gynecologists since the first edition of this book are patients with recent conversion of the tuberculin skin test. The treatment is isoniazid 300 mg/day for one year. Although this drug is contraindicated in the first trimester of pregnancy, it should be prescribed for the second and third trimesters. These patients should have periodic liver function tests performed. In addition, they should receive pyridoxine 10 mg for every 100 mg of isoniazid.

Table 7–11. Antibiotic Prophylaxis for Genitourinary Tract Surgery and Instrumentation

Aqueous crystalline penicillin G, 2,000,000 U IM or IV

or

Ampicillin (1.0 gm IM or IV)

plus

Gentamicin 1.5 mg/kg, not to exceed 80 mg IM or IV
Give initial doses 30 to 60 min prior to procedure. Repeat every 8 hr for two additional doses
If patient is allergic to penicillin:
Vancomycin 1.6 gm intravenously given over 30 to 60 min
Repeat in 12 hr

PRESCRIPTION CHOICES FOR VARIOUS GROUPS OF ANTIBIOTICS FOR OBSTETRICIAN-GYNECOLOGISTS

The penicillins are a popular choice of antibiotics for clinicians. They are effective and have a broad range of activity and a wide margin of safety, i.e., the killing dose for most organisms can be exceeded many times with no fear of toxicity. They are also versatile in that they can be given intravenously, intramuscularly, and orally. Despite this, they should be prescribed less commonly than they were in the 1970's. Better results with clindamycin,[42, 44, 47] and the newer cephalosporins[42, 43, 45, 46] in hospital-acquired infections have decreased the use of penicillin G, and awareness of the significance of *Chlamydia infections* has decreased the outpatient use of ampicillin in the treatment of salpingitis.[69] Despite this, the penicillins are still widely used. The newer penicillins—carbenicillin, ticarcillin, piperacillin, and mezlocillin—all have extended coverage of gram-negative aerobes and anaerobes. Because toxicity is minimal, they will be prescribed frequently. Serious allergic reactions are rare. The newer penicillins, particularly carbenicillin, can have problems, however, the most apparent being an excess sodium load followed by the host response of hypokalemia.[107] In addition, there is an impact on platelet adhesiveness that can result in bleeding.[108] Both of these problems are reversible with discontinuation of the drugs.

The cephalosporins are probably the most frequently prescribed family of antibiotics for the obstetrician-gynecologist. They have all of the advantages of the penicillins, with the additional impact that they have had more studies done in the area of prophylaxis. Like the penicillins, they have little effectiveness in the laboratory against *Chlamydia*. Some of the newer cephalosporins have particular appeal for the obstetrician-gynecologist. Cefoxitin is very stable against beta-lactamases and has good activity against gram-negative anaerobes, particularly *Bacteroides fragilis.*[49] Cefoperazone has a long serum half-life and is appealing for prophylaxis and for treatment,[109] even though its gram-negative anaerobic coverage is not as good as that of cefoxitin.[49] Cefotetin produces in vitro results similar to those of cefoxitin, and it has a long-serum half life, which can be very appealing for use in prophylaxis. There is little toxicity with the newer cephalosporins. Allergic reactions are rare, and renal toxicity is uncommon. Some of the individual cephalosporins have been noted to have some specific problems. Diarrhea has been seen with some frequency with cefoperazone,[109] and bleeding problems have been noted with moxalactam.[110]

The aminoglycosides have been a very popular family of antibiotics for obstetrician-gynecologists. They are used in combination with other antibiotics for coverage of the gram-negative aerobes, and they are bactericidal. Despite these advantages, there are many distinct disadvantages. These agents are not absorbed orally and therefore their prescription is limited to inpatients. Most important, they have a narrow range between therapeutic effectiveness and toxicity. Recently, it has become apparent that the obstetrician-gynecologist prescribing these agents in young healthy women is underdosing 30% or more of the patients,[20, 21] i.e., therapeutic levels have not been achieved with standard doses based upon weight. For the obstetrician-gynecologist, this means that **peak and trough levels must be obtained in all women receiving aminoglycosides.** This is time-consuming and expensive. As a result of pressures to reduce hospital costs, I believe that prescription of aminoglycosides will be largely replaced by the newer cephalosporins or penicillins for coverage of gram-negative aerobes.

Clindamycin has been a widely used antibiotic by obstetrician-gynecologists because of its excellent anaerobic spectrum of activity, particularly against the gram-negative anaerobic rods. I like to call the combination of clindamycin and an aminoglycoside the gold standard of therapy of soft tissue pelvic infections, because it is successful and has been studied in both the animal model[36-39] and in clinical situations.[42,44] Any new approaches to the therapy of soft tissue infections, either with the newer cephalosporins or penicillins, will require prospective comparisons with the clindamycin-aminoglycoside combination. The problem with clindamycin, however, is its gastrointestinal toxicity. Diarrhea can occur, and pseudomembranous enterocolitis has been reported caused by overgrowth of *Clostridium difficile* in the gastrointestinal tract.[111] Every patient that I treat with clindamycin keeps a daily record of the number of bowel movements. If five or more are recorded, the drug is stopped, and culture for *Clostridium difficile* and its toxin is obtained. If the diarrhea persists and the test findings are positive, the treatment of choice is oral vancomycin. **Agents to diminish gastrointestinal peristalsis should not be prescribed for women who develop diarrhea while taking clindamycin.** These can prolong the problem and make it more difficult to treat and cure.

Chloramphenicol is rarely prescribed by the obstetrician-gynecologist. It is a highly effective agent against gram-negative aerobes and anaerobes but has the shortcoming that aplastic anemia can develop after therapy.[112] Although rare, for one per 20,000–100,000 patients this can be fatal, and there is no way of predicting which person is prone to this complication. I believe that the incidence of aplastic anemia is less with the intravenous than the oral route, but cases have been reported with intravenous administration. I only use the intravenous route when I order this antibiotic. Because of this potentially fatal side-effect, **the physician prescribing chloramphenicol should document on the chart the reason that alternative antibiotics have not been prescribed.**

Metronidazole is a highly effective antibiotic against gram-negative anaerobic bacteria. In the laboratory, it is the strongest bactericidal agent against *Bacteroides fragilis,*[49] and it is widely used in the treatment of soft tissue pelvic infections in England. In this country, it has not been widely employed for a number of reasons. There have been concerns because it causes cancer in some experimental animals[113] and is mutagenic for some bacteria.[114] To date, there has been no evidence of an increased risk of cancer in women using this drug.[115] The primary restriction on clinical use is the lack of a large series of studies with the drug in the United States. Another question has been the choice of another antibiotic to use in tandem for aerobic coverage. Although there is more emphasis upon an aminoglycoside,[47] I favor one of the newer cephalosporins, such as cefoxitin, because of its greater effectiveness against many of the gram-positive aerobes.

Erythromycin is what I call an antibiotic reserve. It is safe, and it is the drug of choice in penicillin–allergic pregnant patients who have either gonorrhea or syphilis.[116] In addition, it can be highly effective in eliminating gram-negative aerobes from the urinary tract if the urine can be made alkaline.[22]

REFERENCES

1. Barza, M., Brusch, J., Bergeron, M.G., and Weinstein, L.: Penetration of antibiotics into fibrin loci in vitro. III. Intermittent vs. continuous infusion and the effect of probenecid. J. Infect. Dis., *129*:73, 1974.

2. Chow, A.W., Malkasian, K.L., Marshall, J.R., and Guze, L.B.: The bacteriology of pelvic inflammatory disease: Value of cul de sac cultures and relative importance of gonococci and other aerobic or anaerobic bacteria. Am. J. Obstet. Gynecol., *122*:876, 1975.
3. Riff, L.J., and Jackson, G.G.: Laboratory and clinical conditions for gentamicin inactivation by carbenicillin. Arch. Int. Med., *130*:887, 1972.
4. Feigin, R.D., Moss, K.S., and Shackelford, P.G.: Antibiotic stability in solutions used for intravenous nutrition and fluid therapy. Pediatrics, *51*:1016, 1973.
5. Simberkoff, M.S., Thomas, L., McGregor, D., Shenkein, I., and Levine, B.B.: Inactivation of penicillin by carbohydrate solutions at alkaline pH. N. Engl. J. Med., *283*:116, 1970.
6. Philipson, A.: Pharmacokinetics of ampicillin during pregnancy. J. Infect. Dis., *136*:370, 1977.
7. Schwartz, S.M., Pazin, G.J., Lyon, J.A., Ho, M., and Pasculle, A.W.: A controlled investigation of the pharmacokinetics of gentamicin and tobramycin in obese subjects. J. Infect. Dis., *138*:499, 1978.
8. Conte, J.E., Jr., and Barriere, S.L.: Manual of Antibiotics and Infectious Diseases. Philadelphia, Lea & Febiger, 1981.
9. Regamey, C., Gordon, R.C., and Kirby, W.M.M.: Cefazolin vs. cephalothin and cephaloridine. Arch. Int. Med., *133*:407, 1974.
10. Goosenberg, J., Emich, J.P., and Schwarz, R.H.: Prophylactic antibiotics in vaginal hysterectomy. Am. J. Obstet. Gynecol., *105*:503, 1969.
11. Appel, G.B., and Neu, H.C.: Gentamicin in 1978. Ann. Intern. Med., *89*:528, 1978.
12. Ledger, W.J., Gee, C., and Lewis, W.P.: Guidelines for antibiotic prophylaxis in gynecology. Am. J. Obstet. Gynecol., *121*:1038, 1975.
13. Canha, B.A., and Ristuccia, A.: Use of oral antibiotics in ob/gyn. Inf. Dis. Letters, *4*:61, 1982.
14. Kunin, C.M.: Clinical pharmacology of the new penicillins. I, The importance of serum protein binding in determining antimicrobial activity and concentration in serum. Clin. Pharmacol. Ther., *7*:166, 1966.
15. Ledger, W.J.: Antibiotics in pregnancy. Clin. Obstet. Gynecol., *20*:411, 1977.
16. MacAulay, M.A., Berg, S.R., and Charles, D.: Placental transfer of dicloxacillin at term. Am. J. Obstet. Gynecol. *102*:1162, 1968.
17. Bray, R.E., Boe, R.W., and Johnson, W.L.: Transfer of ampicillin into fetus and amniotic fluid from maternal plasma in late pregnancy. Am. J. Obstet. Gynecol., *96*:938, 1966.
18. Waterman, N.G., Raff, M.J., Scharfenberger, L., and Barnwell, P.A.: Protein binding and concentrations of cephaloridine and cefazolin in serum and interstitial fluid of dogs. J. Infect. Dis., *133*:642, 1976.
19. Condon, R.E., Bartlett, J.G., Nichols, R.L., Schulte, W.J., Gorbach, S.L., and Ochi, S.: Pre-operative prophylactic cephalothin fails to control septic complications of colorectal operations: Results of controlled clinical trial. Am. J. Surg., *137*:68, 1979.
20. Zaske, D.E., Cipolle, R.J., Strate, R.G., Malo, J.W., and Koszalka, M.F., Jr.: Rapid gentamicin elimination in obstetric patients. Obstet. Gynecol., *56*:559, 1980.
21. Zaske, D.E., Cipolle, R.J., Strate, R.G., and Dickes, W.F.: Increased gentamicin dosage requirements: Rapid elimination in 249 gynecology patients. Am. J. Obstet. Gynecol., *139*:896, 1981.
22. Sabath, L.D., Gerstein, D.A., Loder, P.B., and Finland, M.: Excretion of erythromycin and its enhanced activity in urine against gram-negative bacilli with alkalinization. J. Lab. Clin. Med., *72*:916, 1968.
23. Whalley, P.J., Cunningham, F.G., and Martin, F.: Transient renal dysfunction associated with acute pyelonephritis of pregnancy. Obstet. Gynecol., *46*:174, 1975.
24. Whalley, P.J., Martin, F.G., Adams, R.H., and Combes, B.: Disposition of tetracycline by pregnant women with acute pyelonephritis. Obstet. Gynecol., *36*:821, 1970.
25. Schultz, J.C., Adamson, T.S., Jr., Workman, W.W., and Norman, T.D.: Fatal liver disease after intravenous administration of tetracycline in high dosage. N. Engl. J. Med., *269*:999, 1963.
26. Cunin, C.M.: Duration of treatment of urinary tract infections. Am. J. Med., *71*:849, 1981.
27. Williams, J.D., Brumfitt, W., Leigh, D., and Percival, A.: Eradication of bacteriuria in pregnancy by a short course of chemotherapy. Lancet, *1*:831, 1965.
28. Harris, R.E.: The treatment of urinary tract infections during pregnancy. *In* Antibiotics in Obstetrics and Gynecology. Edited by W.J. Ledger. Boston, Martinus Nijhoff, 1982.
29. Harris, R.E., and Gilstrap, L.C., III.: Prevention of recurrent pyelonephritis during pregnancy. Obstet. Gynecol., *44*:637, 1974.
30. Lenke, R.R., Van Dorsten, J.P., and Schifrin, B.S.: Pyelonephritis in pregnancy: A prospective randomized trial to prevent recurrent disease evaluating suppressive therapy with nitrofurantoin and close surveillance. Am. J. Obstet. Gynecol., *146*:953, 1983.
31. Swenson, R.M., Michaelson, T.C., Daly, M.J., and Spaulding, E.H.: Anaerobic bacterial infections of the female genital tract. Obstet. Gynecol., *42*:538, 1973.
32. Ledger, W.J., Norman, M., Gee, C., and Lewis, W.P.: Bacteremia on an obstetric-gynecologic service. Am. J. Obstet. Gynecol., *121*:205, 1975.

33. Landers, D.V., and Sweet, R.L.: Tubo-ovarian abscess: Contemporary approach to management. Rev. Infect. Dis., *5*:876, 1983.
34. Sweet, R.L., Mills, J., Hadley, K.W., Blumenstock, E., Schachter, J., Robbie, M.O., and Draper, D.L.: Use of laparoscopy to determine the microbiologic etiology of acute salpingitis. Am. J. Obstet. Gynecol., *134*:68, 1979.
35. Weinstein, W.M., Onderdonk, A.B., Bartlett, J.G., and Gorbach, S.L.: Experimental intra-abdominal abscesses in rats: Development of an experimental model. Infect. Immun., *10*:1250, 1974.
36. Onderdonk, A.B., Weinstein, W.M., Sullivan-Seigler, N.M., Bartlett, J.G., and Gorbach, S.L.: Experimental intra-abdominal abscess in rats: Quantitative bacteriology of infected animals. Infect. Immun., *10*:1256, 1975.
37. Weinstein, W.M., Onderdonk, A.B., Bartlett, J.G., Louie, T.J., and Gorbach, S.L.: Antimicrobial therapy of experimental intra-abdominal sepsis. J. Infect. Dis., *132*:282, 1975.
38. Louie, T.J., Onderdonk, A.B., J.G., Gorbach, S.L., and Bartlett, J.G.: Antimicrobial therapy of experimental intra-abdominal sepsis. J. Infect. Dis., *135*:S18, 1977.
39. Bartlett, J.G., Louie, T.J., Gorbach, S.L., and Onderdonk, A.B.: Therapeutic efficacy of 29 antimicrobial regimens in experimental intra-abdominal sepsis. Rev. Infect. Dis., *3*:535, 1981.
40. Blanco, J.D., Gibbs, R.S., and Castaneda, Y.S.: Bacteremia in obstetrics: Clinical course. Obstet. Gynecol., *58*:621, 1981.
41. Faro, S.: Group B beta-hemolytic streptococci and puerperal infections. Am. J. Obstet. Gynecol., *139*:686, 1981.
42. Ledger, W.J.: Selection of antimicrobial agents for treatment of infections of the female genital tract. Rev. Infect. Dis., *5*:S98, 1983.
43. Sweet, R.L., and Ledger, W.J.: Cefoxitin: Single-agent treatment of mixed aerobic-anaerobic pelvic infections. Obstet. Gynecol., *54*:193, 1979.
44. DiZerega, G., Yonekura, L., Roy, S., Nakamura, R.M., and Ledger, W.J.: A comparison of clindamycin-gentamicin and penicillin-gentamicin in the treatment of post cesarean endomyometritis. Am. J. Obstet. Gynecol., *134*:238, 1979.
45. Gibbs, R.S., Blanco, J.D., Castaneda, Y.S., and St. Clair, P.J.: A double blind, randomized comparison of clindamycin-gentamicin versus cefamandole for treatment of post-cesarean section endomyometritis. Am. J. Obstet. Gynecol., *144*:261, 1982.
46. Gibbs, R.S., Blanco, J.D., Duff, P., Castaneda, Y.S., and St. Clair, P.J.: A double blind randomized comparison of moxalactam versus clindamycin-gentamicin in treatment of endomyometritis after cesarean section delivery. Am. J. Obstet. Gynecol., *146*:769, 1983.
47. Gall, S.A., Kohan, A.P., Ayers, O.M., Hughes, C.E., Addison, W.A., and Hill, G.B.: Intravenous metronidazole or clindamycin with tobramycin for therapy of pelvic infections. Obstet. Gynecol., *57*:51, 1981.
48. Ledger, W.J., Gee, C.L., Pollin, P., Nakamura, R.M., and Lewis, W.: The use of pre-reduced media and a portable jar for the collection of anaerobic organisms from clinical sites of infection. Am. J. Obstet. Gynecol., *125*:677, 1976.
49. Tally, F.P., Cuchural, G.J., Jacobus, N.V., Gorbach, S.L., Aldridge, K.E., Cleary, T.J., Finegold, S.M., Hill, G.B., Iannini, P.B., McCloskey, R.V., O'Keefe, J.P., and Pierson, C.L.: Susceptibility of the *Bacteroides fragilis* group in the United States in 1981. Antimicrob. Agents Chemother., *23*:536, 1983.
50. Bartlett, J.G.: Recent developments in the management of anaerobic infections. Rev. Infect. Dis., *5*:235, 1983.
51. Brumfitt, W., and Pursell, R.: Trimethoprim-sulfamethoxazole in the treatment of bacteriuria in women. J. Infect. Dis., *128*:S657, 1973.
52. Willman, K., and Pulkkinen, M.O.: Reduced maternal plasma and urinary estriol during ampicillin treatment. Am. J. Obstet. Gynecol., *109*:893, 1971.
53. Boehm, F.H., DiPietro, D.L., and Goss, D.A.: The effect of ampicillin administration on urinary estriol and serum estradiol in the normal pregnant patient. Am. J. Obstet. Gynecol., *119*:98, 1974.
54. Gallagher, J.C., Ismail, M.A., and Aladjem, S.: Reduced urinary estriol levels with erythromycin therapy. Obstet. Gynecol., *56*:381, 1980.
55. Kutscher, A.H., Zegarelli, E.V., Tovell, H.M.M., and Hochberg, B.: Discoloration of teeth induced by tetracycline administered ante partum. J.A.M.A., *184*:586, 1963.
56. Cohlan, S.O., Bevelander, G., and Tiomsic, T.: Growth inhibition of the developing skelton due to tetracycline deposition in bone: Clinical and laboratory investigation. Am. J. Dis. Child., *104*:480, 1962.
57. Lucey, J.F., and Driscoll, J.J., Jr.: Hazard to newborn infants of administration of long acting sulfonamides to pregnant women. Pediatrics, *24*:498, 1959.
58. Hodgman, J.E., and Burns, L.E.: Safe and effective chloramphenicol dosages for premature infants. Am. J. Dis. Child., *101*:140, 1961.
59. Philipson, A.E.L.: Pharmacokinetics of antibiotics in the pregnant woman. *In* Antibiotics in Obstetrics and Gynecology. Edited by W.J. Ledger. Boston, Martinus Nijhoff, 1982.

60. Burke, J.F.: The effective period of preventive antibiotic action in experimental incisions and dermal lesions. Surgery, *50*:161, 1961.
61. Ledger, W.J., Sweet, R.L., and Headington, J.T.: Prophylactic cephaloridine in the prevention of postoperative pelvic infections in premenopausal women undergoing vaginal hysterectomy. Am. J. Obstet. Gynecol., *115*:766, 1973.
62. Allen, J.H., Rampone, J.F., and Wheeless, C.R.: Use of a prophylactic antibiotic in elective major gynologic operations. Obstet. Gynecol., *39*:218, 1972.
63. Karl, R.C., Mertz, J.J., Veith, F.J., and Dineen, P.: Prophylactic antimicrobial drugs in surgery. N. Engl. J. Med., *275*:305, 1966.
64. Ledger, W.J., Cambell, C., Taylor, D., and Willson, J.R.: Adnexal abscess as late complication of pelvic operations. Surg. Gynecol. Obstet., *129*:973, 1969.
65. Ledger, W.J., Gassner, C.B., and Gee, C.: Operative care of infection in obstetrics-gynecology. J. Reprod. Med., *13*:128, 1974.
66. Wong, R., Gee, C.L., and Ledger, W.J.: Prophylactic use of cefazolin in monitored obstetric patients undergoing cesarean section. Obstet. Gynecol., *51*:407, 1978.
67. Osborne, N.G., Wright, R.C., and Dubay, M.: Pre-operative hot conization of the cervix: A possible method to reduce postoperative febrile morbidity following vaginal hysterectomy. Am. J. Obstet. Gynecol., *133*:374, 1979.
68. Long, W.H., Rudd, E.G., and Dillon, M.B.: Intrauterine irrigation with cefamandole nafate solution at cesarean section: A preliminary report. Am. J. Obstet. Gynecol., *138*:755, 1980.
69. Suchet, J.H., Catalan, F., Loffredo, V., Sanson, M.J., Debache, C., Pigeau, F., and Coppin, R.: *Chlamydia trachomatis* associated with chronic inflammation in abdominal specimens from women selected for tuboplasty. Fertil. Steril., *36*:599, 1981.
70. Study Group: An evaluation of metronidazole in the prophylaxis and treatment of anaerobic infections in surgical patients. J. Antimicrob. Chemother., *1*:393, 1975.
71. Brook, I., and Walker, R.I.: Significance of encapsulated *Bacteroides melaninogenicus* and *Bacteroides fragilis* groups in mixed infections. Infect. Immun. *44*:12, 1984.
72. Young, R., Platt, L., and Ledger, W.J.: Prophylactic cefoxitin in cesarean section. Surg. Gynecol. Obstet., *157*:11, 1983.
73. Ford, L.: A double blind study of piperacillin vs cefoxitin. Supp. Inf. Surg., *3*:27, 1984.
74. Webb, D.: Personal communication, 1984.
75. Polk, B.F., Krache, M., Phillippe, M., Munoz, A., Hutchinson, D., Miao, L., and Schoenbaum, S.C.: Randomized clinical trial of perioperative cefoxitin in preventing maternal infection after primary cesarean section. Am. J. Obstet. Gynecol., *142*:983, 1982.
76. Forney, J.P., Morrow, C.P., Townsend, D.E., and Disaia, P.J.: Impact of cephalosporin prophylaxis on conization-vaginal hysterectomy morbidity. Am. J. Obstet. Gynecol., *125*:100, 1976.
77. Creasman, W.T., Hill, G.B., Weed, J.C., Jr., and Gall, S.A.: A trial of prophylactic cefamandole in extended gynecologic surgery. Obstet. Gynecol., *59*:309, 1982.
78. Hodgson, J.E., Major, B., Portmann, K., and Quattlebaum, F.W.: Prophylactic use of tetracycline for first trimester abortions. Obstet. Gynecol., *45*:574, 1975.
79. Sonne-Holm, S., Heisterberg, L., Hebjorn, S., Dyring-Andersen, K., Andersen, J.T., and Hejl, B.L.: Prophylactic antibiotics in first trimester abortions: A clinical controlled trial. Am. J. Obstet. Gynecol., *139*:693, 1981.
80. Pittaway, D.E., Winfield, A.C., Maxson, W., Daniell, J., Herbert, C., and Wentz, A.C.: Prevention of acute pelvic inflammatory disease after hysterosalpingography: Efficacy of doxycycline prophylaxis. Am. J. Obstet. Gynecol., *147*:623, 1983.
81. Polk, B.F., Shapiro, M., Goldstein, P., Tager, I.B., Goren-White, B., and Schoenbaum, S.C.: Randomized clinical trial of perioperative cefazolin in preventing infection after hysterectomy. Lancet, *1*:437, 1980.
82. Shapiro, M., Munoz, A., Tager, I.B., Schoenbaum, S.C., and Polk, B.F.: Risk factors for infection at the operative site after abdominal or vaginal hysterectomy. N. Engl. J. Med., *307*:1661, 1982.
83. Ohm, M.J., and Galask, R.P.: The effect of antibiotic prophylaxis on patients undergoing abdominal hysterectomy. I. Effect of morbidity. Am. J. Obstet. Gynecol., *125*:442, 1976.
84. Grossman, J.H., III, Greco, T.P., Minkin, M.J., Adams, R.L., Hierholzer, W.J., Jr., and Andriole, V.T.: Prophylactic antibiotics in gynecologic surgery. Obstet. Gynecol., *53*:537, 1979.
85. Berkeley, A., Hayworth, S.D., Freedman, K.S., Hirsch, J.C. and Ledger, W.J.: Controlled comparative study of moxalactam and cefazolin for prophylaxis of abdominal hysterectomy. Surg. Gynocol Obstet. In press.
86. Shapiro, M., Townsend, T.R., Rosner, B., and Kass, E.H.: Use of antimicrobial agents in general hospitals. N. Engl. J. Med., *301*:351, 1979.
87. Gordon, H.R., Phelps, D., and Blanchard, K.: Prophylactic cesarean section antibiotics: Maternal and neonatal morbidity before and after cord clamping. Obstet. Gynecol., *53*:151, 1979.
88. Spruill, F.G., Minette, L.J., and Sturner, W.Q.: Two surgical deaths associated with cephalothin. J.A.M.A., *229*:440, 1974.

89. Rudd, E.G., Long, W.H., and Dillon, M.B.: Febrile morbidity following cefamandole nafate intrauterine irrigation during cesarean section. Am. J. Obstet. Gynecol., *141*:12, 1981.
90. Levin, D.K., Gorchels, C., and Andersen, R.: Reduction of postcesarean section infectious morbidity by means of antibiotic irrigation. Am. J. Obstet. Gynecol., *147*:273, 1983.
91. Duff, P., Gibbs, R.S., Jorgensen, J.H., and Alexander, G.: The pharmacokinetics of prophylactic antibiotics, administered by intraoperative irrigation at time of cesarean section. Obstet. Gynecol., *60*:409, 1982.
92. Conover, W.B., and Moore, T.R.: Comparison of irrigation and intravenous antibiotic prophylaxis at cesarean section. Obstet. Gynecol., *63*:787, 1984.
93. Lett, W.J., Ansbacher, R., Davison, B.L., and Otterson, W.N.: Prophylactic antibiotics for women undergoing vaginal hysterectomy. J. Reprod. Med., *19*:51, 1977.
94. Mendelson, J., Portnoy, J., Victor, J.R.D., and Gelfand, M.M.: Effect of single and multidose cephradine prophylaxis on infectious morbidity of vaginal hysterectomy. Obstet. Gynecol., *53*:31, 1979.
95. Hamod, K.A., Spence, M.R., Rosenshein, N.B., and Dillon, M.B.: Single-dose or multidose prophylaxis in vaginal hysterectomy: A comparison of sodium cephalothin and metronidazole. Am. J. Obstet. Gynecol., *136*:976, 1980.
96. Galle, P.C., Urban, R.B., Homesley, H.D., Jobson, V.W., and Wheeler, A.S.: Single dose carbenicillin versus T-tube drainage in patients undergoing vaginal hysterectomy. Surg. Gynecol. Obstet., *153*:351, 1981.
97. Hemsell, D.L., Heard, M.L., Nobles, B.J., and Hemsell, P.G.: Single dose cefoxitin prophylaxis for premenopausal women undergoing vaginal hysterectomy. Obstet. Gynecol., *63*:285, 1984.
98. D'Angelo, L.J., and Sokol, R.J.: Short versus long course prophylactic antibiotic treatment in cesarean section patients. Obstet. Gynecol., *55*:583, 1980.
99. Elliott, J.P., Freeman, R.K., and Dorchester, W.: Short versus long course of prophylactic antibiotics in cesarean section. Am. J. Obstet. Gynecol., *143*:740, 1982.
100. Price, D.J.E., and Sleigh, J.D.: Control of infection due to *Klebsiella aerogenes* in a neurosurgical unit by withdrawal of all antibiotics. Lancet, *2*:1213, 1970.
101. Ledger, W.J., and Puttler, O.L.: Death from pseudomembranous enterocolitis. Obstet. Gynecol., *45*:609, 1975.
102. Stiver, H.G., Forward, K.R., Livingstone, R.A., Fugere, P., Lemay, M., Verschelden, G., Hunter, J.D.W., Carson, G.D., Beresfod, P., and Tyrrell, D.L.: Multicenter comparison of cefoxitin versus cefazolin for prevention of infectious morbidity after nonelective cesarean section. Am. J. Obstet. Gynecol., *145*:158, 1983.
103. Tuomala, R., Steele, L., Sourney, P., Schoenbaum, S.C., and Polk, B.F.: Prospective randomized comparison of cefazolin and moxalactam as prophylaxis in women undergoing abdominal hysterectomy. Infect. Dis. Soc. Ob./Gyn., July 14–18, 1982 meeting, p. 4.
104. Clemens, J.D., Horwitz, R.I., Jaffe, C.C., Feinstein, A.R., and Stanton, B.F.: A controlled evaluation of the risk of bacterial endocarditis in persons with mitral valve prolapse. N. Engl. J. Med., *307*:776, 1982.
105. Kaplan, E.L., Anthony, B.R., Bisno, A., Durack, D., Houser, H., Millard, H.P., Sanford, J., Shulman, S.T., Stillerman, M., Taranta, A., and Wenger, N.: Prevention of bacterial endocarditis. Circulation, *56*:139A, 1977.
106. Durack, D.T., Kaplan, E.L., and Bisno, A.L.: Apparent failures of endocarditis prophylaxis. J.A.M.A., *250*:2318, 1983.
107. Chesney, R.W.: Drug-induced hypokalemia. Am. J. Dis. Child., *130*:1055, 1976.
108. Brown, C.H., III, Natelson, E.A., Bradshaw, M.W., Williams, T.W., Jr., and Alfrey, C.P. Jr.: The hemostatic defect produced by carbenicillin. N. Engl. J. Med., *291*:265, 1974.
109. Strausbaugh, L.J., and Llorens, A.S.: Cefoperazone therapy for obstetric and gynecologic infections. Rev. Infect. Dis., *5*:S154, 1983.
110. Weitekamp, M.R., and Aber, R.C.: Prolonged bleeding time and bleeding diathesis associated with moxalactam administration. J.A.M.A., *249*:69, 1983.
111. Bartlett, J.G., Chang, T.W., Gurwith, M., Gorbach, S.L., and Onderdonk, A.B.: Antibiotic associated pseudomembranous colitis due to toxin producing *Clostridia*. N. Engl. J. Med., *298*:531, 1978.
112. Wallerstein, R.O., Condit, P.K., Kasper, C.K., Brown, J.W., and Morrison, R.R.: Statewide study of chloramphenicol therapy and fatal aplastic anemia. J.A.M.A., *208*:2045, 1969.
113. Roe, F.J.C.: Metronidazole: Review of uses and toxicity. J. Antimicrob. Chemother., *3*:205, 1977.
114. Muller, M.: Action of clinically utilized 5-nitromidazoles on microorganisms. Scand. J. Infect. Dis. (Suppl.), *26*:31, 1981.
115. Friedman, G.D.: Cancer after metronidazole. N. Engl. J. Med., *302*:519, 1980.
116. Centers for Disease Control Morbidity and Mortality Weekly Report Supplement. Sexually transmitted diseases. Treatment Guidelines 1982. *31*:335, 1982.

Chapter 8

COMMUNITY-ACQUIRED GYNECOLOGIC INFECTIONS

Practicing gynecologists must deal with a wide variety of community-acquired infections that are not always obvious to the examining physician. They may encounter the rare patient who has generalized symptoms, such as the skin rash and hypotension of toxic shock syndrome, or the patient who has infectious arthritis caused by *Neisseria gonorrhoeae*. In contrast, the majority of patients present with a rather limited range of symptoms, i.e., they can have vulvar irritation with or without lesions, a vaginal discharge that is annoying, discomfort on urination, or pelvic pain that may or may not be exacerbated by intercourse. These general symptoms can sometimes be related to very specific disease entities. Physicians can often be confused by descriptions in textbook chapters describing these infections in women. These reference sources begin with the diagnosis of a specific entity such as *Candida* vaginitis and then describe one or more distinct management regimens. For the physician seeing these patients for the first time, making the diagnosis can be the most difficult part of the evaluation. Clinicians need to have the background knowledge to do those diagnostic tests that are necessary to establish the cause of the problem so that specific therapy can be prescribed.

VULVAR LESIONS

An increasing number of women present to a gynecologist with newly discovered vulvar lesions. For sexually active women today, an overriding concern is herpes genitalis. This should be a major focus of the examiner. Recent studies of women with recurrent genital herpes have documented the patterns of this disease. Viral shedding begins at the time of the first symptoms, and prodromal symptoms were noted in 85% of women—usually a burning, tingling, or itching in the perineal site at which the lesions subsequently appeared; a few women reported radiating pain.[1] Perineal lesions appeared with pain at the site for a mean of four days, and the healing time of the lesions of 8.2 ± 2.8 days.[1] Findings from daily cultures showed that virus was shed for a mean of 4.8 days from the onset of symptoms, but 16% of women still shed virus after 6 days. Cervical cultures for herpes remained positive in 4% of women in this study during the time they were free of perineal lesions between recurrences.[1] Depending upon the timing of the patient's visit to the physician, the perineal lesions will be at a specific stage of development. The spectrum of clinical response is noted in Figure 8–1.[1] This time frame of signs and symptoms should be kept in mind by the physician as questions to the patient are formulated. At the very least, these women should be asked if

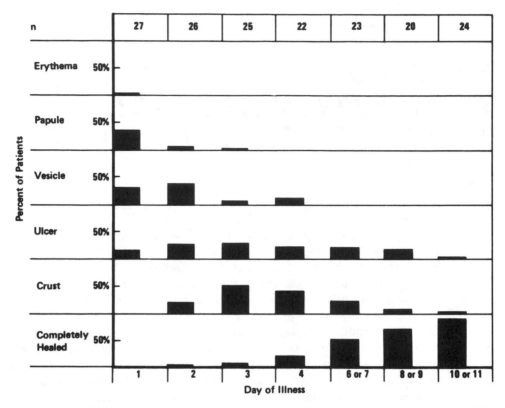

Fig. 8–1. The clinical spectrum of symptoms in patients with genital herpes. (From Guinan, M.E., MacCalman, J., Kern, E.R., Overall, J.C., Jr., and Spruance, S.L.: The course of untreated recurrent genital herpes simplex infection in 27 women. N. Engl. J. Med., *304*:759, 1981. Reprinted by permission of the New England Journal of Medicine.)

this is the first episode, when the symptoms began, what are or were they, and if they noticed any lesions. Confirmation of the diagnosis of herpes genitalis should be made by direct viral culture of the lesion. The clinical diagnosis is not specific, and Pap smear confirmation of multinucleated giant cells is frequently not obtained in women who are culture-positive. For the gynecologist seeing these patients on a continuing basis, I believe it is important to obtain one culture at the time the patient believes she has an episode of recurrent genital herpes, so she is aware of the stage of the disease in which significant quantities of virus are being shed. Blood studies for serum levels of antibody to herpes in women with genital lesions are usually not helpful for a number of reasons. Serum antibodies can be present in a woman who does not have genital herpes because of past oral herpes infection. Alternatively, antibodies may not be present in a woman having her first episode of genital herpes. Finally, there is no correlation between the titer rise of traditional antibody tests and recurrent herpes infections. In fact, one study of genital herpes showed that patients with high titers of neutralizing antibody to herpes virus after the first infection were more likely to have recurrences than those patients without these antibodies.[2] The diagnosis of genital herpes should usually be obvious to the clinician. The woman having her first episode of genital herpes usually has systemic symptoms, i.e., fever and general malaise, as well as local findings. Patients with the first episode of genital herpes who have had oral herpes before may have fewer symptoms.[2] On occasion, the patient with an initial infection has so much discomfort from the lesions that voiding is painful and difficult, and the inguinal lymph nodes are usually palpable and tender.

Herpes is not the only cause of vulvar lesions. Patients can present with vulvar lesions that are painless and "punched out," and in these instances a darkfield examination for spirochetes is clearly indicated. The lesions can be chronic. In these cases, biopsies should be obtained and specific tissue and microbiologic tests done to rule out other diagnoses such as lymphogranuloma venereum or chancroid (see Chapter 3). These other less common infections are frequently reported in studies of populations of African women.[3]

In any woman in whom the clinical diagnosis is not apparent or in whom the symptoms do not disappear with standard therapy, the vulvar lesion should be biopsied to be sure there is no neoplasm. In women of all age groups, the lesions can appear raised and wartlike. Biopsies should be obtained to confirm the clinical diagnosis of Condyloma acuminatum and to rule out the less frequent lesion of Condyloma latum. Prediculosis pubis should be suspected when a patient complains of marked vulvar pruritus, particularly when she has noticed "something moving." Examination of the pubic hair with a magnifying glass usually shows the presence of *Pediculus pubis* crawling on a hair shaft.

There are three other groups of women who can present to the gynecologist with specific vulvar lesions. Physically active women can have trauma to the vulvar area from such episodes as a bicycle seat accident or a boating accident, in which the bruised vulvar area becomes the site of a deep infection, even in cases in which the skin remains intact. Diabetics can develop serious soft tissue infections of the vulva in which there is no prior evidence of trauma.[4] In addition, physicians have to deal on occasion with a patient with a Bartholin's or Skene's gland abscess.

DIAGNOSIS AND TREATMENT OF SPECIFIC VULVAR ENTITIES

Genital Herpes

Too often, physicians responsible for the care of women with genital herpes emphasize the negative aspects of the disease. This often confirms the feeling of unworthiness and low self-esteem some women may have with this illness. Many of these patients feel that they are social outcasts. Frequently, the patient is advised by what she perceives as an unsympathetic physician in words that imply a heavy burden of guilt: "Because of sexual indiscretions, you have acquired an incurable disease that will plague you for the rest of your life. You will have painful recurrent genital infections that will be triggered by either social or personal stresses over which you have no control. You can infect an unsuspecting male sexual contact. If you become pregnant, you are a threat to your unborn baby at the time of delivery and can cause his or her death." To complete this dreary picture of the victim's future life, the patient then hears the prophesy, "you have a greater than normal chance of developing cervical carcinoma." After hearing such negative interpretation, it is not surprising that many patients become severely depressed, are often unable to establish any meaningful adult relationships, and grasp desperately at any of the treatments available for genital herpes, (e.g., the use of

Table 8–1. Effect of Topical Acyclovir on First Episode of Genital Herpes

	Acyclovir-Treated	Placebo-Treated
	N = 26	N = 23
	Results noted in mean days ± S.E. after start of therapy	
Pain	6.0 ± 1.0	8.8 ± 1.0
Viral shedding*	2.8 ± 0.6	6.7 ± 1.0
Time to crusting*	7.1 ± 0.6	10.5 ± 1.1
Time to healing	10.6 ± 0.9	12.3 ± 1.3

*Statistically significant p < 0.01.
(From Corey, L., Nahmias, A.J., Guinan, M.E., Benedetti, J.K., Critchlow, C.W., and Holmes, K.K.: A trial of topical acyclovir in genital herpes simplex infections. N. Engl. J. Med., *306*:1313, 1982. Reprinted by permission of the New England Journal of Medicine.)

vital dyes and fluorescent light[5] or of 2-deoxy-0-glucose[6]) that have not proved effective in controlled studies.

The realistic goals of therapy for the physician of the patient with genital herpes are sympathetic counsel, education of the patient about the disease, and prescription treatment if indicated. If the knowledgeable physician believes that genital herpes is not a hopeless disease, the patient with this ailment can be helped considerably.

Acyclovir, a potent antiviral agent, has an effect upon genital herpes. In a polyethylene glycol ointment for local application to genital herpes lesions in women, it is helpful in the treatment of the first episode of genital herpes.[7] Treated patients have been found to have more rapid healing of the lesions and less viral shedding (Table 8–1).[7] This method of therapy has been approved by the Food and Drug Administration (FDA) and is available for the practicing clinician today. In addition, both intravenous[8] and oral acyclovir have proved effective in symptomatic relief and diminished viral shedding. The results with oral therapy are presented in Table 8–2.[9] There is a suggestion that when given early both the intravenous and oral forms can reduce recurrences of genital herpes, and oral therapy has been approved by the FDA to diminish recurrences. Local acyclovir has not been helpful in the treatment of recurrent genital herpes infection in women; the number of days of virus shedding and of the presence of lesions is unchanged, but oral therapy does diminish the number of recurrences.[10, 11] In the future the physician and the ancillary medical staff must be alert to the early signs of primary herpes so that these women can be seen and receive care. In addition to these new therapeutic developments, recent studies have documented an acceleration of viral growth in culture when prostaglandins have been added.[12]

Table 8–2. Oral Acyclovir Therapy: Duration of Herpes Virus Shedding and Period from Start of Study to Crusting and Healing of All Lesions in Primary Cases

	Acyclovir (N = 16)	Placebo (N = 15)	P Value
	(mean no. of days) (range)		
Duration of shedding	4.9 (2–6)	14.7 (8–26)	< 0.001
Time to crusting	8.8 (4–17)	15 (7–25)	< 0.01
Time to healing	10 (5–17)	16.2 (9–24)	< 0.015

(From Bryson, Y.J., Dillon, M., Lovett, M., Acuna, G., Taylor, S., Cherry, J.D., Johnson, B.L., Wiesmeier, E., Growdon, W., Creagh-Kirk, T., and Keeney, R.: Treatment of first episodes of genital herpes simplex virus infection with oral acyclovir. N. Engl. J. Med., *308*:916, 1983. Reprinted by permission of the New England Journal of Medicine.)

There will be trials carried out in the next few years to see if either the long-term use of antiprostaglandins or their use at the time of prodromal symptoms will decrease the number of recurrences. If this therapeutic approach is successful, it will be a way to modify the long-term course of this disease with medications that to date have shown little toxicity.

There are safe treatments for herpes that can help to relieve symptoms. The physician utilizing local and systemic therapy should be aware that there is scant evidence that any of the adjuvants accelerate the healing of herpes lesions when compared with placebo therapy. Despite this, I am convinced that some patients do note a lessening of symptoms and feel better when some therapy is used. The goal should be to diminish the number of days of discomfort from the herpes lesions on the perineum. Provision of adequate analgesia during an outbreak is indicated. Since antiprostaglandins may diminish viral spread, aspirin or more potent antiprostaglandins such as ibuprofen or Naproxen can be prescribed. If vesicles are present, these should be broken and local medication applied to kill the virus present and to promote the formation of a crust that is usually not associated with pain. A number of agents can be soothing to the patient. These include 1% zinc sulfate solution,[13] 4% boric acid ointment,[14] and antiseptic drying agents like povidone-iodine.[15] I favor the iodine solution because I have had the most experience with it. One regimen that has been discarded by most physicians is ether because it has not been demonstrated to have any benefits[16] and because it is potentially explosive if employed in the office or at home by the patient. The patient can apply the povidone-iodine solution safely at home, and it will result in most patients having less pain from the herpes outbreak. The oral acyclovir preparation is a possibility for recurrent local infections. Statistically, it is more effective than placebo (Table 8–3),[11] but the differences are slight clinically,[17] and there is the added danger that the herpesvirus can become resistant to acyclovir.[18] Because of this, I do not recommend routine use of the oral preparation in recurrent infections. The use of local dyes and fluorescent light is to be condemned. This treatment alters viral DNA and theoretically should prevent replication of the virus and recurrent lesions, but prospective studies have shown no

Table 8–3. Effects of Suppresive Oral Acyclovir on Recurrent Genital Herpes

	ACV-5*	ACV-2†	Placebo
Number of patients (men and women)	51	52	50
Number of patients completing 4 months	45	51	47
Pretreatment recurrences (number/month)	1.03 ± 0.08	0.94 ± 0.06	1.16 ± 0.11
Post-treatment recurrences	0.10 ± 0.24	0.13 ± 0.23	0.84 ± 0.50

* ACV-5—Acyclovir 5 times a day.
† ACV-2—Acyclovir 2 times a day.
(From Douglas, J.M., Critchlow, C., Benedetti, J., Mertz, G.J., Connor, J.A., Hintz, M.A., Fahnlander, A., Remington, M., Winter, C., and Corey, L.: A double-blind study of oral acyclovir for suppression of recurrences of genital herpes simplex virus infection. N. Engl. J. Med., *310*:1551, 1984. Reprinted by permission of the New England Journal of Medicine.)

influence on the healing time of the lesions,[5] and this treatment can be oncogenic in some experimental cell systems.[19] The lack of effect and the potential danger combine to eliminate this local therapy as an alternative for obstetricians-gynecologists.

The gynecologic patient with recurrent herpes genitalis needs to be educated by the physician. An important goal is the patient's awareness of her ability to spread the disease to a sexual partner or to other areas of her body. There is no way to totally avoid the spread of herpes to a sexual partner, but the risks can be considerably reduced. The woman should be taught to examine herself so as to recognize the prodromal signs of the illness and to be aware of the evolution of the genital lesions. There is a limited time frame in which she will be shedding virus from the perineum and is capable of infecting a sexual partner. The patient is also a danger to herself. Although she has systemic antibodies to herpes, scratching an active lesion with a finger that has a break in the skin integument can produce a herpes lesion on the finger or elsewhere on the body if that same finger scratches and breaks the surface. Careful personal hygiene is required. During the time that the patient is free of prodromal symptoms and has no perineal lesions, there should be no risk of perineal contact for herself and no risk for sexual contacts. Some asymptomatic women will shed herpes virus from the cervix,[1] and there is a risk of infecting a male sexual partner. But vaginal spermicidal agents are viricidal for herpes, and if used in conjunction with a condom by the male, they should markedly reduce the risk of spread of herpes in these situations.

Physicians' concern about genital herpes should not be limited to the treatment of patients with the disease, because education is important for the sexually active patient who does not have herpes. The patient with oral herpes (cold sores) is not immune to genital herpes, although herpes antibodies are present in the blood. Genital herpes can be acquired from oral-genital contact if the male has cold sores, and it can be acquired from a male with a past history of herpes who has no visible lesions. A detailed medical history of the male sexual partner is helpful, and the use of condoms or locally applied spermicidal agents or both should decrease the risk for the woman.

Patients with larger individual vulvar lesions should be subject to a systematic workup by the gynecologist. If the lesions appear "punched out," the physician should be suspicious of syphilis and a darkfield examination of secretions of the lesions should be obtained to check for the possibility of spirochetes. This evaluation should be done for all suspicious lesions, even if they are painful, despite the clinical fact that most of the "chancres" are painless. Occasionally, these lesions get secondarily infected and become uncomfortable for the patient. If the darkfield examination is positive for spirochetes, the antibiotic strategy is simple. *Treponema pallidum* is exquisitely susceptible to penicillin, and this organism replicates slowly. The therapeutic goal should be to expose the organism to relatively low levels of penicillin for long periods of time. This is accomplished by the intramuscular injection of benzathine penicillin G, 2,400,000 U. In these patients, an endocervical smear should be obtained for culture of *Neisseria gonorrhoeae*, to make sure that more than one sexually transmitted disease was not acquired; *Neisseria gonorrhoeae* requires a different antibiotic strategy than *Treponema pallidum*.

If the patient has a chronic vulvar lesion, a careful workup of the lesion is required, and tissues should be obtained for culture and microscopic examination, as related in Chapter 3. Selective media should be used to grow *Hemophilus ducreyi* from either the genital ulcers or from aspirate from a fluctuant inguinal node to confirm or rule out the diagnosis of chancroid. The treatment is erythromycin, 500 mg by mouth four times a day, for a minimum of ten days and until the ulcers and lymph nodes have healed. If patients are allergic to erythromycin, they can take trimethoprim-sulfamethoxazole (100–200 mg) twice a day, orally. Both sexual partners should be treated for ten days.[20] *Lymphogranuloma venereum* can be diagnosed by the LGV-complement fixation test.[21] The treatment is tetracycline, 500 mg orally four times a day, or doxycycline, 100 mg orally twice a day, or erythromycin, 500 mg orally four times a day, or sulfisoxazole 1.0 g orally twice a day. All these regimens should be given for at least two weeks.[20] If the lesions are raised and wartlike, the diagnosis is usually that of venereal "warts" or condyloma acuminatum. A biopsy should be obtained in these patients as well as serologic tests to rule out the possibility of an active syphilitic lesion, condyloma latum. The usual diagnosis in these cases is condyloma acuminatum due to papillomavirus. The treatment in the past has focused on local destruction of the lesion. This is normally done by the local application of a 20% podophyllun solution in benzoin. With larger lesions, electrocautery or laser[22] has been employed. There are interesting new developments in the understanding and treatment of condyloma acuminatum. In one recent study of circulating immune complexes in gynecologic patients with a variety of clinical problems (i.e., vaginitis, salpingitis, genital tract malignancy), the highest percentage of patients with immune complexes were those with *Condyloma acuminatum*.[23] In addition, there has been a breakthrough in therapy. Recent studies have shown clinical effectiveness in the control and elimination of massive condyloma lesions that have not responded to local measures of control when interferon has been employed for treatment.[24] Finally, the physician will see some women with pediculosis pubis. The diagnosis is suggested by a history of local itching and rash plus the appearance of the forms on the hair shafts when they are viewed under magnification. The treatment is simple. Personal intimate objects such as bedclothing and undergarments should be thoroughly laundered, and the patient and her sexual partner should be treated with local 1% lindane lotion or cream applied to the infected area and removed by washing the area after nine hours, or with lindane 1% shampoo (Kwell), applied for four minutes and then thoroughly rinsed away.[20] As an alternative, pyrethrins and piperonyl butoxide (nonprescription) can be applied to the infected area and washed off after 10 minutes. None of these regimens is recommended for the pregnant or nursing mother.

There are important treatment considerations in patients with vulvar infections. In those with vulvar trauma, an infection in the resulting hematoma can occur. I have recently managed such a patient who required hospitalization, incision and drainage, and the use of systemic antibiotics. In her case, a coagulase-positive *Staphylococcus* that was resistant to penicillin was isolated in pure culture. A much more serious infection can be seen in diabetics, presenting as a vulvar problem. These women have vulvar infections, anesthesia of the indurated vulvar site, and upon surgical exploration they are found to have a necrotizing fasciitis. The mortality rate in this population is high. A recent report indicated two fatalities in four such women despite extensive debridement of the area and broad-spectrum antibiotic coverage.[4] A wide spectrum of organisms was recovered but *Clostridia* was not isolated. Successful therapy requires early diagnosis and aggressive operative intervention and debridement.

A more common clinical problem is the patient presenting with a Bartholin's or Skene's gland abscess. Although in the past it was thought that *Neisseria gonorrhoeae* was frequently involved in these infections, they have generally been mixed infections with anaerobes as the predominant isolates. The mainstay of treatment is incision and drainage, with antibiotics reserved for those patients whose infection has not been well confined by local host defense mechanisms. This is usually an uncomplicated medical problem.

VAGINAL INFECTIONS

Patients with vaginal or cervical infections will present with a variety of symptoms. Their chief complaint is usually an annoying discharge, but questioning by a sympathetic physician can detail the scope of the problem. Physician attitude has an important bearing on the future welfare of these patients. These infections are not life-threatening, but they should not be dismissed as trivial because they can have a major impact on the patient's quality of life. The physician who takes the time to successfully diagnose and treat these infections will add both to the patient's ability to function normally and to her self-esteem. The questioning at the first visit should be directed toward the cause of the symptoms as well as a sympathetic probe covering the full extent of the problem. If the patient's unspoken concern is a sexually acquired disease, a focus upon vaginal symptoms alone is short-sighted. There are a number of questions that I articulate for my own understanding of the problem in such cases (Table 8–4). The answers to these questions help me to focus on the possible causes of the infection during the physical examination and help in subsequent therapeutic planning after physical diagnosis.

Although the details of the physical and laboratory examinations of these women have been detailed in Chapter 3, every patient with a troublesome vaginal

Table 8–4. Questions to Be Posed to the Patient with Vaginitis

Question	Candida	Trichomonas	Nonspecific	Other (Neisseria gonorrhea)
1. Does the patient have itching?	+ + + +	+ / −	+ / −	+ / −
2. Is the patient aware of an odor?	+	+ +	+ + + +	+
3. Is there vaginal discomfort?	+ + +	+ + + +	+ +	+
4. Is there dyspareunia?	+ + +	+ + + +	+	+ / −
5. Does the patient have a new male sexual partner?	−	+ + +	+	+ + + +
6. Is the patient having sexual relations with a male with symptoms?	+	−	−	+ + + +
7. A relationship of the symptoms to the menstrual cycle?	+ + + +	−	−	−
8. Has there been recent ingestion of local or systemic medicine for these symptoms?	+ + + +	+	+ +	+ +
9. How is the onset of symptoms related to systemic antibiotic use?	+ + + +	−	−	−

+ Presence of symptom—from occasionally + to nearly always + + + +.
− No symptoms.

discharge requires an office laboratory evaluation. Every physician should be familiar with the details of a wet-mount examination of vaginal secretions in separate saline and 10% potassium hydroxide solutions. In addition, a "fishy" amine odor, present when the potassium hydroxide is added to the vaginal secretions, is specific for the diagnosis of nonspecific vaginitis. Routine bacterial cultures are usually not helpful. Physicians should take endocervical specimens for cultures of *Neisseria gonorrhoeae* for all patients for a period of time to determine the yield of positive cultures. If *Neisseria gonorrhoeae* is isolated in a practice population, this routine should be continued. If the patient has a purulent cervicitis, then a culture from the endocervix for *Chlamydia* should be done if possible. With this workup, the diagnosis of the source of the discharge can be made in most cases. The physician should be aware that in some patients, there may be more than one cause of the symptoms. The diagnosis and treatment of individual vaginal infections will be discussed on the basis of specific causes.

Candida albicans Vaginitis

This form of vaginal infection is the most common type of vaginitis seen by gynecologists at present. The diagnosis can be made by seeing mycelia or hyphae on microscopic evaluation of vaginal secretions, particularly after 10% potassium hydroxide solution has been added to the preparation, for this will destroy other cell forms, making the diagnosis much easier. In addition, white cells are usually not seen. If in doubt, a culture using Saboraud's medium will confirm the clinical and microscopic impressions. Many patients with complaints of itching, more marked just before menses, have a red inflamed vulva on examination and will give a history of recent ingestion of antibiotics for an infection elsewhere. Although not proved by prospective study,[25] I believe that discontinuation of oral contraceptives is required in some recurrent episodes of *Candida* vaginitis before a cure can be achieved.

The picture for the treatment of patients with symptomatic *Candida* vaginitis has brightened considerably in the years since the publication of the first edition of *Infection in the Female.* In addition to nystatin, other potent local antifungal agents, including miconazole nitrate and chlortrimazole, have been introduced into clinical practice. They are fungicidal and have the great advantage of being effective as therapy in the shorter time frame of three to seven days rather than the 14-day therapy recommended for the local nystatin preparations. In recurrent infections, the physician can apply gentian violet dye locally to diminish the number of yeast forms in the vagina. In addition to these local forms of therapy, oral ketoconazole has been approved for use in chronic mucocutaneous fungal infections. This gives the physician the opportunity to utilize an oral agent that is far less toxic than amphotericin B in the treatment of these conditions.

Despite these advances, as a group women with recurrent or chronic *Candida* vaginitis are one of the most frustrating in outpatient therapy. This is related in part to their numbers, for they represent the longest number of treatment failures in patients with vaginitis. The major cause of frustration is our inability to cure these women. There are important diagnostic and therapeutic considerations in this group. Those with recurrent or chronic vaginal candidiasis should have their blood glucose levels evaluated, although abnormalities are rarely found. The two-hour postprandial blood glucose test can be used as a screen; if levels are evaluated, it should be followed by an oral three-hour glucose tolerance test. The male sexual partners should be examined to see if they have a balanitis or a local irritation of the penis. Specimens should be cultured, and the males should be treated with local antifungal agents if the culture results are positive. English investigators have observed male sexual partners to be culture-positive in some women with recurrent or chronic *Candida* vaginitis,[26] and I have observed this with ejaculate cultures. In these women, it is important to culture the vaginal secretions to be sure that other yeast forms are not implicated. For example, *Torulopsis glabrata* can be a cause of vaginitis and requires a longer course of oral therapy for cure. Again, this is a rare finding. If all these possibilities have been assessed in women who have not been cured with local therapy, I treat these women with oral ketoconazole, 200 mg twice a day for fourteen days. In one study, this regimen had a high cure rate when followed by long-term suppression.[27] This oral preparation probably reduces bowel carriage of *Candida* as well as having an impact on the vagina, and a cure is achieved in some women. Ketoconazole is not perfect for the treatment of oral candidiasis; a two-week course with this medication was disappointing.[28] Only 25% of treated patients had both resolution of lesions plus eradication of *Candida albicans*.

It is obvious from this discussion that despite all the currently available efforts of diagnosis and treatment, some women will continue to have either recurrent or chronic *Candida* yeast infections. There are two new developments in our understanding of these infections that could help to explain these troubling therapeutic failures. One is the increased awareness that the characteristic of adherence to cells by bacteria and fungi is an important factor in pathogenesis. There is evidence in some women that *Candida* forms can attach to and invade tissue. I recently treated a patient with chronic *Candida* vaginitis and a painful tiny "crack" in the epithelium of the introitus. PAS stains of the microscopic sections revealed tissue invasion with mycelia, and a cure was achieved during hospitalization with a short course of amphotericin B. Similar findings can account for some of the observed treatment failures with local antifungal preparations and are the rationale for using a systemic agent such as ketoconazole or amphotericin B to attempt to achieve a cure in these women. Another new development is the discovery that the lymphocytes of women with recurrent or chronic *Candida* vaginitis do not react to the *Candida* antigen.[29] This failure of response is related to the presence of a suppressor substance in the serum, for serum from these women added to the blood of normally responsive women inhibits their lymphocyte response to *Candida*. This is a limited immunologic deficiency, unlike the complete cellular immuno-suppression that occurs in AIDS, for these women react normally to other antigens such as phytohemagglutinin P and concanavallin A. The reason for the presence of this suppressor substance in these women is not known at present, but there are well-tolerated medications such as antiprostaglandins that lower suppressor substance in the serum. This offers the possibility that modification of this abnormal immune response will result in a clinical cure in some of these patients.

Trichomonas vaginalis Vaginitis

Patients with this symptomatic vaginal infection are not seen as frequently by gynecologists as in the past. This is attributable in part to the marked increase in the number of patients with difficult-to-treat *Candida* vaginal infections, but also perhaps because the availability and widespread use in both males and females of the effective antiprotozoal drug metronidazole has reduced the pool of patients with this troublesome infection. Whatever the reason, the number of women with this problem is less than it was a decade ago.

Patients with this infection have troublesome symptoms, such as a heavy vaginal discharge that may have an odor and vaginal discomfort and burning, particularly after intercourse. In many cases they can relate the onset of symptoms to a specific sexual liaison with a new male partner. The diagnosis is apparent after microscopic examination of the vaginal secretions in saline, in which motile *trichomonads* and white cells are seen.

The therapy is straightforward, although the treatment strategies for this disease have undergone some modifications since the first edition. The systemic agent metronidazole is effective against these protozoa. It is increasingly apparent that many asymptomatic men are carriers of *Trichomonas.* For this reason, I believe it is important for the male sexual partners of these patients to be treated concomitantly with metronidazole. Both the single-dose treatment and the seven-day regimen give equivalent cure rates, and either can be selected by the physician.[30] In the single-dose regimen, both the male and female are given eight 250-mg tablets to be taken at once, so that a total of 2 g is ingested. The advantage of this regimen is its short duration. The disadvantages are that patients can have gastric distress, nausea, and vomiting. Alternatively, patients can be given metronidazole 250 mg four times a day, after meals and at bedtime for seven days. The advantage of this regimen is that each individual dose is better tolerated than the single 2-g dose. The disadvantages are that the prohibition against alcohol (because of the antabuse effect of the drug) and the gastric upset and metallic taste in the mouth may be unacceptable to an asymptomatic male partner, and in many cases result in his discontinuing the therapy before the seven days are completed. There is evidence of lower serum levels of metronidazole when it is given to patients on phenobarbital.[31] Phenobarbital probably lowers serum levels of metronidazole by increasing metronidazole hydroxylation in the liver. In patients taking barbiturates, higher doses of metronidazole may be necessary to achieve therapeutic levels and a cure.

In addition to these problems of patient tolerance of this medication, a new problem in the treatment of patients with *Trichomonas* infections has emerged, that of increasing resistance to metronidazole.[32] Although absolute resistance has not been seen, and these patients can usually be cured with much higher doses of metronidazole—a total of 3.0 g a day for five days—the treatment can be very difficult. One recent case illustrates the complicated therapeutic problems involved. When I first saw this patient, she was living alone and in her history she reported that she had acquired the *Trichomonas* infection from a single sexual liaison eight months earlier. When the vaginal discharge began, she sought medical attention and had been treated on three separate occasions with a five day, a single 2-g dose, and a seven day treatment regimen, which had all failed. Because she knew her diagnosis and was aware of the continuing infection because of the symptoms, she was depressed and avoided any social contacts with males. The treatment required for cure was not easy to achieve. She could not tolerate the daily 3.0-g oral dosage of metronidazole, either as an outpatient or when she was admitted to the hospital and received a concomitant injection of an antiemetic.

A cure was finally achieved with hospital admission and the use of intravenous metronidazole, 4.0 g a day for seven days. On follow-up examination she was ecstatic. In these resistant cases, the male partner is often culture negative and does not require treatment.

There are many consumer concerns about the safety of metronidazole that patients will voice on occasion. Studies in mice[33] and rats[34] have shown metronidazole to be carcinogenic, and it is mutagenic to some strains of bacteria.[35] These are disturbing observations. They have been coupled with the view expressed in *The Medical Letter* that *Trichomonas* vaginitis is a trivial infection,[36] and statements have been made that metronidazole should not be prescribed for women. Much of this argument is semantic, for the infection is only trivial if the definition of significance includes only life-threatening infections. As shown in the previous case report, *Trichomonas* vaginitis can prevent normal adult socialization, and there are no effective alternative therapies to metronidazole. There are comforting observations for physicians prescribing this drug. The doses producing cancers in mice and rats are 1,500 to 3,000 times the human dose. In addition, similar results in animals have been reported with the widely used antitubercular drug isoniazid.[37] Finally, long-term follow-up studies in humans to date have shown no increased incidence of cancer.[38] Metronidazole should be prescribed for patients with *Trichomonas* vaginitis.

Nonspecific Vaginitis or Bacterial Vaginosis

This is an extremely confusing syndrome for most clinicians. Most of the confusion has resulted from controversy in the literature. Conflicting statements appear. For example, physicians are instructed that nonspecific vaginitis is caused by a specific organism, *Hemophilus vaginalis*,[39] now called *Gardnerella vaginalis*. At the opposite extreme, other investigators find no correlation between the presence of this organism and symptoms.[40] Diagnostic criteria vary widely, particularly in the assessment of the importance of the "clue" cell on microscopic examination of the vaginal smear. Finally, a wide range of treatments have been advocated for this syndrome, including either local therapy or a variety of systemic antibiotics. What follows is my approach to the patient with bacterial vaginosis.

A separate group of women who have a distinct clinical syndrome labeled nonspecific vaginitis are seen by the gynecologist. These patients complain of a foul odor, and upon examination of the often greyish vaginal discharge, a fishy odor is observed when 10% potassium hydroxide is added to the vaginal secretions. Although recent investigators have been enthusiastic about the specificity of "clue" cells in confirming the diagnosis,[41] I have been impressed with the frequency with which I see a few of these cellular forms in women who are asymptomatic. For me, the unpleasant odor that results when 10% KOH is added to the secretion is diagnostic. This disease is associated with a heavy growth of both *Gardnerella vaginalis* and anaerobic bacteria. *Gardnerella vaginalis* in small numbers can be isolated from asymptomatic women.[40] The treatment of this disease has been controversial. Triple sulfa vaginal cream and ampicillin have been recommended, but these have an unacceptably high failure rate.[42] The most effective treatment is metronidazole 500 mg twice a day for seven days.[42] The exact role of the male sexual partner in this disease is not clear at present. Currently I do not treat males initially, but the male partners of women with recurrent disease receive therapy as well.

Postmenopausal Vaginitis

This is a diagnosis of exclusion by the clinician. Although some of these women have a troublesome discharge, the most common complaint is discomfort, especially during intercourse. Careful clinical and microscopic examinations of the vaginal secretions show no evidence of other microscopic entities, and there should be a paucity of the large superficial squamous cells on vaginal smear. Any lesions or suspicious-appearing areas at the introitus or in the vagina should be biopsied. If no tissue abnormalities are noted, these women can be treated with either oral conjugated estrogens, 0.625 mg per day, or alternatively with a local vaginal estrogen cream. The physician using estrogen in these women should be prepared to sample the endometrium at regular intervals to detect any cellular abnormalities, or to add a progestational agent to the regimen.

CERVICITIS

A small percentage of the women with a troublesome vaginal discharge will have a cervicitis. This should be considered in patients complaining of a vaginal discharge with clinical evidence of cervicitis when the other causes of vaginitis have not been found. In these patients, a culture of the endocervical tissue should be obtained for *Neisseria gonorrhoeae* as well as for *Chlamydia* and *Ureaplasma urealyticum* if these tests are available. The treatment for the culture-positive patient is similar for any of these isolates, either tetracycline 500 mg orally four times a day for seven days or doxycycline 100 mg orally twice a day for a similar period of time.[20] In these cases, the male sexual partner should be treated concomitantly. In the culture-positive women, a serologic test for syphilis should also be obtained. If it is negative, this tetracycline therapy is probably adequate for incubating syphilis. If positive, a fluorescent treponemal antibody absorption test (FTA-ABS) should be obtained. If this is positive, a careful history of syphilis exposure needs to be elicited to determine whether the infection has occurred within the past year. The treatment recommendations for asymptomatic syphilis from the Centers for Disease Control are noted in Table 8–5.[20] The success rate, i.e., elimination of symptoms and the cervicitis, is close to 100% when the causative organism is a gonococcus[43] and 92% when it is *Chlamydia.*[43] In these patients with persistent cervicitis, I have been unimpressed with local therapy, particularly cryosurgery, in obtaining a cure.

ENDOMETRITIS

This is another uncommon cause of a foul-smelling vaginal discharge. It should be suspected when other causes of vaginitis have not been found, particularly in

Table 8–5. Treatment Recommendations of CDC for Asymptomatic Syphilis

Less than One Year's Duration	Unknown or More Than One Year's Duration
Benzathine penicillin G, 2.4 million U IM or Tetracycline 500 mg by mouth, four times a day for 15 days or Erythromycin 500 mg by mouth, four times a day for 15 days	Benzathine penicillin G, 2.4 million U IM once a week for 3 weeks (7.2 million U) or Tetracycline 500 mg by mouth, four times a day for 30 days or Erythromycin 500 mg by mouth, four times a day for 30 days

the patient who has used an intrauterine device for long periods of time.[44] The best treatment is removal of the device. In addition to this, some women can become colonized with *Actinomyces bovis.* This should be suspected in every patient with an intrauterine device in place who has clumps of debris present on the Papanicolau smear.[45] This finding should result in the physician's removal of the intrauterine device, for the endometritis can progress to salpingitis and pelvic abscess formation. How long these devices need to be removed before the woman can utilize this form of contraception again is not known at the present time.

ACUTE URETHRAL SYNDROME

A few patients will present to the gynecologist with the acute urinary symptoms of urgency, frequency, and dysuria. This syndrome has been called the acute urethral syndrome, and these women should be carefully evaluated with a urine culture of clean-voided urine. The pioneering work of Stamm and colleagues[46] in women with these symptoms demonstrated that a colony count of less than 10^5 of *Escherichia coli* per mm^3 of urine correlates well with bladder bacteria (see Chapter 3). It is important for the physician to write on the laboratory request for the urine culture that the patient has the acute urethral syndrome so that any *Escherichia coli* growth of less than 10^5/ml will not be thrown out as a contaminant by laboratory personnel. Other differential diagnoses include urethritis due to *Neisseria gonorrhoeae, Chlamydia,* or *Ureaplasma urealyticum.* If available to the clinician, cultures should be obtained for these organisms, for their treatment requires antimicrobial therapy that varies from that employed for urinary tract infections. In general, these lower urinary tract infections can be treated with either a sulfa drug or with nitrofurantoin orally for 10 days (see Chapter 7), with a posttreatment culture as a test for cure. For those patients with either gonococcal or nongonococcal urethritis, the treatment of choice is either tetracycline 500 mg by mouth, four times a day for seven days, or doxycycline 100 mg by mouth, twice a day for seven days. Alternatively, these patients can receive erythromycin 500 mg by mouth, four times a day for seven days.[20] The sexual partners of these women should be treated concomitantly.

OTHER URINARY TRACT INFECTIONS

Patients with other urinary tract infections are infrequently seen by the gynecologist. The criteria for laboratory diagnosis have been noted in Chapter 3, and antibiotic strategies outlined in Chapter 7. Those women who either fail to respond to therapy or have recurrent infections need a more complete urinary tract evaluation to rule out the possibilities of stones or congenital abnormalities.

SALPINGO-OOPHORITIS

My view of the clinical presentation of salpingitis has changed radically since the publication of *Infection in the Female* in 1977. In that first edition, my criteria for diagnosis were strict and followed the guidelines noted in Table 8–6. There were

Table 8–6. Older Criteria for the Diagnosis of Salpingitis

1. Acute pelvic pain
2. Fever above 38°C
3. Bilateral tender adnexal swellings or masses
4. Elevated white blood cell count and sedimentation rate

many reasons for this, but the most important one was based upon the immediate clinical response of patients. If the views expressed there were to be used as a guide for the diagnosis of salpingitis, I did not want to hear from a reader that an afebrile patient with pelvic pain had been given antibiotics based upon my recommendations and then was later found to have an ectopic pregnancy. These cases with other pathologic conditions had more impact on my consciousness than patients with tubal blockages who had minimal symptoms with untreated salpingitis. There have been two major discoveries that have altered my views on the clinical and laboratory presentation of women with this disease. The first and most important is that the old criteria were inaccurate. Studies in Sweden[47] and the United States[48] have employed laparoscopy to document the diagnosis in women admitted to the hospital with clinical evidence of salpingitis. These studies have shown that many women with a clinical diagnosis of salpingitis had normal pelvic findings on laparoscopy. When the frequency of the classic signs noted in Table 8–6 were documented in these women with either salpingitis or a normal pelvis, some surprising observations were made (Table 8–7).[47] The observations in Table 8–7 are important for the practitioner who is seeing an individual patient with lower abdominal and pelvic pain. This table makes it obvious that the physician adhering to the old criteria will not make the proper diagnosis in the majority of cases. It is also clear that the diagnosis of salpingitis is a difficult one, for the variance between the two populations is not clear-cut. This point needs to be emphasized. Even though the differences between the two populations noted in Table 8–7 have statistical significance when the criteria of fever, adnexal mass or swelling, or elevated sedimentation rate are compared, they do not have clinical significance. For example, the majority of women with salpingitis do not have elevated temperatures or adnexal swellings or masses (see Table 8–7).[47] The elevated sedimentation rate seems helpful at first glance, except that it is nonspecific. It is also present in the majority of women with normal pelvic findings on laparoscopy. New diagnostic criteria are needed to reflect the clinical picture of women with salpingitis. Another reason for the modification of diagnostic criteria here is related to improved diagnostic and therapeutic techniques available to the practicing physician. Sensitive tests can be performed for the presence of human chorionic gonadotropin, while ultrasonography and laparoscopy have made it much easier to diagnose an ectopic pregnancy at an early stage. Many older requirements of prolonged observation in patients with pelvic pain by serial hematocrit are no longer necessary. In addition to these diagnostic advances, there

Table 8–7. The Classic Signs and Laboratory Findings of Salpingitis Observed in Women with a Laparoscopic Diagnosis of Salpingitis and Those with a Normal Pelvis

Classic Signs and Laboratory Findings	Salpingitis Patients (%)	Normal Patients (%)	Statistical Significance
1. Acute pelvic pain	94	94	No
2. Fever above 38°C	41.3	19.6	Yes
3. Tender adnexal swelling or mass	49.4	24.5	Yes
4. Elevated sedimentation rate	75.9	52.7	Yes

(From Jacobson, L., and Westrom, L.: Objectivized diagnosis of acute pelvic inflammatory disease. Am. J. Obstet. Gynecol., *105*:1088, 1969.)

is abundant evidence that early antibiotic therapy in women with pelvic infections will produce the best therapeutic results.[49]

There also have been tremendous changes in our understanding of the microbiologic invaders in acute salpingitis. These will alter our future antibiotic strategies. In the past decade, there have been delays in the evaluation of new antimicrobial regimens because of adherence to traditional theories on pathophysiology. The classic theory of salpingitis equated the early symptoms of the initial episode with the gonococcus, which presumably elicited tissue changes that permitted secondary invasion by other organisms, particularly anaerobes. This focus upon the gonococcus was the basis for the preoccupation with single antibiotic therapy of salpingitis in the 1972 Centers for Disease Control guidelines contained in the first edition of this book, employing either a penicillin or a standard tetracycline alone. Persistent attempts to match this single pathogen concept in the initiation of infection to the reality of the observed microbiologic studies of salpingitis utilizing laparoscopy and performed by Sweet and co-workers have failed.[48] These investigators made a number of significant microbiologic findings that have important implications for clinicians. The most relevant observation is that these infections are invariably multibacterial. In addition to *Neisseria gonorrhoeae,* the clinician has to consider other aerobes and anaerobes as well as *Chlamydia* and *Ureaplasma urealyticum.* Some of these data fit the classic theory. The isolation of *Neisseria gonorrhoeae* occurs most frequently during the first clinical episode and decreases in frequency in women who have had other episodes of salpingitis previously. Although this parallels traditional teaching, the clinician should be aware that in many women having their first episode of salpingitis, cultures will not be positive for *Neisseria gonorrhoeae.* The most striking variance between theory and microbiologic data has been found in the recent laparoscopic studies. The reiterated theory in most gynecologic texts that the gonococcus is the initial invader that prepares the pelvic organs for other secondary bacterial invaders has not been confirmed. In fact, contemporary studies show the highest recovery of other organisms when cultures were done within 24 hours of the onset of symptoms.[48] If the time interval was longer, fewer different species of organisms were recovered. These data highlight the multibacterial etiology of salpingitis and demonstrate the shortcomings of a single microbiologic focus such as gonococcal salpingitis.[49] This is important to remember, for there has been what I consider to be an inordinate emphasis on *Chlamydia* in the current Centers for Disease Control recommendations. While this family of organisms is important in salpingitis, I personally do not feel it should have any greater weight for the clinician than anaerobes. This does not negate *Chlamydia,* which does play an important role in the pathophysiology of salpingitis. Swedish investigators utilizing laparoscopy to obtain a fimbrial biopsy in women with a milder clinical form of the disease than is seen in the United States isolated the organism in 30% of the cases.[50] In the evaluation of women in the United States with more severe forms of salpingitis, this organism has rarely been recovered from fallopian tube secretions or peritoneal fluid. However, serum antibody response to *Chlamydia,* a fourfold or higher rise in titer, was noted in 20.3% of such women,[51] and the organism has been grown from endometrial biopsies in patients with salpingitis.[52] It is likely that *Chlamydia* is more frequently involved in the milder clinical cases of salpingitis, which can progress to tubal damage and pelvic adhesion formation.

One study from France demonstrated the recovery of this organism from pelvic adhesions.[53] All of these evaluations highlight the multibacterial nature of salpingitis.

There have been a number of observations made on the frequency and severity of salpingitis in sexually active women. The physician should be aware of these but should not attempt to apply these data as absolutes in individual patients. The mechanisms are not understood, and population trends may have no significance for the individual patient. Young women are at risk, for those under the age of 25 are more likely to have salpingitis[54] (Figure 8–2). Despite this increased frequency, the severity of the infection seems not as great, for the incidence of postinfection infertility is less in this group than in older women[54] (Table 8–8). The explanation for these differences is not clear. Some physicians have equated the increased frequency of infection in young women with early sexual experiences with multiple male sexual partners. This is a possibility, but the high rate of divorce in the United States in women over the age of 25 is frequently followed by a period of increased sexual activity with different male partners. Despite this, the marked difference in the attack rate by age persists.

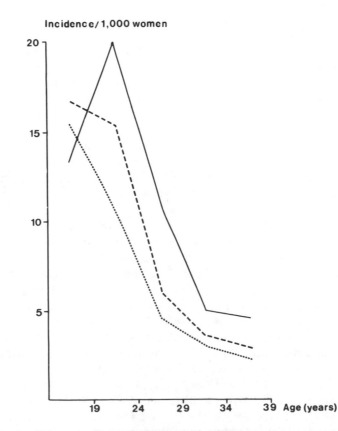

Fig. 8–2. Graph showing the higher incidence of salpingitis in younger women in a range from 19 to 39 years of age. (From Westrom, L.: Incidence, prevalence and trends of pelvic inflammatory disease and its consequences in industrialized countries. Am. J. Obstet. Gynecol., *138*:880, 1980.)

Table 8–8. Percentage of Women with Infertility Because of Tubal Occlusion after One, Two, Three or More Episodes of Salpingitis

No. of Infections	% Postsalpingitis Infertility in Age Groups		
	15–24 yr	25–39 yr	Total
1	9.4	19.2	11.4
2	20.9	31.0	23.1
3+	51.6	60.0	53.9

(From Westrom, L.: Incidence, prevalence and trends of pelvic inflammatory disease and its consequences in industralized countries. Am. J. Obstet. Gynecol., *138*:880, 1980.)

Another theory advanced is that anatomic changes in the cervix in young women make it less effective in preventing the upward spread of organisms.[55] There are also different incidences of salpingitis related to the type of contraception employed. Some methods of contraception are clearly protective. Those women using oral contraceptives[56] or a barrier form of contraception such as a diaphragm, foam, or jelly[57] or whose partners use a condom have a lower frequency of salpingitis than women not employing any protection. There is evidence that women using intrauterine devices may be more at risk for pelvic infection. There is a higher frequency of salpingitis when intrauterine devices are employed,[58] especially when the population is nulligravidas under the age of 25.[59] One recent study of infertile women with evidence of prior pelvic inflammatory disease showed a greater than expected prior use of intrauterine devices in this population.[60] In addition, there are special problems of pelvic infection seen in intrauterine device users. Although rare, infection with the group A beta-hemolytic *Streptococcus* has been associated with death in women employing this form of contraception.[61] There is also an association between intrauterine devices and pelvic infections caused by the gram-positive anaerobic bacillus *Actinomyces*.[62] Finally, unilateral tubo-ovarian abscesses are more common in patients who have chosen an intrauterine device as their method of contraception.[63] Despite the majority opinion that intrauterine devices increase the risk of infection, there are still many unresolved questions. There has been a heavy emphasis placed upon the presence of the tail of the device in the vagina as providing a conduit for bacteria to the upper genital tract.[64] At least one study showed no difference in the infection rate in the same population of women when a tailed device was compared with one entirely within the uterine cavity.[65] An alternative to the theory of the tail as a vehicle for bacteria to enter the upper genital tract has been provided by Toth and associates, who demonstrated the capability of spermatozoa to transport bacteria through a fluid medium.[66] In support of the importance of spermatozoa in carrying infectious bacteria, the highest frequency of pelvic infections has been noted in women who use no form of contraception or use an intrauterine device that does not block the ascent of spermatozoa, while the lowest rates have been in those using barrier methods and oral contraceptives that effectively block the upward passage of spermatozoa. In addition, there is a low rate of pelvic infections in the female partners of males with azospermia.[67] There are other questions as well. Although many physicians use the intrauterine device as a marker for more serious pelvic infections, there is no evidence that the severity of the infection—as measured by the fever index response to systemic antibiotics—was any different in women using other methods of contraception than the response in women employing this form of contraception

(Figure 8–3).[68] In addition to this observation, a method of contraception associated with an inordinately high rate of pelvic infection also would be expected to be associated with a high rate of infertility when the method is discontinued. The reported data have not been conclusive in this regard. Figure 8–4 shows a similar rate of subsequent fertility with intrauterine devices, as compared to oral and injectable contraceptives.[69] More data are needed to clarify this important point. All of the observations should be part of the physician's data base, either in the evaluation of patients suspected of having salpingitis or when reading claims in the literature on the diagnosis and treatment of salpingitis.

All of these population trends assume a role of secondary importance for the physician examining a patient with lower abdominal discomfort, for clinical decisions have to be made on the basis of findings in that one person. Although the diagnosis is difficult in many instances, there is no excuse for a strategy of

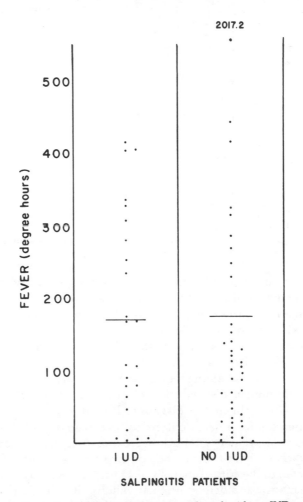

Fig. 8–3. The fever indices of patients with salpingitis with and without IUDs who were treated with antibiotics. The solid line represents the mean. There are no statistical differences between the two groups. (Reprinted with permission from the American College of Obstetricians and Gynecologists. From Ledger, W.J., Moore, D.E., Lowensohn, R.I., and Gee, C.L.: A fever index evaluation of chloramphenicol or clindamycin in patients with serious pelvic infections. Obstet. Gynecol., *50*:523, 1977.)

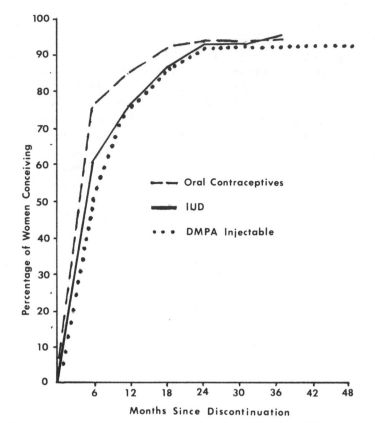

Fig. 8–4. The percentage of women conceiving after discontinuation of three methods of contraception; oral contraceptives, intrauterine devices, and Depo-Provera. Twenty-four months after the methods were stopped, the percentage of women who had conceived was exactly the same. (From Purdthaisong, T.: Return of fertility after use of the injectable contraceptive Depo Provera; updated data analysis. J. Biosocial Sci., *16*:23, 1984.)

observation and withholding of antibiotics to await the better delineation of signs and the results of laboratory tests. The evidence is clear that the earlier antibiotics are prescribed, the better the clinical results will be.[49] What is the best method of making the diagnosis in individual patients?

The diagnosis of salpingitis should be made more frequently than in the past, because the criteria are not as strict as those noted in Table 8–5. The physician should suspect tubal infection in every sexually active woman who presents with lower abdominal discomfort. Unfortunately, there are no clinical or laboratory findings that clinch the diagnosis. Recently, a group of American gynecologic investigators formulated criteria for the diagnosis of acute salpingitis in the vast majority of women who are not exposed to laparoscopy (Table 8–9).[70] I have reservations about these criteria on two counts. Academically, they have not been subjected to the critical analysis of a prospective study with laparoscopy to confirm the diagnosis and determine their validity. It is likely that some of the individual criteria of diagnosis have a heavier weight of significance than others. Clinically, I am concerned that rigid adherence to these criteria will mean that some women with salpingitis will not be diagnosed. Since the publication of the first edition of this book, I have seen many women in New York City with either tubal damage

Table 8–9.   Criteria for the Diagnosis of Acute Salpingitis (Without Laparoscopy)

A. Three of the following signs or symptoms must be present:
 1. Lower abdominal pain and tenderness, with or without rebound tenderness.
 2. Cervical motion tenderness
 3. Adnexal tenderness
B. In addition, one or more of the following conditions must be present:
 1. Fever equal to or greater than 38°C
 2. White blood cell count equal to or greater than 10,000/cu mm
 3. Inflammatory pelvic mass documented by clinical examination or sonogram or both
 4. Culdocentesis reveals white blood cells and bacteria on Gram stain of peritoneal fluid
 5. Gram-negative intracellular diplococci found on Gram stain of material from cervix

(Reprinted with permission from the American College of Obstetricians and Gynecologists. From Hager, W.D., Eschenbach, D.A., Spence, M.R., and Sweet, R.L.: Criteria for diagnosis and grading of salpingitis. Obstet. Gynecol., *61*:113, 1983.)

or pelvic adhesions who have no recollection of experiencing the clinical symptoms noted in Table 8–9.[70] This is particularly true for those patients with salpingitis in whom *Neisseria gonorrhoeae* is not recovered. The clinician should be suspicious that the patient may have salpingitis if she has symptoms of menorrhagia, dysuria, or dyspareunia. One recent study underscored this point. In a laparoscopic evaluation of women with infertility, 80 patients were found to have a hydrosalpinx.[71] Of these 80 women, only 20 (25%) could recall a previous episode of acute pelvic pain. It is not known how many women with these symptoms have no evidence of salpingitis. The important thing is that the utilization of these criteria (see Table 8–9)[70] will yield a clinical diagnosis of salpingitis more often than dependence upon the classic criteria (see Table 8–5).

In many patients who are suspected of having salpingitis, whether according to the criteria listed in Table 8–9 or because they have menorrhagia, dysuria, or dyspareunia, there are two diagnostic tests that are especially helpful. The first is needle culdocentesis, and it is noted as one of the additional criteria in Table 8–9. This has been an extremely valuable diagnostic test for me, particularly in the evaluation of the afebrile patient with pelvic pain. To be of most value, the test should be done properly, with the patient positioned with the head elevated a few degrees to utilize gravity in order to keep peritoneal fluid in the cul-de-sac for aspiration. A careful pelvic examination should be performed before the aspiration to be sure the cul-de-sac is free. If fluid is obtained, it should be examined with the Gram stain for the presence of bacteria. Bacteria are normally not present in peritoneal fluid. The clinician must be aware that bacteria are not specific for salpingitis, for they are also present in patients with appendicitis, but the clinical history should distinguish these patients. In addition, the peritoneal fluid can be examined for isoamylases, which are specific for the fallopian tube.[72] Although a positive needle culdocentesis for bacteria is usually specific, the absence of peritoneal fluid does not rule out the possibility of salpingitis for adhesions, or a misplaced needle can yield a "dry tap." The advantage of needle culdocentesis is that a positive test denotes infection. In addition to the culdocentesis, Westrom has recommended the use of microscopic examination of a wet mount of vaginal secretions.[73] There are many advantages to this test. It is simple to perform, and the patient has none of the discomfort associated with needle culdocentesis. In addition, it is confirmatory when positive. Westrom has stated he had never seen a patient with salpingitis found on laparoscopy who has not had inflammatory cells present on microscopic examination of vaginal secretions.

This is another confirmatory test that is not invasive and is particularly helpful in the febrile patient with pelvic pain.

The role of laparoscopy in the diagnosis of salpingitis has not been established as yet. Studies in Sweden have shown the feasibility of laparoscopy in every patient admitted with a diagnosis of acute salpingitis and have also demonstrated a high percentage of women (35%) in whom the admission diagnosis was incorrect.[47] In the United States, there has not been acceptance of routine laparoscopy in patients suspected of having salpingitis.[74] There are a number of reasons for this. The majority of these women are not admitted to the hospital, there are not sufficient operating room facilities to provide this service, and there is a risk, albeit minimal, with laparoscopy. Because of this, American physicians have been more selective with laparoscopy. I believe laparoscopy should be performed in women in whom the diagnosis of salpingitis is in doubt, particularly in the patient who has had repeated courses of antibiotics for pelvic pain. Some of these women will have other pelvic disease such as endometriosis, or have extensive pelvic adhesions. Both of these conditions are not helped by antibiotic therapy. Hormones may be indicated for the first, while operative intervention may be needed for the relief of the discomfort associated with both conditions. This limited use of laparoscopy can change. If increasing numbers of women are admitted to the hospital for the care of salpingitis, a higher number will probably undergo laparoscopy, particularly if it can be demonstrated that this increases the likelihood of more successful therapy in the long run.

There are a number of laboratory studies that should be obtained in women suspected of having salpingitis before treatment is begun. From a microbiologic point of view, aerobic endocervical cultures should be done for *Neisseria gonorrhoeae* and the group A beta-hemolytic streptococci as well as for *Ureaplasma urealyticum* if the latter culture is available. The swab should be kept in place in the endocervical canal for at least 15 seconds. The recovery of either *Neisseria gonorrhoeae* or *Chlamydia* will dictate treatment of the male sexual partner as well. In addition, a culture for test of cure will be necessary. If the culture is positive for *Neisseria gonorrhoeae,* the patient should have both a rectal and an endocervical sample cultured seven days after the completion of therapy, for this will pick up one third of the treatment failures not obvious on endocervical culture alone.[75] If peritoneal fluid is obtained by needle culdocentesis, a portion should be sent for culture for *Neisseria gonorrhoeae,* aerobes and anaerobes, plus *Ureaplasma urealyticum* if possible. I believe culdocentesis fluid cultures are indicated because they are the only samples available from near the site of infection—the fallopian tube—even though there is poor correlation between the bacteria isolated from peritoneal fluid and fluid aspirated from the fallopian tube.[76] Since there has been the rare isolation of *Chlamydia* from peritoneal fluid,[76] the best sample for the isolation of *Chlamydia* from the genital tract of women with salpingitis seems to be an endometrial biopsy after careful cleaning of the endocervix.[52] In addition to these microbiologic studies, a number of other studies should be done. These include a complete blood count and a sedimentation rate, for these can help in providing other criteria for the diagnosis (see Table 8–9).[70] All these patients should have a serologic test for syphilis performed as well. If the test is negative and they receive an antibiotic regimen for salpingitis that includes either a penicillin, a cephalosporin, or a tetracycline, they probably have had adequate therapy for incubating syphilis. If the serologic test is positive, they will need an FTA-ABS test performed, and if this is positive, they should receive therapy for syphilis, depending upon whether it was acquired less than or more than a year previously (see Table 8–5).[20]

It is impossible to indicate the best antibiotic strategy in patients with acute salpingitis, for the critical studies on the impact of therapy have not been done. The clinician should have two goals when antibiotics are prescribed. The immediate aim is the relief of symptoms. This is easy to measure: the patient should either become afebrile or remain afebrile, with rapid resolution of both pelvic and abdominal pain. There are a great many data available on this immediate response, and valid judgments on antibiotic selection can be made on this basis. However, the most important measure for the patient and the physician is the status of the pelvis after therapy. Clinicians recognize that a certain portion of women will have blocked tubes or pelvic adhesions or both that will prevent pregnancy after what seems to be successful antibiotic treatment for acute salpingitis. Westrom has recently documented this (see Table 8–8).[54] The reader should also be aware that none of the treatment regimens recommended by the Centers for Disease Control provide information on this crucial point. In addition, the physician should recognize that seemingly logical conclusions from microbiologic data or from the patient's initial response to therapy may not be correct. There are a number of examples of misguided logic in the past, but this is best illustrated by a study by Falk published in 1966.[77] His prestudy hypothesis was that if blocked tubes or adhesion formation represented an inflammatory response to pelvic infection, then the use of an anti-inflammatory agent (adrenocortical steroids) in pharmacologic doses might be beneficial. The immediate clinical response in the patients treated with steroids and antibiotics was better than in the patients treated with antibiotics alone. Patients with a fever became afebrile more quickly, those with adnexal swelling had this disappear more rapidly, women with abdominal pain had this resolve sooner, and those without an appetite had this return more quickly. If the study had been terminated at the end of this initial evaluation, steroids would now be routinely employed in patients admitted to the hospital for the treatment of salpingitis. Fortunately, this Swedish investigator followed this initial course of therapy with laparoscopy three to four months later. The results were both interesting and surprising. The frequency of blocked tubes and adhesion formation was the same in both groups of women. Because of these important observations, steroids are not indicated for the therapy of acute salpingitis, for they do not improve long-term results. In addition to laparoscopy, there is another way to evaluate treatment. This involves the long-term documentation of the fertility of women treated for salpingitis. Until follow-up studies are done, either by laparoscopy or assessment of subsequent fertility, any judgment of the best treatment of salpingitis remains conjecture, not fact.

There are other observations that will help to guide the therapy of patients with acute salpingitis. There is a big difference in the prognosis of therapy in an early versus a well-established infection. In one study, patients were defined as having early infections if they had symptoms for less than five days and had no masses on pelvic examination, while those with well-established infections had a history of five or more days of symptoms or a finding of a pelvic mass or both.[49] Those patients with well-established infections were more likely to fail to respond to systemic antibiotics and more frequently required operative care for the pelvic abscesses. Similar observations by Monif have been the basis for his clinical classification of salpingitis.[78] In addition, there is good evidence that different approaches to therapy will give better initial responses of the patient to antibiotic therapy. Table 8–10[49] details an improved initial response of patients with acute salpingitis to the second and third generation cephalosporins when compared with the 1972 Centers for Disease Control recommendations of treatment with either a penicillin or a tetracycline alone. Whether these superior initial results will be accompanied by better future pelvic health and more subsequent pregnancies is not known at this time, since these newer cephalosporins do not provide antimicrobial coverage of *Chlamydia*.

The criteria for admitting patients to the hospital for the treatment of salpingitis are in a state of flux at present. Admission to the hospital implies the use of parenteral antibiotics reaching higher serum and tissue levels than would be achieved with most oral antibiotics. Theoretically, this should improve the chances for a clinical cure. However, whether this strategy improves the long-term prognosis for pregnancy is not known, for the studies needed to establish this point have not been done. In addition, our hospital care system, particularly in urban areas, does not have the bed capacity to handle this added influx of patients. In an attempt to provide a scientific rationale for the admission of a limited number of patients to the hospital, Table 8–11 [20,79] lists old and new criteria for the admission of the patient to the hospital. Although they are helpful, there are objections to the guidelines. No prospective study has been done to see if adherence to these criteria identifies a group of women who would benefit the most from hospitalization. Two of the criteria in some of the older recommendations were particularly bothersome. First, the emphasis upon a temperature above 38°C as a criterion for admission, despite the rationale that this identified more seriously ill patients. If salpingitis is classified as either gonococcal or nongonococcal, those patients with oral temperatures above 38°C are more likely to have gonococcal salpingitis. Women with gonococcal salpingitis and no masses have a better initial response to antibiotics and a lower incidence of post-treatment tubal obstruction than those with nongonococcal salpingitis.[80] In effect, this criterion identifies a low risk population for admission and treatment with parenteral antibiotics, whereas the higher risk afebrile population is more likely to be treated as outpatients. This makes no therapeutic sense. Second, I am not certain that a woman with an intrauterine device in place requires hospital admission for parenteral

Table 8–10. Comparison of Traditional Antibiotic Regimens and Second and Third Generation Cephalosporins in the Treatment of Women with Salpingitis Seen Early in the Course of Infection*

Antibiotic Regimen	No. Patients	No. (%) Cured	Alternative Therapy	
			Antibiotics	Surgical Intervention
Traditional	640	537 (83.9%)	Not stated	Not stated
Second and third generation cephalosporins	85	82 (96.5%)	2 (2.4%)	1 (1.2%)

*Differences between the two groups were statistically significant in terms of cure (X^2 with Yates correction = 7.9; $p < 0.01$). (From Ledger, W.J.: Selection of antimicrobial agents for treatment of infections of the female genital tract. Rev. Infect. Dis., 5:598, 1983.)

Table 8–11. Criteria for Admission of Patients to the Hospital for Treatment of Salpingitis

Old	New (1982)	Comments
1. The diagnosis is uncertain	1. The diagnosis is uncertain	1. Remains the same
2. None	2. Surgical emergencies such as appendicitis and ectopic pregnancy must be excluded	2. New
3. A pelvic abscess is suspected	3. A pelvic abscess is suspected	3. Remains the same
4. Upper peritoneal signs	4. Severe illness precludes outpatient management	4. Modified
5. The patient is pregnant	5. The patient is pregnant	5. Remains the same
6. Nausea and vomiting preclude oral antibiotics	6. The patient is unable to follow or tolerate an outpatient regimen	6. Modified
7. Failure to respond to oral antibiotics within 48 hours	7. Patient has failed to respond to outpatient therapy	7. Modified
8. None	8. Clinical followup after 48–72 hours of antibiotic therapy cannot be arranged	8. New
9. Temperature 38°C or higher	9.	9. Dropped
10. Presence of an IUCD	10.	10. Dropped

antibiotic therapy. The data portrayed in Figure 8–3 give no hint that the immediate prognosis is any more serious in a woman with an intrauterine device in place.[68] I am encouraged that both of these criteria were absent in the latest recommendations from the CDC.[20] Although the studies have not been done, I would prefer to admit as many patients as possible to the hospital to give them what I consider optimal therapy in the form of parenteral antibiotics.

With this background, no physician should care for women with salpingitis without awareness of the Centers for Disease Control recommendations. These are listed in Table 8–12.[20] Of necessity, these should be the framework for any planned antibiotic strategy.

There are objections to these recommendations that will remain until clinical trials with long-term followup have been performed. All the regimens represent an attempt to provide antibacterial coverage of the more commonly isolated organisms, including *Neisseria gonorrhoeae, Chlamydia, Ureaplasma urealyticum,* and aerobes and anaerobes in the multibacterial infection of salpingitis. All have shortcomings, and my major objection is that some of the regimens have focused their antibacterial activity on *Neisseria gonorrhoeae* and *Chlamydia* while not providing the best agents against gram-negative aerobes and all anaerobes. Since it is important for the prescribing physician to be aware of the shortcomings of every regimen, each one will be discussed in detail.

The first inpatient CDC regimen in Table 8–12, doxycycline and cefoxitin, provides optimal coverage for the patient with an infection caused by *Neisseria gonorrhoeae,* including penicillinase-producing strains, and *Chlamydia trachomatis.* It does not provide the best coverage for gram-negative anaerobes based upon antibacterial susceptibility studies done by Tally and associates.[81] The second regimen for hospitalized patients, clindamycin plus either gentamicin or tobramycin, provides the broadest spectrum of activity against anaerobes and facultative gram-negative rods. However, it is not the best treatment for *Chlamydia trachomatis* and *Neisseria gonorrhoeae,* and this combination is also not effective against many strains

Table 8–12. Antibiotic Treatment for Salpingitis

Recommended Inpatient Therapy

1. Doxycycline 100 mg IV twice a day, plus cefoxitin 2.0 g IV four times a day. Continue the intravenous antibiotics for at least four days and at least 40 hours after the patient defervesces. Continue doxycycline 100 mg by mouth twice a day after discharge from the hospital to complete 10–14 days of therapy.
2. Clindamycin 600 mg IV four times a day plus gentamicin or tobramycin 3.0 mg/kg IV followed by 1.5 mg/kg IV three times a day in patients with normal renal function. Continue IV drugs at least four days and at least 48 hours after the patient defervesces. Continue clindamycin 450 mg by mouth four times a day after discharge from the hospital to complete 10–14 days of therapy.
3. Doxycycline 100 mg IV twice a day plus metronidazole 1.0 g IV twice a day. Continue IV drugs for at least four days and at least 48 hours after patient defervesces. Then continue both drugs at same dosage orally to complete 10–14 days of therapy.

Recommended Ambulatory Treatment

Cefoxitin 2.0 g IM or amoxicillin 3.0 g by mouth, or ampicillin 3.5 g by mouth, or aqueous procaine penicillin G 4.8 million U IM at two sites, each along with probenecid 1.0 g by mouth, followed by doxycycline 100 mg twice a day for 10–14 days. Tetracycline hydrochloride 500 mg by mouth four times a day can also be used but is less active against certain anaerobes and requires more frequent dosing, both drawbacks in the treatment of salpingitis.

of enterococci. The third inpatient antibiotic combination of doxycycline and metronidazole provides the best antibiotic treatment for both gram-negative anaerobes and *Chlamydia trachomatis*. It is not optimal therapy for gram-positive anaerobes and gram-negative aerobes, and it is a poor choice for the patient with an infection caused by penicillinase-producing *Neisseria gonorrhoeae,* the coagulase-positive staphylococci, or the group A beta-hemolytic streptococci.

The suggested outpatient treatment regimens are also not comprehensive. The single-dose therapy of cefoxitin has not been tested for effectiveness in women with salpingitis in which penicillinase-producing *Neisseria gonorrhoeae* is involved, and all the penicillin alternatives are ineffective against this strain, which is being isolated with greater frequency, particularly in urban centers. This single-dose therapy combined with doxycycline provides less than optimal treatment of infections caused by gram-positive pathogens such as the coagulase-positive staphylococci, the group A beta-hemolytic streptococci, all gram-negative aerobes, and both gram-positive and gram-negative anaerobes. The physician should be aware of these gaps in microbiologic coverage when ordering the initial antibiotic regimen in women with acute salpingitis so that appropriate antibiotics can be added if the patient fails to respond to the initial choice. Patients with a pelvic mass who are suspected of having a pelvic abscess are a high-risk population. They should receive the best anaerobic coverage, which I believe is provided by a regimen utilizing either clindamycin or metronidazole. It is not known whether second or third generation cephalosporins or the newer penicillins such as piperacillin or mezlocillin will provide equivalent clinical results, because their coverage of *Bacteroides fragilis* in the laboratory is not as complete as that of clindamycin and metronidazole.[81] In addition to the anaerobic coverage provided by clindamycin and metronidazole plus an aminoglycoside—either gentamicin or tobramycin—some physicians will also add penicillin G or ampicillin to broaden the antibacterial spectrum to include the enterococci. Although widely used, there is no evidence that this triple coverage is any more effective in achieving a medical cure in patients with a pelvic mass when therapy is begun than treatment with two antibiotics. Heparin has theoretical appeal in the medical treatment of women because of its demonstrated effectiveness in releasing more active free antibiotic in the presence of pus.[82] However, this laboratory phenomenon has never been examined in prospective clinical studies to determine if it would be more effective.

The role of the concomitant treatment of the male sexual partner of these women has not yet been clearly established. Treatment of the male is clearly indicated when the woman has positive cultures for either *Neisseria gonorrhoeae* or *Chlamydia*. The male has not been routinely treated in the past when there are other microbiologic causes of nongonococcal salpingitis in the woman. The observations of Toth and co-workers on the role of spermatozoa as a vehicle for the transport of bacteria to the upper genital tract may modify this pattern of no treatment for the male.[66]

OPERATIVE THERAPY FOR SALPINGITIS

There has been a continuous evolution in the philosophy of operative therapy for patients with salpingitis. A number of factors have influenced changes in present operative care of these women. Laparoscopy, with its attendant minimal postoperative morbidity, has made it much easier to visualize the pelvis of a patient with an uncertain diagnosis who has acute or recurrent pelvic pain. Better understanding of the role of anaerobes in pelvic abscess formation has altered antibiotic strategies so that fewer patients need extirpative care for this problem. Further, the operation for pelvic infection now involves less extensive removal of tissue. This is due in part to the awareness that less extensive surgery, such as drainage of a pelvic abscess[83] and supracervical hysterectomy[84] instead of a mandatory total abdominal hysterectomy[85] and unilateral removal of the adnexa in patients with unilateral tubo-ovarian abscesses,[63] has been followed by a low incidence of postoperative complications. Finally, the development of in vitro fertilization has meant that future pregnancy is still possible for women with damaged tubes that are not amenable to operative care. Automatic removal of uterus, tubes, and ovaries in every woman with blocked tubes and pelvic pain is no longer acceptable surgical therapy. Any discussion of operative care must proceed logically from the point of accepted standard care, with the understanding that there is still much disagreement in our literature on some of the indications for surgery.

The patient with a ruptured tubo-ovarian Abscess is seriously ill and requires operative intervention. The diagnosis of this uncommon condition is important, for the longer the interval between the apparent rupture and the exploration, the greater the possibility of serious postoperative morbidity and death.[86] A ruptured tubo-ovarian abscess should be suspected in patients who, in addition to the usual lower abdominal findings, have point tenderness and rebound tenderness in the upper abdomen and a pulse rate that is more rapid than would be expected from the temperature. In women with these physical findings, a rapid confirmatory diagnostic test is needle culdocentesis of the posterior cul-de-sac, which invariably yields a free flow of purulent material. An exploratory laparotomy should be performed in these women, and I believe a vertical abdominal skin incision should be done for adequate exploration of the intra-abdominal cavity. If a ruptured tubo-ovarian abscess is found, individual operative judgment will dictate the extent of surgery. Older studies stressed the necessity for the removal of tubes, ovaries, and a total hysterectomy with no intraperitoneal drainage performed.[85]

However, recent reports have indicated that alternative treatments, either a supracervical hysterectomy[84] or no hysterectomy at all,[87] are associated with results equivalent to those with complete extirpation. In the presence of a ruptured tubo-ovarian abscess, the surgeon should meticulously remove all the intraperitoneal purulent material by direct aspiration and lavage. Since the inflamed peritoneum is an efficient surface for absorption of substances that reach the intravascular space,[88] the lavage solution should contain potassium rather than normal saline alone, for massive volume lavage with normal saline has been known to result in postoperative hypokalemia. I advocate short-term postoperative use of intraperitoneal drains in these grossly contaminated cases. The pelvic peritoneum can be drained through the vagina, with the drain removed within 48 hours of the operation. The abdominal wound requires meticulous preventive care to avoid serious infection or dehiscence or evisceration or both. I favor Smead-Jones closure of the peritoneum and fascia together with monofilament nylon (Figure 8–5),[89] with secondary closure of the skin three to four days postoperatively. These patients are usually very ill in the postoperative period and require large volumes of intravenous fluids with monitoring by central intravascular lines, and they should receive a combination of antibiotics effective against gram-negative aerobes and anaerobes. I use clindamycin and an aminoglycoside in this situation, but metronidazole in combination with other antibiotics is an alternative, as are the newer cephalosporins and penicillins.

There is more unanimity of feeling in management of the other extreme of this syndrome, acute salpingitis without abscess formation. If a laparoscopy has been performed for an uncertain diagnosis or a laparotomy done for suspected appendicitis and acute salpingitis is found, no extirpative therapy is needed. It is very important to make this point to general surgeons, who face this situation on occasion when an exploration for acute appendicitis reveals acute salpingitis. Too often there is a tendency to believe that extirpation is necessary in the face of acute pelvic inflammation with purulent material exuding from the fimbria, but this is not the case. These patients should be treated with systemic antibiotics.

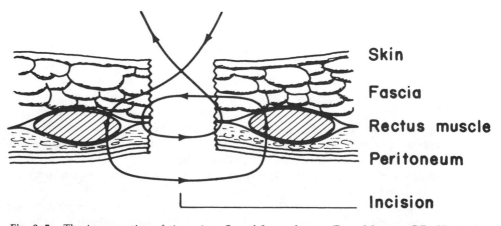

Fig. 8–5. The incorporation of tissue in a Smead-Jones closure. (From Morrow, C.P., Hernandez, W.L., Townsend, D.E., and Di Saia, P.J.: Pelvic celiotomy in the obese patient. Am. J. Obstet. Gynecol., *127*:335, 1977.)

Controversy exists about the care of some pelvic abscesses. Formerly, I favored laparotomy in all these women to avoid subsequent operations, but I have modified this stand. If a patient has a pelvic abscess that is accessible to extraperitoneal drainage through the vagina, this should be performed. Most initially respond quickly to this treatment; 14 of 38 (36.8%) required a subsequent laparotomy for failure of response or persistent pelvic pain, and 10% subsequently had an intrauterine pregnancy.[83] Rivlin found that 5 out of 40 (12%) of the potentially fertile women became pregnant.[90] Despite my new enthusiasm for colpotomy, I agree with Mickal and Sellman that fewer of these procedures are being performed now than 10 to 15 years ago.[91] I believe this is largely because of an increased awareness of the frequent involvement of gram-negative anaerobic bacteria in pelvic abscess formation and the earlier use of antibiotics that are effective against these organisms. The diagnosis of pelvic abscess, best treated by colpotomy drainage, should be made when a bulging cul-de-sac mass is found that extends beyond the external os of the cervix into the vagina. These patients should be taken to the operating room for reevaluation under general anesthesia. A needle should be inserted into the mass and an attempt made to determine the content by aspiration. If purulent material is obtained, a scalpel should be used to incise the abscess wall and blunt dissection done to complete the drainage. The patients should be treated with antibiotics effective against gram-negative aerobes and anaerobes. Usually, this procedure is curative. However, there are occasional therapeutic failures. Figure 8–6 documents the course of a patient with a pelvic abscess that was drained through a colpotomy incision at arrow 1, and *Bacteroides fragilis,* susceptible to both chloramphenicol and clindamycin in the laboratory, was cultured from a specimen of the content of the abscess.[92] When the patient remained febrile, subtotal hysterectomy and bilateral salpingo-oophorectomy were performed at arrow 2. Intact tubo-ovarian abscesses were present, and *Bacteroides fragilis,* which again was susceptible to chloramphenicol and clindamycin in the laboratory, was grown from samples of the abscesses.

The most controversial consideration in the operative care of women with salpingo-oophoritis and unruptured tubo-ovarian abscesses is the timing of laparotomy and intraoperative strategies. There have been wide swings in operative strategies that reflect changes in medical knowledge and therapy. The traditional gynecologic approach was to avoid acute-phase operation. This decision was based on sound clinical observations from the preantibiotic era. In 1909, Simpson reported a drop in operative mortality from 20% to less than 1% by avoiding operation in the acute phase and by delaying operation until the patient remained afebrile for at least three weeks with repeated pelvic examinations.[93] This policy was successfully followed by other urban gynecologic services. In 1927, Miller reported a 4.2% mortality rate in patients undergoing acute-phase operation compared with less than 1% in those who had no clinical evidence of acute infection.[94] It is likely that the mortality following acute-phase operation in these preantibiotic era studies resulted from operative intervention in patients with an active group A beta-hemolytic streptococcal infection.

Despite good results with the conservative approach, physicians became disenchanted with it when antibiotics became available, for a number of reasons. The process of waiting for the resolution of an acute inflammatory process sometimes involved weeks or even months of hospitalization for the patient. Antibiotics

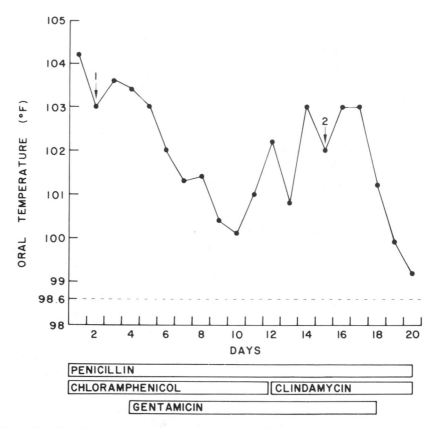

Fig. 8–6. The clinical course of treatment of a patient with a pelvic abscess. See text for details. (From Ledger, W.J.: Anaerobic infections. Am. J. Obstet. Gynecol., *123*:111, 1975.)

shortened the patient's hospital stay, but the problem of a recurrent infection remained before the scheduled admission to the hospital. A great impetus for a new aggressive operative approach was provided by Anderson and Bucklew in 1962.[95] They reported seven women in whom intraperitoneal rupture of tubo-ovarian abscess occurred while they were undergoing antibiotic therapy as in-patients. They suggested that there might be a place for an acute-phase operation to avoid this dreaded complication, and their results were good. This use of the acute-phase operation was expanded by Kaplan and associates.[96] They justified their aggressive surgical intervention in patients who showed only partial or no response to systemic antibiotics after 48 hours of hospitalization on the basis of the high percentage of these women who eventually required surgery. Their results were impressive, with few demonstrable serious postoperative complications. My own experience has been similar, for acute-phase operation with appropriate antibiotic coverage can be performed with little serious postoperative morbidity[97] (Figure 8–7).

Although acute-phase operation can be performed safely, it is less frequently necessary at present. This is probably related to awareness of the importance of gram-negative anaerobic bacteria in pelvic abscess formation and the more frequent early use of antibiotics such as clindamycin, metronidazole, chloramphenicol, carbenicillin, ticarcillin, pipercillin, mezlocillin, and cefoxitin, which are

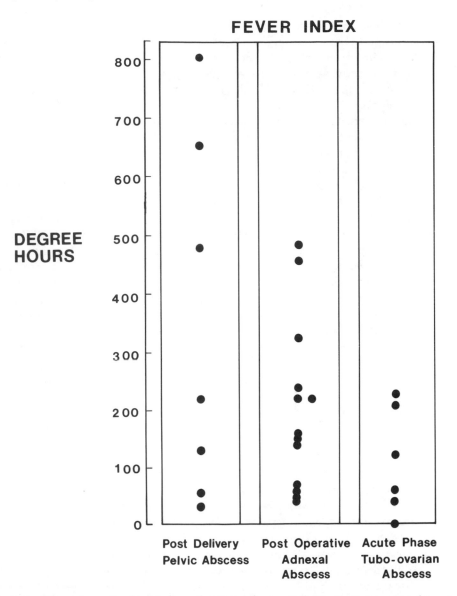

FEVER INDEX

Post Delivery Pelvic Abscess

Post Operative Adnexal Abscess

Acute Phase Tubo-ovarian Abscess

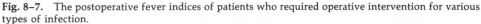

Fig. 8–7. The postoperative fever indices of patients who required operative intervention for various types of infection.

effective against gram-negative anaerobes. I had a similar experience to that of Anderson and Bucklew[95] in the early 1960s, when inpatients would rupture a tubo-ovarian abscess after five or more days of inpatient therapy with penicillin G and an aminoglycoside. I have not seen this occur when antibiotics effective against *Bacteroides fragilis* were used from the start of therapy. In addition to this, most patients with salpingitis respond to systemic antibiotics. Less than 5% of women with salpingitis seen early in the course of the infection required operative therapy for failure of response. In patients with well-established pelvic infections and with an indurated pelvic mass, many still respond to antibiotics alone. My experience with this group indicates that close to 50% eventually require operative intervention.[49] There are widely reported ranges of clinical response. Franklin and colleagues found surgery necessary in only 25%,[98] and even lower figures have been cited in the clinical experience of many infectious disease experts.[99] In contrast, a study by Hager from 1970 to 1974 demonstrated operative care needed in 90% of such patients.[100] In this study, antibiotics most effective against *Bacteroides fragilis* were not employed, and this may account for the difference. In my own past experience, the women needing operative intervention are usually older, for those patients needing operative therapy had a mean age of 34 years as compared with 24 years for all those admitted to the hospital with salpingo-oophoritis.[84] The few patients who do not respond to systemic antibiotics tolerate the operative procedure without mortality when covered with appropriate antibiotics but frequently have a complicated postoperative course and are quite ill. Appropriate time limits (72 hours or more) for antibiotic therapy should be allowed for observation, but the patient should be administered systemic antibiotics effective against gram-negative aerobes and anaerobes, and supplemental care includes hyperalimentation.[101] My own decision to perform an acute-phase laparotomy is based upon the lack of clinical response in the patient with persistent fever and not on the presence of a pelvic mass. Pelvic masses that are complexes can be observed by clinical and ultrasonographic examination and frequently disappear over a period of weeks with resolution of the infection. In patients with persistent fever and no masses, a trial of heparin to rule out septic thrombophlebitis is indicated as well as a trial without antibiotics to ensure that the patient does not have a drug fever. In one recent evaluation of 12 patients with drug-induced fever without antibiotics, fever disappeared in a median time of 26 hours.[102] Thus, these clinical determinations of response can be made in 24 to 28 hours. In postmenopausal women with tubo-ovarian abscesses, the incidence of gynecologic and gastrointestinal malignancy is high.[103] A thorough workup to rule out this possibility is needed.

Another unresolved question is the extent of the surgical removal of adnexal tissue. Since most patients with upper genital tract infections have bilateral abscesses, the decision at the time of operation for bilateral removal is easy. There are exceptions. Many patients have unilateral inflammatory disease, and they tolerate unilateral salpingo-oophorectomy without short-term or long-term complications.[63] In an attempt to delineate pathologic adnexa, Weiner and Wallach tried to correlate abnormal uterine bleeding in women with pelvic inflammatory disease and the finding of abnormal ovaries.[104] This clinical correlation with pathologic findings suggests that unilateral adnexal operations can be performed without placing the patient at excessive risk for subsequent operations. This decision must be made with the realization that rarely, in 5% or fewer cases, reoperations will be necessary because of unrecognized ovarian involvement.

There are exciting new operative strategies in patients with salpingitis who have either persistent pelvic pain or infertility. These involve surgical procedures in which pelvic organs are not removed. Laparoscopy is the first step in the workup. I do not always follow this with a same-day laparotomy, for I believe that the patient should have a full disclosure of the findings and then make a decision about subsequent surgical needs. This means administration of two anesthetics, but I believe that patients are best served by an opportunity for discussion about planned operative procedures. In these patients, I usually discover pelvic adhesions and occasionally a hydrosalpinx with no fimbria present. At laparotomy for the second operative procedure, the adhesions are lysed with electrocautery and heparin solution irrigation is used. Following the completion of the operation, high molecular weight dextran is placed in the pelvis prior to closure. There is good experimental and clinical evidence that this diminishes subsequent adhesion formation.[105, 106] However, dextran does support the growth of bacteria and should not be employed in a patient with an active infection. If the fimbria are absent and a hydrosalpinx is present, a fimbrioplasty can be performed. The results of relief of pelvic pain and successful subsequent pregnancy have been gratifying. These adhesions are filmy, not the thick ones seen in the past when antibiotic therapy was not specifically directed against gram-negative anaerobes. If it can be demonstrated that *Chlamydia* are frequently recovered from these adhesions, it is possible that tetracycline will be used in these patients both intra- and postoperatively.

PELVIC THROMBOPHLEBITIS

Infrequently, a severe inflammatory disease may be associated with septic thrombophlebitis. In an old review of this condition, before the significance of anaerobes was recognized by Collins and coworkers, 3 of the 70 patients had pelvic inflammatory disease.[107] The relationship of pelvic infections caused by anaerobic organisms to septic pelvic thrombophlebitis had been noted. However, when antibiotics effective against anaerobes are used, the requirement for specific therapy for this condition is rare. The diagnosis should be suspected in the patient who remains febrile despite good anaerobic bacterial antibiotic coverage and who has no evidence of a pelvic abscess on examination. This combination is rare, and usually an abscess is found during exploratory laparotomy. In such patients, I make no attempt to explore the ovarian veins or inferior vena cava to place ligatures. In addition, I have not routinely used anticoagulation following operation, but this should be a consideration for future studies. The surgical removal of the site of infection and the appropriate antibiotic coverage usually suffice for cure.

NONSEXUALLY ACQUIRED PELVIC INFECTIONS

Pelvic Tuberculosis

One of the great medical deceivers is pelvic tuberculosis, which can appear in varied forms. It is a disease with highly variable levels of risk that seem to be dependent on the socioeconomic status of the patient. Most private practitioners will never see a case during their professional careers, and only an occasional patient will be seen on large gynecologic units serving the urban poor. In contrast, a third world country may have a significant percentage of women with pelvic tuberculosis seeking gynecologic care. This disease should be part of the differential diagnosis of women of childbearing age who have unexplained infertility, abnormal uterine bleeding, or persistent adnexal masses and an atypical history and response to chemotherapeutic agents when pelvic inflammatory disease has been diagnosed. In the United States, this disease is most frequently encountered in foreign-born women,[108] and it is on the rise as the result of the great influx of southeast Asian and Caribbean refugees. Although it usually is blood-borne, with the pulmonary tract being the primary site of infection, the diagnostic tests do not fit an expected sequence. These patients usually have a positive reaction to the tuberculin skin test, but less than 50% have a chest roentgenogram showing gross lesions compatible with tuberculosis, for host defense mechanisms have limited the progression of the disease in the lungs.[109] The diagnosis of tuberculosis is usually not suspected by the clinician and becomes apparent with the discovery of granulomas and giant cells in biopsy specimens of endometrium or sections of tubes removed for pelvic inflammatory disease, or by the gross appearance of tubes studded with tubercles at laparotomy. When microscopic or gross findings are present, confirmation of the diagnosis is ultimately based on microscopic testing. Late secretory or menstrual endometrial samples or operative samples can be cultured on artificial media or by guinea pig inoculation for the presence of tubercle bacilli.

The most remarkable changes in gynecologic care of pelvic inflammatory disease have been related to the availability of chemotherapeutic agents for pelvic tuberculosis. Prior to this, the diagnosis of pelvic tuberculosis was equated with 100% infertility, with cure accomplished only by surgical extirpation of the pelvic organs. The introduction of effective systemic chemotherapeutic agents has meant that the majority of patients with this disease can be treated successfully with systemic agents, and operation can be reserved for those who remain culture-positive for bacilli or who have persistent pelvic masses. Of great interest is the observation that successfully treated women occasionally become pregnant. Pregnancies are rare, and the pregnancy wastage, that is, abortion and ectopic pregnancy rates, is high, but a few viable infants have been delivered following successful chemotherapy. Since patients with pelvic tuberculosis are infrequently seen by the obstetrician-gynecologist, consultation with the infectious disease service is indicated because the treatment requires the use of such unfamiliar drugs as rifampin, ethambutol, and isoniazid. It is important to know that treatment is not casual once this condition is diagnosed, and women with this disease often receive a combination of chemotherapeutic agents for a minimum of one year.

MANIFESTATIONS OF INFECTIONS IN OTHER SYSTEMS

Neisseria Gonorrhoeae Infections

Pharyngeal Gonorrhea. Pharyngeal gonorrhea is seen with some frequency in female patients and is related to the practice of fellatio. It is so common that some urban clinics obtain results of a pharyngeal culture as a test of cure in patients who previously have had positive results of endocervical culture for gonorrhea. This procedure may have great clinical significance in some populations, for pharyngeal gonococcal infections are more difficult to eliminate than anogenital gonorrhea because the ampicillin and amoxicillin regimens are ineffective.[20] For patients who do not respond to aqueous penicillin G, a tetracycline treatment schedule of 500 mg orally four times a day for ten days should be employed.

Gonorrheal Arthritis. Infectious arthritis caused by gonococci is occasionally seen by the gynecologist. It is the most common disseminated gonococcal infection, occurring in 47 of 55 (85.5%) of women in a recent study.[110] The next most frequent symptom in patients with a disseminated infection is a rash, present in 43.6%.[110]

Gonococcal arthritis should be suspected in any sexually active woman with clinical signs of infectious arthritis. Endocervical, blood, and joint fluid cultures from the involved joint should be performed to confirm the diagnosis. The effective treatment schedules are 10,000,000 U of aqueous crystalline penicillin G administered intravenously until improvement occurs, followed by 2 g of oral ampicillin or amoxicillin daily to complete seven days of therapy. Injections can be avoided if oral ampicillin (3.5 g) or amoxicillin 3.0 g and probenecid 1.0 g are given, followed by 500 mg of oral ampicillin or amoxicillin four times a day for at least seven days. For the penicillin-allergic patient, alternative regimens include an oral dose of tetracycline 2 g a day for at least seven days. If the infection is caused by penicillinase-producing gonorrhea, use cefoxitin 1.0 g or cefotaxime 500 mg given intravenously four times a day for at least seven days. All these regimens should be prolonged in the rare case showing no clinical improvement.[20]

Gonococcal Meningitis and Endocarditis. Meningitis and endocarditis are rare and serious forms of disseminated gonococcal infection. Patients with meningitis and endocarditis require at least 10,000,000 U of intravenously administered aqueous penicillin a day for four weeks. They can be seriously ill, and at least one death has been reported in a patient with a documented *Neisseria gonorrhoeae* endocarditis.[111] The diverse manifestations of disease caused by this pathogen should be considered in the evaluation of the female patient with systemic symptoms.

Hepatitis

The gynecologist will see some women with liver disease. Usually, they will complain of malaise, loss of appetite, and in smokers, a loss of the desire to smoke. Sometimes the diagnosis will be more apparent because of obvious signs of jaundice. One frequent cause of this type of problem is hepatitis caused by hepatitis viruses A, B, or non-A, non-B. A frame of reference is needed for the gynecologist seeing these women as outpatients. The most frequently encountered problems will be related to the hepatitis B virus. Table 8–13 lists the prevalence of hepatitis B in various population groups.[112] This virus can be acquired by close personal contact. The high risk groups that gynecologists will see in their practice include women who are sexually active with bisexual men, recent immigrants from southeast Asia, and health care workers in high risk areas within the hospital, such as on a renal dialysis unit. There are two types of tests that are useful in the evaluation of these women. The first indicates the presence of hepatitis surface antigen HBsAg, which points to past infection with hepatitis B. In most patients, this is present in the serum for a few weeks and then disappears. Within the core of the virus are the HB core antigen and C antigen. The presence of these antigens in the serum beyond 10 weeks correlates well with the patient's continued carriage of the virus and capability of infecting the physician and other health workers as a chronic carrier. Another group of tests measure antibodies to these antigens. These core antibody tests are helpful as markers of hepatitis in patients who no longer have HBsAg in the serum but do not yet show HBsAb. There are other causes of hepatitis. Rarely, secondary syphilis will be associated with hepatitis. The diagnosis should be considered in patients whose reagin tests for syphilis have a high titer and who have a positive FTA-ABS test. The diagnosis is likely when the evaluation of a liver profile reveals elevated serum aminotransferase

Table 8–13. Expected Hepatitis B Virus Prevalence in Various Population Groups

Population	Prevalence of Serologic Markers of HBV Infection	
	HBsAG (%)	All Markers (%)
High Risk		
Immigrants or refugees from areas of high HBV endemicity	13	70–85
Clients in institutions for the mentally retarded	10–20	35–80
Users of illicit parenteral drugs	7	60–80
Homosexually active males	6	35–80
Household contacts of HBV carriers	3–6	30–60
Patients on hemodialysis units	3–10	20–80
Intermediate Risk		
Prisoners (male)	1–8	10–80
Staff of institutions for the mentally retarded	1	10–25
Health-care workers (frequent blood contact)	1–2	15–30
Low Risk		
Health-care workers (no or infrequent blood contact)	0.3	3–10
Healthy adults (first-time volunteer blood donors)	0.3	3–5

(From Inactivated hepatitis B virus vaccine. MMWR, *31*:317, 1982.)

and sometimes elevated alkaline phosphatase. A biopsy of the liver usually shows inflammatory cells. Fortunately for these women, systemic therapy with benzathine penicillin is curative. Finally, some women with mononucleosis will have an associated hepatitis. A heterophile test should be done and the diagnosis considered in a woman who manifests an immediate rash when given ampicillin for a sore throat.

Toxic Shock Syndrome

Toxic shock syndrome (TSS) is a serious illness that should be suspected in any woman presenting with the sudden onset of high fever and gastrointestinal symptoms, followed by the development of hypotension and shock. When initially seen, these women often have an erythematous "sunburnlike" rash, followed later by blistering and desquamation, particularly of the palms and skin. To focus the diffuse organ system involvement of this syndrome, the characteristics of cases have been defined by the Centers for Disease Control (Table 8–14).[113]

There are a number of interesting observations that suggest the cause of this syndrome. *Staphylococcus aureus* is involved, probably by means of toxin release and absorption and not as a result of the invasion of the organism, because bacteremia is rare. Indeed, the original case study definition eliminated those patients with positive blood cultures (see Table 8–14). The exact nature of the toxin or toxins released by this organism is not known. Schlievert and associates have championed the concept of a unique pyrogenic exotoxin C[114] and another group has described an enterotoxin F.[115] A recent study of Shutzer and co-workers has found lysogenicity or the presence of template bacteriophages in 11 of 12 strains of *Staphylococcus* recovered from patients with toxic shock syndrome, and only 1 of 8 control strains showed this.[116] This would account for the appearance of this new syndrome. The demographics of this disease are fascinating. As of April 8, 1982,[117]

Table 8–14. Toxic Shock Syndrome Case Definition

1. Fever (temp ≥ 38.9°C (102°F))
2. Rush (diffuse macular erythroderma)
3. Desquamation, 1–2 weeks after onset of illness, particularly of palms and soles
4. Hypotension (systolic blood pressure ≤ mm Hg for adults or < 5th percentile by age for children < 16 years of age, or orthostatic syncope)
5. Involvement of 3 or more of the following organ systems:
    A. Gastrointestinal (vomiting or diarrhea at onset of illness)
    B. Muscular (severe myalgia or creatine phosphokinase level ≥ two times upper normal limits)
    C. Mucous membrane (vaginal, oropharyngeal, or conjunctival hyperemia)
    D. Renal (BUN or creatinine ≥ 2 times upper normal limits or ≥ 5 white blood cells per high power field in the absence of a urinary tract infection)
    E. Hepatic (Total bilirubin, SGOT, or SGPT ≥ two times upper limits of normal)
    F. Hematologic (Platelets ≤ 100,000/mm³)
    G. CNS (Disorientation or alterations in consciousness without focal neurologic signs when fever and hypotensions are absent)
6. Negative results on the following tests if obtained
    A. Blood, throat, or cerebrospinal fluid cultures
    B. Serologic tests for Rocky Mountain spotted fever, leptospirosis, or measles

(From Follow-up on toxic shock syndrome, MMWR, *29*:441, 1980.)

96% of the cases involved women, of whom at least 92% had had the onset during a menstrual period. Some earlier studies showed a predominance of cases in which the Rely tampon, a superabsorbent brand, was involved.[113] Of great interest are the marked differences in the geographic distribution of the cases.[117] Utah and Minnesota have had the highest number of cases in terms of their population base, and recently the number of cases has been diminishing in Utah while remaining constant in Minnesota.[117] The reason for this discrepancy is not clear. TSS can be associated with any infection involving the coagulase-positive *Staphylococcus,* and this syndrome has been seen following childbirth, pregnancy termination, infected abdominal wounds, and any infected skin lesions.[117] It seems clear that the systemic manifestations are caused by a toxin or toxins produced by coagulase-positive staphylococci, and the regional variation in incidence could be related to the geographic colonization patterns of this toxin-producing bacteria.

Physicians have a number of measures at their disposal to deal with toxic shock syndrome. As a preventive measure, particularly in high risk areas like Minnesota and Utah, women can be advised that their risk is probably diminished by not using tampons or wearing them intermittently during each menstrual period. The physician should be aware of the possibility of toxic shock syndrome in every seriously ill patient who has a high temperature, a rash, and hypotension. Vaginal cultures should be obtained for the coagulase-positive *Staphylococcus* and therapy begun with a semisynthetic penicillin or a beta-lactam antibiotic. Intravascular lines should be used to monitor fluid requirements.

Acquired Immune Deficiency Syndrome

Acquired immune deficiency syndrome (AIDS) is significantly influencing the practice of gynecologists. On the surface, this would seem to deviate from the facts, for unlike TSS, AIDS has been recognized mostly in males and particularly in the homosexual community. To date, the four groups in whom nearly all the cases have been reported have been homosexuals in urban areas, heterosexual intravenous drug abusers, Haitian immigrants, and hemophiliacs. The distribution of the syndrome has many similarities to the distribution of hepatitis B (see Table

8–13) and fits the hypothesis that AIDS is caused by a biologic agent transmissible by a number of routes, particularly sexual contact and intravenous injection. Recently, a virus has been implicated.[118] The most disturbing part of this syndrome is its lethality, for no survivors have been reported to date. There are many reasons for concern about AIDS in women. It is clear that the incubation period of this syndrome can be years, and this raises concern about large numbers of asymptomatic people in urban communities who will be sources of infection through intimate contact or through the donation of blood products. There are two potential sources of infection in women. Recently, a report demonstrated the transmission of AIDS to women from sexual contact with men with AIDS[119] who were drug abusers. This is a sexually transmitted disease that the gynecologist must be on the lookout for in the future. Finally, there is concern about the spread of this agent through the use of blood products in urban hospitals.[120] Already there is tremendous pressure for autotransfusion in elective gynecologic procedures so that patients will not be receiving blood from unknown donors. Finally, there will be questions from health personnel about the hepatitis B vaccine. The volunteer source of the inactivated virus vaccine is a population with a high incidence of AIDS. Although the manufacturing process eliminates the possibility of virus survival and to date there have been no AIDS cases in vaccine recipients in people whose lifestyles do not put them at risk for AIDS, the fear of receiving this immunization persists.

ANTIBIOTIC THERAPY OF ASYMPTOMATIC INFERTILE COUPLES

There has always been controversy about the treatment of asymptomatic couples to prevent infertility. In the first edition of this book, I was dubious about the value of the treatment of women who had been colonized by *Mycoplasma* organisms because no pathologic lesions in the genital tract had been identified, and I quoted one clinical study in which this treatment had not been of value.[121] I have modified this position somewhat because of new discoveries in this area. Toth and co-workers[66] have demonstrated the capability of spermatozoa serving as carriers for bacteria through liquid media, and Friberg has shown that *Escherichia coli* bind to spermatozoa.[122] In addition, one recent study by Toth and associates showed an increase in the fertility rate when couples, both positive for *Mycoplasma,* were treated with antibiotics.[123] There is evidence that asymptomatic men can have bacteriospermia, and this is associated with an increase in the number of abnormal spermatozoa forms. The treatment of these asymptomatic males and females eliminates the carriage state for the male and produces a better quality of sperm. More prospective controlled studies will be needed to establish this as accepted gynecologic therapy, for some well-controlled studies have shown no benefit with this form of treatment.[124]

REFERENCES

1. Guinan, M.E., MacCalman, J., Kern, E.R., Overall, J.C., Jr., and Spruance, S.L.: The course of untreated recurrent genital herpes simplex infection in 27 women. N. Engl. J. Med., *304*:759, 1981.
2. Reeves, W.C., Corey, L., Adams, H.G., Vontver, L.A., and Holmes, K.K.: Risk of recurrence after first episode of genital herpes. N. Engl. J. Med., *305*:315, 1981.
3. Meheus, A., Van Dyck, E., Ursi, J.P., Ballard, R.C., and Piot, P.: Etiology of genital ulceration in Swaziland. Sex. Transm. Dis., *10*:33, 1983.
4. Addison, W.A., Livengood, C.H., III, Hill, G.B., Sutton, G.P., and Fortier, K.J.: Necrotizing fasciitis of vulvar origin in diabetic patients. Obstet. Gynecol., *63*:473, 1984.

5. Meyers, M.G., Oxman, M.N., Clark, J.E., and Arndt, K.A.: Failure of neutral red photodynamic inactivation in recurrent herpes simplex virus infections. N. Engl. J. Med., *293*:945, 1975.

6. Corey, L., and Holmes, K.K.: The use of 2-deoxy-O-glucose for genital herpes. Letter to the Editor. J.A.M.A., *243*:29, 1980.

7. Corey, L., Nahmias, A.J., Guinan, M.E., Benedetti, J.K., Critchlow, C.W., and Holmes, K.K.: A trial of topical acyclovir in genital herpes simplex infections. N. Engl. J. Med., *306*:1313, 1982.

8. Mindel, A., Adler, M.W., Sutherland, S., and Fiddian, A.P.: Intravenous acyclovir for primary genital herpes. Lancet, *1*:697, 1982.

9. Bryson, Y.J., Dillon, M., Lovett, M., Acuna, G., Taylor, S., Cherry, J.D., Johnson, B.L., Wiesmeier, E., Growdon, W., Creagh-Kirk, T., and Keeney, R.: Treatment of first episodes of genital herpes simplex virus infection with oral acyclovir. N. Engl. J. Med., *308*:916, 1983.

10. Straus, S.E., Takiff, H.E., Seidlin, M., Bachrach, S., Lininger, L., DiGiovanno, J.J., Western, K.A., Smith, H.A., Lehrman, S.N., Creagh-Kirk, T., and Alling, D.W.: Suppression of frequently recurring genital herpes. N. Engl. J. Med., *310*:1545, 1984.

11. Douglas, J.M., Critchlow, C., Benedetti, J., Mertz, G.J., Connor, J.A., Hintz, M.A., Fahnlander, A., Remington, M., Winter, C., and Corey, L.: A double-blind study of oral acyclovir for suppression of recurrences of genital herpes simplex virus infection. N. Engl. J. Med., *310*:1551, 1984.

12. Baker, D.A., Thomas, J., Epstein, J., Possilico, D., and Stone, M.L.: The effect of prostaglandins on the multiplication and cell to cell spread of herpes simplex virus type 2 in vitro. Am. J. Obstet. Gynecol., *144*:346, 1982.

13. Wahba, A.: Topical application of zinc solutions: A new treatment for herpes simplex infection. Acta Derm. Venereol., *60*:175, 1980.

14. Raab, B., and Lorincz, A.L.: Genital herpes simplex-concepts and treatment. J. Am. Acad. Dermatol., *5*:249, 1981.

15. Friedrich, E.G., and Masukawa, T.: Effect of povidone-iodine on herpes genitalis. Obstet. Gynecol., *45*:337, 1975.

16. Corey, L., Reeves, W.C., Chiang, W.T., Vontver, L.A., Remington, M., Winter, C., and Holmes, K.K.: Ineffectiveness of topical ether for the treatment of genital herpes simplex virus infection. N. Engl. J. Med., *299*:237, 1978.

17. Nilsen, A.E., Aasen, T., Halsos, A.M., Kinge, B.R., Tjotta, E.H.L., Wikshom, K., and Fiddian, H.P.: Efficacy of oral acyclovir in the treatment of initial and recurrent genital herpes. Lancet. *2*:571, 1982.

18. Crumpacker, C.S., Schnipper, L.E., Marlowe, S.I., Kowalsky, P.N., Hershey, B.J., and Levin, M.T.: Resistance to antiviral drugs of herpes simplex virus isolated from patient treated with acyclovir. N. Engl. J. Med., *306*:343, 1982.

19. Rapp, F., Jui-Lien, H.L., and Jerkofsky, M.: Transformation of mammalian cells by DNA containing viruses following photodynamic inactivation. Virology, *55*:339, 1973.

20. Centers for Disease Control. MMWR Supplement. Sexually transmitted diseases. Treatment Guidelines 1982. *31*:335, 1982.

21. Grayston, J.T., and Wang, S.P.: New knowledge of chlamydiae and the diseases they cause. J. Infect. Dis., *132*:87, 1975.

22. Calkins, J.W., Masterson, B.J., Magrina, J.F., and Capen, C.V.: Management of condyloma acuminata with the carbon dioxide laser. Obstet. Gynecol., *59*:105, 1982.

23. Witkin, S.S., and Ledger, W.J.: Circulating immune complexes in sera of patients with gynecologic disorders. Surg. Gynecol. Obstet., *159*:413, 1984.

24. Gall, S.: Personal communication, 1983.

25. Spellacy, W.N., Zaias, N., Buhi, W.C., and Birk, S.A.: Vaginal yeast growth and contraceptive practices. Obstet. Gynecol., *38*:343, 1971.

26. Oriel, J.D., Partridge, B.M., Denny, M.J., and Coleman, J.C.: Genital yeast infections. Br. Med. J., *4*:761, 1972.

27. Sobel, J.D.: Management of recurrent vulvovaginal candidiasis with intermittent ketoconazole prophylaxis. Obstet. Gynecol., *65*:435, 1985.

28. Hughes, W.T., Bartley, D.L., Patterson, G.G., and Tufenkeji, H.: Ketoconazole and candidiasis: A controlled study. J. Infect. Dis., *147*:1060, 1983.

29. Witkin, S.S., Yu, I.R., and Ledger, W.J.: Inhibition of *Candida albicans*—induced lymphocyte proliferation by lymphocytes and sera from women with recurrent vaginitis. Am. J. Obstet. Gynecol., *147*:809, 1983.

30. Hager, W.D., Brown, S.T., Kraus, S.J., Kleris, J.S., Perkins, G.J., and Henderson, M.: Metronidazole for vaginal trichomoniasis: Seven day vs. single dose regimen. J.A.M.A., *244*:1219, 1980.

31. Mead, P.B., Gibson, M., Schentag, J.T., and Ziemniak, J.A.: Letter to the editor. Possible alteration of metronidazole metabolism by phenobarbital. N. Engl. J. Med., *306*:1490, 1982.

32. Muller, M., Meingassner, J.G., Miller, W.A., and Ledger, W.J.: Three metronidazole resistant strains of *Trichomonas vaginalis* from the United States. Am. J. Obstet. Gynecol., *138*:808, 1980.

33. Rustia, M., and Shubik, P.: Induction of lung tumors and malignant lymphomas in mice by metronidazole. J. Natl. Cancer Inst., *48*:721, 1972.

34. Rustia, M., and Shubik, P.: Experimental induction of hepatomas, mammary tumors and other tumors with metronidazole in non inbred Sas: MRC(WI) BR rats. J. Natl. Cancer Inst., *63*:863, 1979.
35. Voogd, C.E., VanderStel, J.J., and Jacobs, J.J.: Mutagenic action of nitroimidazoles. I. Metronidazole, nimorazole, dimetridazole, ronidazole. Mut. Res., *26*:483, 1974.
36. Is Flagyl dangerous? Med. Lett., *17*(13):53, 1975.
37. Finegold, S.M.: Summary of Conference. Metronidazole. Excerpta Medica, vol. 438, 1978.
38. Beard, C.M., Noller, K.L., O'Fallon, W.M., Karland, L.T., and Dockerty, M.B.: Lack of evidence for cancer due to use of metronidazole. N. Engl. J. Med., *301*:519, 1979.
39. Gardner, H.L., and Dukes, C.D.: *Haemophilus vaginalis* vaginitis. Am. J. Obstet. Gynecol., *69*:962, 1955.
40. McCormack, W.M., Hayes, C.H., Rosner, B., Evrard, J.R., Crockett, V.A., Alpert, S., and Zinner, S.H.: Vaginal colonization with *Corynebacterium vaginale (Haemophilus vaginalis).* J. Infect. Dis., *136*:740, 1977.
41. Amsel, R., Totten, P.A., Spiegel, C.H., Chen, K.C.S., Eschenbach, D., and Holmes, K.K.: Nonspecific vaginitis. Am. J. Med., *74*:14, 1983.
42. Pheifer, T.A., Forsyth, P.S., Durfee, M.A., Pollock, H.M., and Holmes, K.K.: Non specific vaginitis: Role of *Haemophilus vaginalis* and treatment with metronidazole. N. Engl. J. Med., *298*:1429, 1978.
43. Stamm, W.E., Guinan, M.E., Johnson, C., Starcher, T., Holmes, K.K., and McCormack, W.M.: Effect of treatment regimens for *Neisseria gonorrhoeae* on simultaneous infection with *Chlamydia trachomatis.* N. Engl. J. Med., *310*:545, 1984.
44. Burnhill, M.S.: Syndrome of progressive endometritis associated with intrauterine contraceptive devices. Adv. Fam. Plann., *8*:144, 1972.
45. Petitti, D.B., Yamamoto, D., and Morgenstern, N.: Factors associated with *Actinomyces*-like organisms on Papanicolau smear in users of intrauterine contraceptive devices. Am. J. Obstet. Gynecol., *145*:338, 1983.
46. Stamm, W.E., Counts, G.W., Running, K.R., Fihn, S., Turck, M., and Holmes, K.K.: Diagnosis of coliform infection in acutely dysuric women. N. Engl. J. Med., *307*:463, 1982.
47. Jacobson, L., and Westrom, L.: Objectivized diagnosis of acute pelvic inflammatory disease. Am. J. Obstet. Gynecol., *105*:1088, 1969.
48. Sweet, R.L., Draper, D.L., and Hadley, W.K.: Etiology of acute salpingitis: Influence of episode number and duration of symptoms. Obstet. Gynecol., *58*:62, 1981.
49. Ledger, W.J.: Selection of antimicrobial agents for treatment of infection of the female genital tract. Rev. Infect. Dis., *5*:S98, 1983.
50. Mardh, P.-A., Ripa, T., Svensson, L., and Westrom, L.: *Chlamydia trachomatis* infection in patients with acute salpingitis. N. Engl. J. Med., *296*:1377, 1977.
51. Eschenbach, D.A., Buchanan, T.M., Pollock, H.M., Forsyth, P.S., Alexander, E.R., Lin, J., Wang, S., Wentworth, B.B., McCormack, W.M., and Holmes, K.K.: Polymicrobial etiology of acute pelvic inflammatory disease. N. Engl. J. Med., *293*:166, 1975.
52. Sweet, R.L., Schachter, J., and Robbie, M.O.: Failure of beta-lactam antibiotics to eradicate *Chlamydia trachomatis* in the endometrium despite apparent clinical cure of acute salpingitis. J.A.M.A., *250*:2641, 1983.
53. Henry-Suchet, J., Catalan, F., Loffredo, V., Serfaty, D., Siboulet, A., Perol, Y., Sanson, M.J., Debache, C., Pigeau, F., Coppin, R., DeBrux, J., and Poynard, T.: Microbiology of specimens obtained by laparoscopy from controls and from patients with pelvic inflammatory disease or infertility with tubal obstruction. *Chlamydia trachomatis* and *Ureaplasma urealyticum.* Am. J. Obstet. Gynecol., *138*:1022, 1980.
54. Westrom, L.: Incidence, prevalence and trends of pelvic inflammatory disease and its consequences in industrialized countries. Am. J. Obstet. Gynecol., *138*:880, 1980.
55. Arya, O.P., Mallinson, H., and Goddard, A.D.: Epidemiological and clinical correlates of *Chlamydial* infection of the cervix. Br. J. Vener. Dis., *57*:118, 1981.
56. Senanayake, P., and Kramer, D.G.: Contraception and the etiology of pelvic inflammatory disease: New perspectives. Am. J. Obstet. Gynecol., *138*:852, 1980.
57. Kelaghan, J., Rubin, G.L., Ory, H.W., and Layde, P.M.: Barrier-method contraceptives and pelvic inflammatory disease. J.A.M.A., *248*:184, 1982.
58. Osser, S., Liedholm, P., and Sjoberg, N-O.: Risk of pelvic inflammatory disease among users of intrauterine devices, irrespective of previous pregnancy. Am. J. Obstet. Gynecol., *138*:864, 1980.
59. Westrom, L., Bengtsson, L., and Mardh, P.: The risk of developing pelvic inflammatory disease in women using intrauterine devices as compared to non-users. Lancet, *2*:221, 1976.
60. Gump, D.W., Gibson, M., and Ashikaga, T.: Evidence of prior pelvic inflammatory disease and its relationship to *Chlamydia trachomatis* antibody and intrauterine contraceptive device use in infertile women. Am. J. Obstet. Gynecol., *146*:153, 1983.
61. Marshall, B.R., Hepler, J.K., and Jinquji, M.S.: Fatal *Streptococcus pyogenes* septicemia associated with an intrauterine device. Obstet. Gynecol., *41*:83, 1973.
62. Hager, W.D., and Majmudar, B.: Pelvic actinomycosis in women using intrauterine contraceptive devices. Am. J. Obstet. Gynecol., *133*:60, 1979.

63. Golde, S.H., Israel, R., and Ledger, W.J.: Unilateral tubo-ovarian abscess: A distinct entity. Am. J. Obstet. Gynecol., *127*:807, 1977.
64. Sparks, R.A., Purrier, B.G.A., Watt, P.J., and Elstein, M.: The bacteriology of the cervical canal in relation to the use of an intrauterine device. *In* The Uterine Cervix in Reproduction. Edited by V. Insler and G. Bettendorf. Stuttgart, George Thieme Publishers, 1977, pp. 271-277.
65. Willson, J.R., Ledger, W.J., Bollinger, C.C., and Andros, G.J.: The Margulies intrauterine contraceptive device. Am. J. Obstet. Gynecol., *92*:62, 1965.
66. Toth, A., O'Leary, W.M., and Ledger, W.J.: Evidence for microbial transfer by spermatozoa. Obstet. Gynecol., *59*:556, 1982.
67. Toth, A., Lesser, M.L., and Labriola, D.: The development of infections of the genitourinary tract in the wives of infertile males and the possible role of spermatozoa in the development of salpingitis. Surg. Gynecol. Obstet., *159*:565, 1984.
68. Ledger, W.J., Moore, D.E., Lowensohn, R.I., and Gee, C.L.: A fever index evaluation of chloramphenicol or clindamycin in patients with serious pelvic infections. Obstet. Gynecol., *50*:523, 1977.
69. Purdthaisong, T.: Return of fertility after use of the injectable contraceptive Depo Provera; updated data analysis. J. Biosocial Sci., *16*:23, 1984.
70. Hager, W.D., Eschenbach, D.A., Spence, M.R., and Sweet, R.L.: Criteria for diagnosis and grading of salpingitis. Obstet. Gynecol., *61*:113, 1983.
71. Rosenfeld, D.L., Seidman, S.M., Bronson, R.A., and Scholl, G.M.: Unsuspected chronic pelvic inflammatory disease in the infertile female. Fertil. Steril., *39*:44, 1983.
72. Westrom, L., Skude, G., and Mardh, P.-A.: Amylases of the genital tract. Am. J. Obstet. Gynecol., *126*:657, 1976.
73. Westrom, L.: Clinical manifestation and diagnosis of pelvic inflammatory disease. J. Reprod. Med., *28*:703, 1983.
74. Ledger, W.J.: Laparoscopy in the diagnosis and management of patients with suspected salpingo-oophoritis. Am. J. Obstet. Gynecol., *138*:1012, 1980.
75. Schroeter, A.L., and Reynolds, G.: The rectal culture as a test of cure of gonorrhea in the female. J. Infect. Dis., *125*.499, 1972.
76. Sweet, R.L., Mills, J., Hadley, K.W., Blummenstock, E., Schachter, J., Robbie, M.O., and Draper, D.L.: Use of laparoscopy to determine the microbiologic etiology of acute salpingitis. Am. J. Obstet. Gynecol., *134*:68, 1979.
77. Falk, V.: Treatment of acute non-tuberculous salpingitis with antibiotics alone and in combination with glucocorticoids. Acta Obstet. Gynecol. Scand., *44*:Suppl. 6, 1965.
78. Monif, G.R.G.: Clinical staging of acute bacterial salpingitis and its therapeutic ramifications. Am. J. Obstet. Gynecol., *143*:489, 1982.
79. Sweet, R.L.: Diagnosis and treatment of salpingo-oophoritis. Mediguide to Ob/Gyn, *2*:1, 1983.
80. Westrom, L.: Effect of acute pelvic inflammatory disease on fertility. Am. J. Obstet. Gynecol., *121*:707, 1975.
81. Tally, F.P., Cuchural, G.J., Jacobus, N.V., Gorbach, S.L., Aldridge, K.E., Cleary, T.J., Finegold, S.M., Hill, G.B., Iannini, P.B., McCloskey, R.V., O'Keefe, J.P., and Pierson, C.L.: Susceptibility of the *Bacteroides fragilis* group in the United States in 1981. Antimicrob. Agents Chemother., *23*: 536, 1983.
82. Bryant, R.E., and Hammond, D.: Interaction of purulent material with antibiotics used to treat *Pseudomonas* infection. Antimicrob. Agents Chemother., *6*:702, 1974.
83. Rubenstein, P.R., Mishell, D.R., Jr. and Ledger, W.J.: Colpotomy drainage of pelvic abscess. Obstet. Gynecol., *48*:142, 1976.
84. Ledger, W.J., Gassner, C.B., and Gee, C.: Operative care of infection in obstetrics-gynecology. J. Reprod. Med., *13*:128, 1974.
85. Collins, C.G., Nix, F.G., and Cerha, H.T.: Ruptured tubo-ovarian abscess. Am. J. Obstet. Gynecol., *72*:820, 1956.
86. Vermeeren, J., and Telinde, R.: Intra-abdominal rupture of pelvic abscesses. Am. J. Obstet. Gynecol., *68*:402, 1954.
87. Rivlin, M.E., and Hunt, J.A.: Ruptured tubo-ovarian abscess. Is hysterectomy necessary? Obstet. Gynecol., *50*:518, 1977.
88. Robinson, S.C.: Observations on the peritoneum as an absorbing surface. Am. J. Obstet. Gynecol., *83*:446, 1962.
89. Morrow, C.P., Hernandez, W.L., Townsend, D.E., and DiSaia, P.J.: Pelvic celiotomy in the obese patient. Am. J. Obstet. Gynecol., *127*:335, 1977.
90. Rivlin, M.E.: Clinical outcome following vaginal drainage of pelvic abscess. Obstet. Gynecol., *61*:169, 1983.
91. Mickal, A., and Sellmann, A.H.: Management of the tubo-ovarian abscess. Clin. Obstet. Gynecol., *12*:252, 1969.
92. Ledger, W.J.: Anaerobic infections. Am. J. Obstet. Gynecol., *123*:111, 1975.
93. Simpson, F.F.: The choice of time for operation for pelvic inflammation of tubal origin. Surg. Gynecol. Obstet., *9*:45, 1909.

94. Miller, C.J.: The rational treatment of tubal disease. Surg. Gynecol. Obstet., *45*:110, 1927.
95. Anderson, G.V., and Bucklew, W.B.: Abdominal surgery and tubo-ovarian abscesses. West. J. Surg. Obstet. Gynecol., *70*:67, 1962.
96. Kaplan, A.L., Jacobs, W.M., and Ehresman, J.B.: Aggressive management of pelvic abscess. Am. J. Obstet. Gynecol., *98*:482, 1967.
97. Ledger, W.J.: The surgical care of severe infections in obstetric and gynecologic patients. Surg. Gynecol. Obstet., *136*:753, 1973.
98. Franklin, E.W., III, Hevron, J.E., and Thompson, J.D.: Management of the pelvic abscess. Clin. Obstet. Gynecol., 16(2):66, 1973.
99. Landers, D.V., and Sweet, R.L.: Tubo-ovarian abscess: Contemporary approach to management. Rev. Infect. Dis., *5*:876, 1983.
100. Hager, W.D.: Followup of patients with tubo-ovarian abscess(es) in association with salpingitis. Obstet. Gynecol., *61*:680, 1983.
101. Kamm, R., and Hibbard, L.T.: Hyperalimentation in the management of overwhelming pelvic infection. Obstet. Gynecol., *44*:246, 1974.
102. Young, E.J., Fainstein, V., and Musher, D.M.: Drug-induced fever: Cases seen in the evaluation of unexplained fever in a general hospital population. Rev. Infect. Dis., *4*:69, 1982.
103. Heaton, F.C., and Ledger, W.J.: Post-menopausal tubo-ovarian abscess. Obstet. Gynecol., *47*:90, 1976.
104. Weiner, S., and Wallach, E.E.: Ovarian histology in pelvic inflammatory disease. Obstet. Gynecol., *43*:431, 1974.
105. DiZerega, G.S., and Hodgen, G.D.: Prevention of postoperative tubal adhesions. Am. J. Obstet. Gynecol., *136*:173, 1980.
106. Pfeffer, W.H.: Adjuvants in tubal surgery. Fertil. Steril., *33*:245, 1980.
107. Collins, C.G., MacCallum, E.A., Nelson, E.W., Weinstein, B.B., and Collins, J.H.: Suppurative pelvic thrombophlebitis. Surgery, *30*:298, 1951.
108. Klein, T.A., Richmond, J.A., and Mishell, D.R., Jr.: Pelvic tuberculosis. Obstet. Gynecol., *48*:99, 1976.
109. Schaefer, G.: Tuberculosis of the female genital tract. Clin. Obstet. Gynecol., *13*:965, 1970.
110. Al-Suleiman, S.A., Grimes, E.M., and Jonas, H.S.: Disseminated gonococcal infection. Obstet. Gynecol., *61*:48, 1983.
111. Tanowitz, H.B., Adler, J.J., and Chirito, E.: Gonococcal endocarditis. N.Y. State J. Med., *72*:2782, 1972.
112. Inactivated hepatitis B virus vaccine. MMWR, *31*:317, 1982.
113. Follow-up on toxic shock syndrome. MMWR, *29*:441, 1980.
114. Schlievert, P.M., Shands, K.N., Dan, B.B., Schmid, P., and Nishimura, R.D.: Identification and characterization of an exotoxin from *Staphylococcus aureus* associated with toxic shock syndrome. J. Infect. Dis., *143*:509, 1981.
115. Bergdoll, M.S., Crass, B.A., Reiser, R.F., Robbins, R.N., and Davis, J.P.: A new staphylococcal enterotoxin F, associated with toxic shock syndrome *Staphylococcus aureus* isolates. Lancet, *1*:1017, 1981.
116. Schutzer, S.E., Fischetti, V.A., and Zabriskie, J.B.: Toxic shock syndrome and lysogeny in *Staphylococcus aureus.* Science, *220*:316, 1983.
117. Toxic shock syndrome, United States, 1970–1982. MMWR, *31*:201, 1982.
118. Gallo, R.C., Salahoddin, S.Z., Popovic, M., Shearer, G.M., Kaplan, M., Haynes, B.F., Palker, T.J., Redfield, R., Oleske, J., Salai, B., White, G., Foster, P., and Markham, P.D.: Frequent detection and isolation of cytopathic retroviruses (HTLV-111) from patients with AIDS and at risk for AIDS. Science, *224*:500, 1984.
119. Harris, C., Small, C.B., Klein, R.S., Friedland, G.H., Moll, B., Emeson, E.E., Spigland, I., and Steigbigel, N.H.: Immunodeficiency in female sexual partners of men with the acquired immunodeficiency syndrome. N. Engl. J. Med., *308*:1181, 1983.
120. Curran, J.W., Lawrence, D.N., Jaffe, H., Kaplan, J.E., Zyla, L.D., Chamberland, M., Weinstein, R., Lui, K.J., Schonberger, L.B., Spira, T.J., Alexander, W.J., Swinger, G., Ammann, A., Solomon, S., Auerbach, D., Mildean, D., Stoneburner, R., Jason, J.M., Havellos, H.W., and Evatt, B.L.: Acquired immunodeficiency syndrome (AIDS) associated with transfusion. N. Engl. J. Med., *310*:69, 1984.
121. Harrison, R.F., Delouvois, J., Blades, M., and Hurley, R.: Doxycycline treatment and human infertility. Lancet, *1*:605, 1975.
122. Friberg, J., and Fullan, N.: Attachment of *Escherichia coli* to human spermatozoa. Am. J. Obstet. Gynecol., *146*:465, 1983.
123. Toth, A., Lesser, M.L., Brooks, C., and Labriola, D.: Subsequent pregnancies among 161 couples treated for T-*mycoplasma* genital tract infection. N. Engl. J. Med., *308*:505, 1983.
124. Gump, D.W., Gibson, M., and Ashikaga, T.: Lack of association between genital mycoplasmas and infertility. N. Engl. J. Med., *310*:937, 1984.

Chapter 9

HOSPITAL-ACQUIRED GYNECOLOGIC INFECTIONS

Hospital-acquired infections are a significant problem for gynecologic patients. One surveillance study of a gynecology service revealed that 14% of the patients admitted to the hospital received antibiotics for a hospital-acquired infection during their stay.[1] This figure can vary from service to service, depending upon the mix of patients. For example, women with more extensive operations have a higher rate of infection,[1] and infections are more common in women of lower socioeconomic classes.[2] In another view of this problem, one nationwide survey of patients undergoing abdominal and vaginal hysterectomy, in a period of time before prophylactic antibiotics were employed, revealed that nearly 50% received systemic antibiotics during their hospitalization.[3] These are high figures, higher than have been noted in the reported data on hospital-acquired infections.[4, 5]

The increased frequency of hospital-acquired infections on a gynecology service is not unexpected. Admission to the hospital results in the patient's acquisition of a hospital bacterial flora[6] that is more antibiotic-resistant. Further, all the physician's surgical endeavors have significant risk factors for the patient. General anesthesia has a suppressant effect on the patient's cellular response to antigens, which may increase host susceptibility to bacterial pathogens.[7] This abnormal laboratory response is reflected clinically in some operative procedures that have an associated higher infection rate when general compared with regional anesthesia is used.[8] This impaired response is present at the time of operation, which is a critical time in the initiation of infection, for experimental studies of antibiotic prophylaxis demonstrate a limited time frame in which this preventive therapy works.[9] Postoperative soft tissue infections are the result of the interplay of several factors that are initiated in the operating room. This focus is important for the physician, for Cruse has demonstrated in his studies that wound infections are initiated in the operating room and are the responsibility of the operating surgeon.[10] He has stated, "it is better to have a perfect surgeon with poor aseptic technique than perfect aseptic technique and a poor surgeon."[10] In addition to these observations, Maki and co-workers could find no difference in hospital-acquired infection rates among different hospitals, even though samples of environmental bacteria varied considerably between an older and a brand new hospital.[11]

Operations create the milieu for soft tissue infections. There is trauma with poorly perfused tissue produced by the crush injuries of clamping, and in addition suture ligation adds a foreign body to the wound. The extent of the tissue trauma is related to both the operative skill of the gynecologist and the extent of the operation. Bacterial contamination of the wound is necessary for an infection to occur, and this is usually endogenous, from the patient herself. For example, in many gynecologic procedures, the vagina, a microbiologically contaminated area, is exposed during the operation. Blood products such as ferric iron[12] and hemoglobin[13] enhance the virulence of contaminating organisms, particularly the gram-negative aerobes. Many gynecologic operations are performed to correct stress urinary incontinence, and the operative trauma diminishes the patient's ability to void in the immediate postoperative period. Thus, prolonged periods of indwelling catheterization of the bladder are often required, with an increased risk of ascending urinary tract infection.

Operative trauma can result in infections in other body systems. Some post-operative respiratory problems are initiated by breathing dysfunction from the discomfort of an abdominal incision, which inhibits the deep inspiratory sigh or yawn that acts to prevent this problem. Less common but more serious is aspiration pneumonia, which can occur during or immediately after an operation.

Advances in operative techniques, radiotherapy, chemotherapy, and intravenous hyperalimentation have led to improved cure rates in patients with gynecologic malignancies. However, these extensive therapies, which are either invasive or suppress the patient's immune response, are often accompanied by difficult-to-treat hospital-acquired infections. The stress of operative intervention creates an environment in which infection can occur. Knowledge of the factors involved in hospital-acquired infections should be used to institute measures of preventive care.

PREVENTIVE CARE

Preoperative Screening for Community-Acquired Infections

The gynecologist should make an active effort to screen for community-acquired infections prior to elective operation. The effects of anesthesia and operative manipulations may permit an unrecognized infection to progress to one of serious clinical significance or to be a source of bacterial contamination at the operative site or the sites of intravascular or urinary tract catheters.

A preoperative fever or respiratory symptoms or both should be closely evaluated to be certain there is no incubating upper or lower respiratory tract infection. If this is present and not recognized, serious postoperative pneumonia can result.

The urinary tract is a common site of postoperative infections. Surveys of sexually active women usually reveal 5 to 10% with significant bacteriuria who are asymptomatic. If unrecognized, bacteriuria can be the source of major post-operative febrile disease in the patient, with postoperative problems of voiding. Urinary tract screening should be performed in patients prior to admission to the hospital for elective operations, and those with significant bacteriuria should have appropriate therapy until the bacteria have been cleared from the tract. I favor the use of nitrofurantoin, unless the bacteria isolated are resistant, for this agent has minimal impact on the gastrointestinal flora.

There should be a close evaluation of the lower genital tract prior to the performance of a hysterectomy. A patient with active acute cervicitis will shed more bacteria into the operative wound site at the time of hysterectomy than a patient with an uninfected cervix. The source of the cervicitis may be *Chlamydia,* which requires antibiotics such as tetracycline or erythromycin for a cure. There is evidence that patients with genital tract malignancies have colonization with a greater number of bacteria, and this can be a source of postoperative infection.[14] The potential focus of increased microbiologic contamination is present during the healing of the cervix after electrocautery, cryosurgery, and cone biopsy procedures. Elective hysterectomy following any of these procedures is best performed when the cervix has healed completely, although one pre-prophylaxis study indicated that there was no increase in serious infection if the interval between conization and hysterectomy was less than 48 hours.[15] The almost universal use of systemic antibiotics has modified this dictum of waiting for cervical healing. One recent study showed no difference in the incidence of infection when this interval was longer than 40 hours, but this study included the long-term use of antibiotics, i.e., more than 5 days, in 93.6% of the patients having conization and then a hysterectomy.[16]

In addition to the recognition of obvious cervical infections, some population groups undergoing elective gynecologic operations should be screened for the presence of *Neisseria gonorrhoeae*. It has been demonstrated that women with a positive endocervical culture for *Neisseria gonorrhoeae* have a higher than expected incidence of postoperative pelvic infections following elective termination of pregnancy.[17] It is mandatory to screen these women with cultures before the procedure and to treat the *Neisseria gonorrhoeae* infection before the invasive procedure is done. There is also evidence that patients in the childbearing age group with abnormal uterine bleeding have a higher than expected incidence of positive endocervical cultures for this organism.[18] Although it is not proved, this may reflect gonococcal endometritis with a greater possibility of postoperative infection following elective gynecologic surgical procedures. This is more than a theoretical consideration. There was one death on the gynecologic service of the University of Michigan from the intraperitoneal rupture of a postoperative adnexal abscess. A research study of transfundal uterine aspiration at the time of operation showed a positive growth of *Neisseria gonorrhoeae*. This asymptomatic woman had upper genital tract colonization with this organism, and she became febrile immediately postoperatively. Perioperative prophylactic antibiotics were not employed. Despite many courses of postoperative antibiotics, she eventually became acutely ill and failed to survive the operation for a ruptured postoperative adnexal abscess.[19] The decision about routine screening for *Neisseria gonorrhoeae* depends upon the experience of the service. In many urban settings, it would be appropriate to screen all women for the presence of *Neisseria gonorrhoeae*.

There can also be bacterial contamination of the upper genital tract from recent invasive procedures. An endometrial biopsy or a curettage procedure contaminates the uterine cavity, and the same time intervals for subsequent operation that have been applied to conization should be enforced here as well or prophylactic antibiotics used. It is also important to note that use of the intrauterine device has been associated with histologic evidence of salpingitis[20] and has been related to postoperative abscess formation when laparoscopic elective fulguration has been employed.[21] In patients with an intrauterine device who desire the disruption of normal tubal function, there are two options. The first is to remove the device for at least one cycle before the elective operative procedure. Alternatively, in the patient who is concerned about a pregnancy because of a lack of an effective alternative contraceptive, a prophylactic antibiotic may be employed and the device left in place.

Elderly patients admitted to the hospital from nursing homes have a high potential for serious postoperative infections. Some of these women will need gynecologic care for pelvic malignancy, pelvic relaxation, or stress urinary incontinence. One survey of 532 patients in nursing homes showed a prevalence rate of infection of 16.2%.[22] These infections included infected decubitus ulcers, conjunctivitis, symptomatic urinary tract infections, and lower respiratory tract infections. Of special interest to the gynecologist was the observation that 25% of the patients with indwelling urinary catheters had asymptomatic bacteriuria, and such difficult to treat organisms as *Proteus vulgaris* and *Providencia stuartii* were isolated. Prior to the admission of nursing home patients for elective gynecologic operations, they should be screened carefully by physical examination to be sure they have no respiratory infections or decubitus ulcers. In addition, a urine culture should be obtained to see if they have significant bacteriuria, and appropriate preadmission antibiotic therapy should be begun if there is significant bacteriuria.

Prevention by Surveillance

A primary goal for the management of patients with hospital-acquired gynecologic infections is to establish a system of prevention, for this is preferable to treatment of an established infection. It is important that preventive measures be based on firm data gathered in the hospital by a system of surveillance and not on the whims or biases of decision-making bodies within the obstetric-gynecology department. Also, a broad information base is available that can be utilized to determine policies for the care of hospitalized patients.

HOSPITAL PERSONNEL

A starting place for the prevention of hospital-acquired gynecologic infections is the establishment of acceptable work habits by members of the professional staff who have daily contact with patients. This should not be a new standard for the obstetrician-gynecologist. In the nineteenth century, Semmelweiss and Holmes recognized the role of the physician as a source of contagion in childbirth fever, and antibiotics have not eliminated this unwanted role for hospital personnel. A number of studies have documented the importance of the asymptomatic physician in the spread of hospital-acquired epidemics. In one outbreak of group A beta-hemolytic streptococcal infections, the common initiating source was traced to an anesthesiologist who was an asymptomatic anal carrier of this organism.[23] In another, a series of coagulase-positive staphylococcal wound infections were related to the contamination of the beard of a resident in general surgery.[24]

Physicians with long hair are potentially greater shedders of dangerous bacteria like the gram-positive, coagulase-positive *Staphylococcus.* Long hair styles in both women and men and beards and mustaches in men are a personal prerogative, but exposure of hair in the operating room is not. In some instances of an epidemic of hospital-acquired staphylococcal infections, mandatory antistaphylococcal shampoos may be necessary. These gynecologists must always use operating room caps and masks that provide complete hair coverage.

Firm but reasonable rules must be established to prevent the medical staff from inadvertently acting as asymptomatic carriers of infection. The wearing of scrub suits by house or attending staff members outside of the operating room suite should be discouraged in all hospitals. All approved obstetric-gynecologic programs require a considerable amount of service work by the house staff. The overworked, overtired junior house staff officers often feel more comfortable on work rounds in a scrub suit, particularly when they face more than 24 hours of continued duty. This practice by itself is acceptable, but the constant pressure of time may cause these physicians to forego changing into a fresh scrub suit before entering the operating room after inspection of wound dressings on rounds. This practice can result in cross-contamination.

Surgeons should be discouraged from taking showers just before beginning the operative schedule. British investigators found that this practice increased the shedding of bacteria by individual members of the operative team.[25] Another staff source of hospital-acquired infections can be from medical attendants who develop skin infections that are hidden from view. These persons disseminate huge quantities of potentially dangerous pathogens such as the coagulase-positive *Staphylococcus,* and because of this, they should not be directly involved in patient care. Nursing, house, and attending staff should not be expected to be altruistic. Their voluntary report of the presence of an infected skin lesion can be delayed because of the economic loss of salary when they are relieved of clinical responsibilities. Hospitals should set up some form of compensation so that economic pressure will not be a factor in the decision of a health care team member to report a lesion.

ENVIRONMENT

There are many possibilities for environmental contamination of the patient during hospitalization that in turn can result in a postoperative infection. Usually, problems of this nature occur in intensive care units, an environment in which many invasive procedures are performed against a backdrop of rapid turnover of both medical care personnel and patients. If a new pathogen is introduced into this setting, an epidemic of infections can result. One example of this was an outbreak of *Serratia marcescens* bacteremias traced to contaminated pressure transducers in an intensive care unit.[26] Another clustering of hospital-acquired infections due to *Pseudomonas cepacia* was linked to colonization by this organism of a widely used local anesthetic solution.[27] There can be other threats from the hospital environment. One evaluation of hospital salads showed heavy colonization with *Pseudomonas.*[28] This dietary entrée should not be given to immunosuppressed patients. One persistent outbreak of hospital-acquired Legionnaire's disease pneumonias was related to the contamination of the hospital air-conditioning system.[29] The hospital environment can also be contaminated by patients with hospital-acquired infections. Patients with wound infections caused by the coagulase-positive staphylococci can be a source of widespread colonization of the hospital environment and of other patients as well. Historically, the puerperal infections described by Semmelweiss were probably caused by the group A beta-hemolytic streptococci and were spread from one patient to another by poor physician practices.[30] Recently, patients with psuedomembranous enterocolitis caused by *Clostridium difficile* have been shown to be a source of cross-contamination in hospital-acquired infections.[31] The possibility of an environmental source of infection should be considered when there is the sudden appearance of a number of infections with the same, unusual bacterial isolate.

Blood products are potentially dangerous substances unique to the hospital environment. In the past, a major concern was hepatitis, but the availability of markers in the blood of those infected with hepatitis B has markedly diminished this risk.[32] These markers include hepatitis B surface antigen and its antibody, hepatitis B core antibody, and hepatitis B antigen and its antibody. Among immunocompromised patients, there is concern about the acquisition of cytomegalovirus.[33] Recently, there has been increasing concern by patients about the risk of obtaining acquired immune deficiency syndrome (AIDS) from blood transfusions. Although its occurrence from this source is rare, AIDS has been reported in patients who received blood transfusions[34] and in some hemophiliacs who were given pooled blood products. Despite the infrequency of its transmission in this manner, the lethality of AIDS has resulted in the refusal of any blood products by many patients. Even though the etiologic agent has been definitely identified and a screening test for antibody to this virus developed, I do not expect this concern to wane in urban areas. The criteria for elective transfusions will remain strict, and other options will be sought. Patients undergoing elective surgery can give their own blood prior to admission, which will then be available to them if needed. Obviously this is not an option in women who require extensive pelvic surgery necessitating the use of more than one unit of blood.

OPERATIVE TECHNIQUES

A major consideration in the judgment of the competence of a surgical service is the incidence of postoperative infections in surgical incisions. Prevention of these infections should be the goal of every physician. A high incidence of postoperative infections in surgical wounds is equated with less successful surgical techniques. This judgment is particularly valid when all cases with gross operative field contamination by bacteria are eliminated, and only the rate of wound infection in clean operations is evaluated.

Intraoperative procedures can influence the rate of postoperative infection. Some widely employed techniques may not be beneficial. Over the years, many gynecologists have employed the local injection of vasoconstrictors to diminish intraoperative bleeding, particularly with myomectomy and vaginal hysterectomy. One recent study evaluated this intervention in 200 women undergoing vaginal hysterectomy. All received prophylactic antibiotics. One hundred of these women had a local injection of vasoconstrictor. This population had 11 postoperative vaginal cuff infections compared with two in the population that did not receive the vasoconstrictor.[35] These differences are statistically significant. A locally injected vasoconstrictor is not indicated in gynecologic operations.

Many other factors can be involved in the production of postoperative infection of wounds. The most comprehensive studies of the influence of hospital practices on this rate have been performed by Cruse.[10] He eliminated all patients whose operations were performed in a contaminated operative field, so that the influences of technique would be maximized. In the patients who underwent elective clean operations, he assessed the factors related to an increased incidence of postoperative infection. Some of the discoveries are not amenable to preventive measures by the physician; for example, there were increased postoperative infection rates of wounds in elderly patients. However, other influences that could be changed were noted. The longer the operative procedure, the greater the incidence of postoperative infection. Clearly, efficient use of operating room time is necessary.

Besides concern about the efficient use of surgical skills, a number of related events can be altered by concerned physicians. One example has been the repeated observation that prolonged preoperative hospitalization is related to an increased postoperative infection rate. This may not be a cause-and-effect relationship, for patients with a greater number of medical problems may require a more detailed preoperative workup and a longer hospitalization. However, most surveys indicate that the colonization rate of patients with more resistant hospital-acquired bacteria, particularly gram-negative organisms, increases with the length of hospital stay.[6] The planning of a gynecologic service should provide for outpatient diagnostic studies, if possible, to enable brief preoperative hospitalization before elective operation.

Many commonly employed operating room rituals to prevent infection cannot be demonstrated to be effective. Cruse evaluated many techniques, and his study had some unexpected findings.[10] The care of the surgeon's hands did not constitute an important factor in wound infections. Also, the infection rate following clean surgery was no different whether a providone-iodine, hexachlorophene, or chlorhexidine scrub was used. Surprisingly, there was also no increased infection rate when the surgeon's gloves were punctured doing the operation. Some aspects of patient care were found to be beneficial. A preoperative shower by the patient with hexachlorophene lowered the infection rate. The elimination of razor-shaving the patient's abdomen the night before the operation reduced the number of postoperative infections,[10] and this has been confirmed by Seropian and Reynolds.[36] Adhesive plastic skin drapes were associated with a higher wound infection rate than linen drapes.[10] The use of electrocautery was associated with a higher infection rate, and routine drainage of a wound also increases the risk of infection.[10] These observations in clean surgical cases suggest that all these procedures should be abandoned by the gynecologic surgeon. In contrast, there are recent studies that demonstrate a benefit with some ancillary procedures. In operations on obese women, closed suction drainage through a separate stab wound is associated with a lower infection rate.[37] T-tube closed suction drainage of the vaginal cuff after hysterectomy reduces the number of postoperative pelvic infections.[38]

Prophylactic Antibiotics

This strategy of care has a dramatic effect upon the postoperative infection rate. This is particularly true in the case of vaginal hysterectomy and is the reason that two recent studies have emphasized the relative safety of the vaginal approach as compared with the abdominal.[39, 40] In addition to vaginal hysterectomy, prophylactic antibiotics have been employed in tubal ligation, reconstructive tubal surgery, abdominal hysterectomy, and the more extensive oncologic operations. The guidelines for the use of prophylactic antibiotics have been detailed in Chapter 7 on antibiotics.

Patient Factors

Factors in postoperative infection rates in soft tissue that are important but difficult to measure are the social class of the patient and the operative skill of the surgeon. Some gynecologic studies indicate that the postoperative infection rate is higher on a clinic service.[2] It is probably true that the nutritional status of the patient plays a role in the differences. In addition, it was noted by Richardson and associates that careful attention to operative techniques can have a dramatic impact on the postoperative morbidity rate.[41]

COMMON SITES OF PRE- AND POST-OPERATIVE INFECTIONS

Respiratory Problems

Preoperative respiratory disabilities should be ascertained and correlated, if possible, before operation. To date, I am unaware of any controlled study demonstrating any benefit from preoperative respiratory care on a gynecologic service, but I have no question of its benefit. In a society with widespread urban air pollution and many cigarette smokers, a careful preoperative evaluation of the respiratory tract is important. A history of smoking or the finding of rales or wheezing on examination is an indication for a preoperative arterial pO_2 determination. If it is low, appropriate respiratory therapy, with diminishment of smoking, postural drainage, and intermittent positive-pressure breathing, can improve preoperative respiratory function. This is especially important in the older, debilitated patient who is a candidate for an extensive pelvic operation.

Urinary Tract Infections

A common site of postoperative infection in gynecologic patients is the urinary tract, usually because of the patient's inability to void and the necessity for long-term drainage of the bladder with a urethral catheter. The catheter creates around itself an easily traversed avenue for potentially dangerous microorganisms that normally reside on the female perineum to enter the urinary tract. In addition, the collected urine is an excellent culture medium for any microbes contaminating the collecting system. Many modifications of the indwelling urethral catheter system have been made to decrease the risk of ascending urinary tract infection. A closed drainage system seems to decrease the incidence of urinary infection, and acceptable commercial systems are available.[42]

One alternative to the transurethral catheter is a transabdominal suprapubic catheter system. A number of evaluations demonstrated a decrease in the rate of postoperative urinary tract bacteriuria when a suprapubic catheter was used.[43, 44] An alternative approach, widely used by practicing gynecologists, is systemic prophylactic chemotherapy to prevent urinary tract infection in patients with catheters in place. One study has demonstrated systemic antibiotics to be effective, utilizing antibiotics with limited activity outside of the urinary tract.[45]

DIAGNOSIS AND TREATMENT

Onset of Fever Within 48 Hours After Operation

The early onset of fever following a gynecologic operation presents a difficult diagnostic problem for the physician. A major concern is sepsis, and the usual response is to search for both the site of infection and the organisms involved. Identification of the organism recovered on blood culture usually is not available for two to three days, and clinical findings that locate the site of infection at this early stage may be vague or absent. A rational approach to diagnosis in these patients requires some knowledge of the possible causes of early elevations in temperature.

CONTAMINATED INTRAVENOUS INFUSION

A major concern in these patients is the possibility of a contaminated intravenous infusion. This occurs infrequently, but when it does it provides a continuous source of microbiologic stress for the patient if the contamination of the intravenous infusion is not recognized and the patient continues to receive it. Very little contaminated solution needs to be infused for symptoms to appear. Sack demonstrated sepsis and endotoxic shock in a series of patients who each received a few milliliters of a common source of contaminated intravenous barbiturate for the induction of anesthesia.[46]

A number of diagnostic and therapeutic steps should be followed in patients who are suspected of having an infection from a contaminated intravenous infusion. The intravenous bottle should be inspected under adequate lighting for cracks, and the solution should be inspected for cloudiness. A portion of the intravenous fluid from the bottle and tubing should be spread on a slide, allowed to dry, and a Gram stain applied. The presence of bacteria on microscopic examination is diagnostic, and the staining characteristics of the organisms should aid the physician in the initial selection of antibiotics. The tubing and intravenous bottle should be changed in every patient with early onset of pyrexia, and separate specimens for culture should be obtained from the tubing and bottles. One nationwide epidemic of bloodstream infections related to contaminated intravenous fluids was eventually traced to contaminated caps on intravenous bottles manufactured at a single plant.[47]

Confirmation of the diagnosis of contaminated intravenous fluids occurs with the recovery of organisms in the microbiology laboratory. Frequently, uncommon pathogens (*Erwinia, Enterobacter cloacae,* and *Pseudomonas stutzeri*) that are less susceptible to commonly used antibiotics are discovered.[47] This syndrome of contaminated intravenous fluid can be fatal, particularly in the elderly debilitated patient. Prompt resolution of the sepsis usually can be brought about by early recognition of the syndrome, the immediate discontinuation of the contaminated infusion, and the administration of bacterial agents such as carbenicillin and gentamicin in separate bottles. Steroids can also be administered for septic shock if necessary.

Fungemia has occurred in some patients receiving hyperalimentation from contamination of the intravenous feeding. An early warning of this problem is the appearance of fungal forms in the patient's urine. If fungemia persists after the infusion has been stopped, systemic therapy with amphotericin B or ketoconazole will be necessary for cure.

EARLY ABDOMINAL WOUND INFECTIONS

Another uncommon early postoperative infection is a wound infection. Physicians need to be alert for this possibility because of the seriousness of the problem. There are two major types of early wound problems that need to be considered by the obstetrician-gynecologist. One is related to aerobic organisms such as the group A beta-hemolytic streptococci as well as the coagulase-positive staphylococci. This should be suspected in early onset wound problems in which the presentation is a copious serous drainage from the wound, an inflammation of the wound edge, and a high temperature.[48] These patients must be seen immediately and evaluated thoroughly by the physician. The wound should be opened to the fascia to be sure that it is intact, for serous drainage can be a warning sign of a wound dehiscence. If a Foley catheter is not in place, it should be inserted and dye utilized in a bladder irrigation solution to be certain there has been no unrecognized bladder injury. A portion of the serous drainage should be sent for culture and a Gram stain used on the secretions. The findings of gram-positive cocci should confirm the diagnosis, and the patient should be treated with an antibiotic like cefoxitin, which is effective against both the group A and group B beta-hemolytic streptococci and the coagulase-positive staphylococci; the latter are sometimes present in addition. If a semisynthetic penicillin other than methicillin is prescribed, high doses of penicillin G should be employed as well because of the high protein binding of the semisynthetic agents. The latter will cover *Staphylococcus,* while the former provides higher serum and tissue levels against the *Streptococcus.* These patients should be observed hourly to be sure there is no spreading of the inflamed wound edge, for this can be a sign of a synergistic necrotizing infection, which is the other serious early wound infection. In the synergistic infections, anaerobic bacteria, particularly *Clostridia,* are often involved. These are very dangerous infections because of their rapid spread and high mortality rate. Close clinical assessment is important because the early sign of rapid spread of local inflammation is followed by dusky discoloration, with a portion of the wound turning black and some vesicle formation. A common early finding is skin anesthesia. The advancing inflammatory edges must be evaluated every hour. If rapid spread is found, the patients must be taken immediately to the operating room for extensive debridement of the wound. The skin and fascia must be incised and debrided until fresh bleeding is encountered.[49]

Ureteral Damage

Another rare but serious problem of postoperative infections is related to unrecognized ureteral damage at the time of operation. If extravasation of urine occurs, these patients can have a high spiking fever early in the postoperative period. Figure 9–1 shows the postoperative temperature record of a patient who had operative damage to the ureter and required a nephrostomy and subsequent reimplantation of the ureter into the bladder. At arrow 1 the patient had a vaginal hysterectomy and received three 1-g intramuscular doses of prophylactic cephaloridine at six-hour intervals. Her bladder was inadvertently lacerated during the operation and was immediately repaired. Because of the early onset of fever and right costovertebral angle pain, an intravenous pyelogram was obtained at arrow 2; this demonstrated the spill of urine from the right ureter into the retroperitoneal space. At arrow 3 a nephrostomy was performed, and the ureter was reimplanted into the bladder. This rare complication provides additional support to the concept that antibiotic prophylaxis be limited to the day of operation. As is evident from Figure 9–1, the early temperature rise first alerted the physician to the problem. The prolonged use of systemic antibiotics as prophylaxis might have masked this patient's febrile response and delayed the correct diagnosis and the appropriate operative intervention.

Early Onset Sepsis

Specific microorganisms can be recovered from the bloodstream of patients with early onset of high postoperative fevers. The pathophysiology of these infections is predicted on the basis of the virulence and rapidly invasive properties of organisms involved. The human host has little time to react to the spread of such infections, and this fact should be acknowledged in the evaluation of patients with early postoperative elevations of temperature. There often are no localizing signs upon examination. Broad-spectrum antibiotics should be employed until

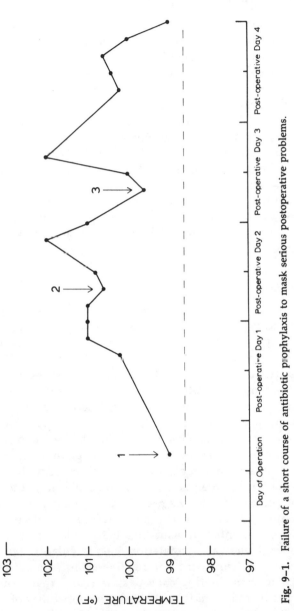

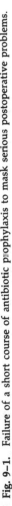

Fig. 9–1. Failure of a short course of antibiotic prophylaxis to mask serious postoperative problems.

culture results are available. This broad-spectrum coverage can be achieved with a combination of clindamycin and an aminoglycoside or the use of a second or third generation cephalosporin or one of the newer penicillins.

Unrecognized Established Infections

The sudden onset of postoperative fever can also result from the operative manipulation of the site of an asymptomatic infection that becomes symptomatic in the immediate postoperative period. This is not an uncommon situation on an urban gynecologic service, where unsuspected pelvic inflammatory disease can be present at the time an elective hysterectomy is performed. Intra- and postoperative antibiotics have usually sufficed, often a cephalosporin alone. Another clinical situation in which unexpected infection may be found is in the patient undergoing tuboplasty. Frequently these women are given perioperative prophylactic antibiotics, but despite this coverage many become febrile in the immediate postoperative period. Because of the frequent involvement of *Chlamydia* in this specific clinical situation, the use of tetracycline or doxycycline is indicated.

In addition to the genital tract, the urinary tract can be involved with early infection. This is particularly true in the patient with untreated asymptomatic bacteriuria who has a major pelvic operation and requires catheterization postoperatively. Usually, these patients present with a low-grade fever.

Intrauterine Manipulation

Another group of women who may manifest early rises in temperature in the postoperative period are those who develop pelvic infections following intrauterine manipulation. Most of these infections are not serious problems, for they usually respond to systemic antibiotics. Clinically, this is often seen on the oncology service after a radium implant and is an indication for the immediate removal of the radium and for treatment with systemic antibiotics—either a combination of clindamycin and an aminoglycoside, or a second or third generation cephalosporin, or a newer penicillin. These antibiotics cover most gram-positive and gram-negative aerobes and anaerobes but are not the best choice for infections with *Chlamydia.* Another clinical consideration is the patient who develops a pelvic infection following dilatation and curettage. The observation by Curran and co-workers of an association between abnormal uterine bleeding and positive results of endocervical culture for *Neisseria gonorrhoeae* can be a major factor in this syndrome.[18] Examination should be performed carefully to rule out the possibility of a perforation and an infected hematoma before placing complete reliance on systemic antibiotics. Unless an extrauterine mass is enlarging or the patient continues to show a drop in hematocrit reading, there is no immediate reason for a laparotomy in these women. In this clinical situation, I favor the use of agents such as clindamycin or metronidazole to cover the possibility of a *Bacteroides fragilis* infection in addition to an aminoglycoside. Occasionally, a patient fails to respond to systemic antibiotics and a laparotomy is necessary to drain or remove an infected hematoma. The operation should be limited to the site of infection. The pelvic organs can be conserved when they are not physically involved in the infectious process.

HOSPITAL-TERMINATED PREGNANCY

Early infections following termination of pregnancy in the hospital are usually not serious clinical problems. Figure 9–2 shows the febrile response of patients with an infection following termination of pregnancy and an associated bacteremia.[50] The febrile response is less than with other hospital-acquired infections. If no pelvic masses are palpated, these women can be treated with a newer cephalosporin, for example cefoxitin, or a newer penicillin, such as piperacillin or mezlocillin alone. If fever persists, a major concern should be retained secundines, and an inspection for this should be done and a curettage performed if intrauterine tissue is present.

Hospital termination of pregnancy can occasionally be associated with a serious infection manifested by early spiking fever. Sepsis, confirmed by positive results of blood culture and laboratory evidence of disseminated intravascular coagulation, has been reported following the instillation of hypertonic saline solution.[51] Severe sepsis and death have been reported following the use of hypertonic glucose and have led to the virtual abandonment of this procedure in the United States.[52] There seems to be a disproportionally higher than expected recovery of *Staphylococcus aureus* from the bloodstream of patients receiving saline infusion, and this high

HOSPITAL ACQUIRED INFECTIONS

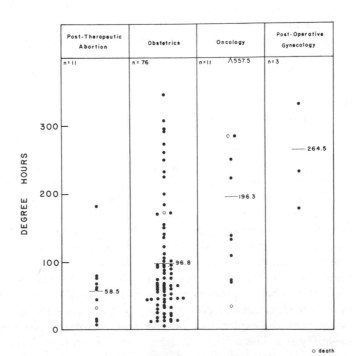

Fig. 9–2. Fever indices in degree hours of patients with bacteremia secondary to a hospital-acquired infection. The bar indicates the mean fever index for each group. (Reprinted with permission from the American College of Obstetricians and Gynecologists. From Ledger, W. J., Kriewall, T. J., and Gee, C.: The fever index. A technique for evaluating the clinical response to bacteremia. Obstet. Gynecol., 45:603, 1975.)

rate has been associated with patient mortality.[53] Treatment should include antibiotic coverage effective against this gram-positive aerobe with either one of the cephalosporins or the semisynthetic penicillins, combined with efforts to evacuate the uterus. The early onset of sepsis has not been limited to women receiving intraamniotic hypertonic injection. It has also been present in women who have had a pregnancy terminated by hysterotomy. Sepsis and intravascular coagulation followed by death seem to be more common among elderly multiparas, who will need heroic measures for cure, including multiple antibiotic coverage, steroids, and immediate laparotomy to remove the infected pelvic organs.[54] This degree of illness has led to the abandonment of this technique of termination of pregnancy in most urban medical centers.

Other attempts to terminate an unwanted pregnancy may result in an early onset of sepsis resulting from damage to the uterus or other vital organs in the peritoneal cavity. The initiating event is uterine perforation, and the unrecognized operative damage sets the stage for serious postoperative illness, which may take a number of forms. This is particularly dangerous in women who are more than 12 weeks pregnant.[55] There may be lateral uterine perforation, with laceration of a uterine vessel and subsequent infection of a hematoma of a broad ligament. Operative intervention is essential for these patients, because infected hematomas are usually not perfused by systemically administered antibiotics.[56] Another type of serious operative damage occurs when a suction aspirator is unknowingly placed through the uterine wall and the suction causes bowel damage. The peritoneal cavity has an efficient system of reaction to bacterial insult, but it is unable to tolerate continued fecal contamination. If there is a suggestion of perforation by a suction aspirator when suction is applied or if a patient shows signs of sepsis in the immediate postsuction curettage period, with point tenderness and rebound tenderness, then abdominal exploration with close inspection of the large and small bowel is indicated. Anaerobes make up the majority of large bowel bacteria, and this should be a factor in the selection of antibiotics for these patients.

RESPIRATORY TRACT

The respiratory tract is a common source of early postoperative fevers. Atelectasis is not uncommon in postoperative gynecologic patients, particularly following an abdominal surgical approach. These patients typically are febrile (although their temperatures are usually not above 101° F orally), have a tachycardia, and frequently have a low pO_2 on arterial blood sampling.[57, 58] Usually, basilar rales can be heard on auscultation of the chest, but roentgenogram examination shows no abnormal findings. This febrile condition does not require systemic antibiotics for resolution. It responds to maneuvers designed to increase deep inspiration and to clear the upper respiratory tract of the retained secretions. Most of the early temperature elevations in gynecologic patients have been attributed to atelectasis. This has been the explanation for the large number of posthysterectomy patients who satisfy the classic obstetric definition of febrile morbidity but do not require systemic antibiotics to become afebrile. Prophylactic antibiotics can influence this temperature response, for some studies of vaginal[59] and abdominal hysterectomy[60] have shown a reduction in the incidence of standard temperature morbidity when perioperative prophylaxis was used. Other sites of infection should be considered by the physician if the temperature elevation persists beyond the first 48 hours postoperatively. In elderly debilitated patients who have undergone extensive operative procedures, particularly those on the oncology service, more complicated respiratory care, including intermittent positive-pressure breathing, may be helpful, although the benefits of this maneuver in gynecologic patients have not been proved by prospective study.

A temperature elevation above 101° F orally and more extensive pulmonary findings than those of atelectasis on auscultation should alert the examining physician to the possibility of aspiration pneumonia or massive atelectasis caused by improper placement of the endotracheal tube. Figure 9–3 shows the chest x-ray of a woman with a high fever in the immediate postoperative period in whom the endotracheal tube was improperly placed throughout the operation. If there is extensive pulmonary involvement, antibiotics such as penicillin or erythromycin should be used in addition to supportive pulmonary care. Aspiration pneumonia occurs infrequently in gynecologic patients; it is a more common problem following major operations in obstetric patients. In addition, a massive pulmonary embolism can occur in the immediate postoperative period, indicated by a temperature elevation as well as respiratory distress.

Onset of Fever Later than 48 Hours After Operation

The fevers that develop more than 48 hours after operation are the most important for the physician to understand. The largest number of patients with postoperative infections who require antibiotics first manifest infection several days after operation, even though the operation is usually the initiating factor. Most of the bacterial pathogens involved in the infection are endogenous and do not have the pathogenicity of group A beta-hemolytic streptococci. A period of

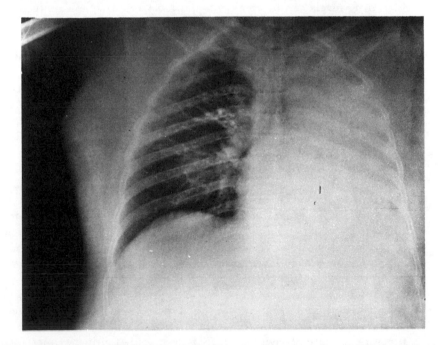

Fig. 9–3. Total collapse of left lung as a result of improper placement of an endotracheal tube during operative procedure.

incubation for bacterial multiplication is needed before the patient's symptoms become evident. Recognition of the operation as the initiating event is crucial to the care of patients with these infections.

URINARY TRACT

A common site of infection during postoperative hospitalization is the urinary tract. The factors involved in the appearance of these infections have been noted previously. The ready accessibility of urine because of indwelling catheter drainage permits reliance on culture for diagnosis. The principles of diagnosis and care of postoperative urinary tract infections are simple but are often not followed by physicians. Diagnosis should be based on the finding of bacteria in the immediate microscopic examination of freshly obtained urine or on the positive results of a culture. One recent study showed that less than 10^5 bacteria in the urine of women with an indwelling catheter was indicative of a subsequent infection.[61] Both red and white blood cells may occasionally be seen in the urine of a woman following operative trauma to the bladder wall. Upper urinary tract symptoms, in particular costovertebral angle tenderness, can never be ignored in a postoperative patient. The tenderness may reflect ureteral damage or obstruction, and an intravenous pyelogram (IVP) or ultrasonographic examination should be done. These studies are also valuable to perform in a patient who maintains a prolonged postoperative temperature in the 100° to 102° F range with no evidence of a pelvic infection on examination. If the results of these studies are normal and ureteral and bladder integrity is maintained, the gynecologist can initiate antimicrobial care for the urinary tract infection. The physician's task is eased by a number of favorable considerations. Most antibacterial agents are concentrated in the urine so that high drug levels can be achieved, and most microorganisms recovered from gynecologic patients with hospital-acquired urinary tract infections are not highly resistant to these agents. In addition, only a small percentage of gynecologic patients have a history of repeated urinary tract infections after multiple treatment with antimicrobial agents.

With all of the aforementioned factors in mind, successful treatment of significant bacteriuria in the postoperative gynecologic patient can usually be accomplished by administration of agents such as the sulfas or the nitrofurans. There are a number of advantages to such therapy. The rate of success is equivalent to that reported with the administration of more powerful systemic agents such as ampicillin or a cephalosporin. The limited activity of the sulfas or nitrofurans outside the urinary tract prevents the masking of symptoms of a postoperative infection in the pelvis or in an abdominal wound and the delay in recognition until after the patient has been discharged from the hospital. More important, this restricts the use of more powerful systemic antibiotic agents on the gynecology service and eases the pressure towards the selection of resistant microorganisms. A treatment regimen of 10 days is given. If there is still significant bacterial growth on urine culture after two days of therapy, the susceptibility pattern of the recovered organisms should be evaluated and alteration in therapy made on this basis. Finally, results of a culture should be obtained a few days after the cessation of therapy. This conservative antibiotic treatment should not be adhered to in the care of patients with a history of repeated urinary tract infections while receiving antimicrobial care or in oncologic patients; these patients frequently have more resistant microorganisms and may require powerful systemic antibiotics.

THIRD DAY SURGICAL FEVER

One disease of medical progress seen during postoperative hospitalization has been described by Altemeier and associates as the third day surgical fever.[62] As the name implies, it is manifested by a high spiking fever on about the third postoperative day in a patient who has undergone an extensive surgical procedure and is still receiving intravenous fluids. The sepsis is secondary to invasion of the bloodstream by normal microorganisms of the skin that have passed through the fluid-reactive material around the plastic intravenous line into the blood. The diagnosis can be suspected in any patient who has had an indwelling intravenous catheter in place for 48 hours or longer and has a tender inflamed superficial vein proximal to the intravenous line. The basis of therapy is removal of the catheter. Culture of fluid obtained from the catheter tip and of blood from an alternate venous site should be performed. Antibiotics are usually not necessary, for these patients become afebrile and asymptomatic when the intravenous catheter is removed. This disease is preventable and is the result of a cavalier attitude toward the principles of surgical antisepsis in the care of an indwelling intravenous line.

Insertion of a large bore intravenous line to ensure massive fluid infusion during operation is the usual cause of third day surgical fever. Since there is no plan for long-term intravenous feeding, insertion of the line follows principles of skin antisepsis used in the past for ordinary intravenous infusion. When the physician responsible for postoperative care decides to continue to utilize this intravenous line, the patient's symptoms will often appear on the third or fourth day after operation. The key to therapy is prevention, which can take one of two forms. In the preoperative patient in whom prolonged postoperative intravenous feeding is contemplated, the indwelling intravenous catheter should be inserted with strict adherence to surgical antisepsis. The most simple preventive measure is to prohibit the use of intravenous lines for longer than 48 hours after operation.[63] Two recent studies showed no advantage when these intravenous lines were changed every 24 hours as compared with every 48 hours.[64, 65] If these guidelines are followed, this syndrome will be eliminated. If they are not followed or an infected superficial phlebitis is present in spite of them, removal of the intravenous catheter is often sufficient for cure. A smear of the exudate from the skin around the entry site of the catheter should provide hints for the initial selection of antibiotics before results of culture are available. Because of concern about the coagulase-positive staphylococci, a cephalosporin or a semisynthetic penicillin should be used for therapy.

ABDOMINAL WOUNDS

Abdominal wound infections are usually diagnosed during postoperative hospitalization. Wound hemostasis, the quantity of bacterial contamination, and the amount of foreign material left in the wound determine whether a postoperative wound infection will develop. The infection rates of clean versus contaminated field operations vary widely (Table 9–1).[1] With these probabilities in mind, it is difficult to support the use of a running subcuticular stitch to close the abdominal wound in a clean contaminated field of operation such as is found in an abdominal hysterectomy. This type of closure prevents egress of serum from the wound in the immediate postoperative period and makes drainage difficult if it becomes necessary later on. One study of postappendectomy wound closure showed the

Table 9–1. Rates of Infection in Clean and Contaminated Operative Fields

Surgical Procedure	Total No. of Cases	Wound Infections	Percentage
Clean operative field			
Adnexal operation	257	12	4.7
Herniorrhaphy	259	11	4.2
Contaminated operative field			
Total abdominal hysterectomy	337	35	10.4
Colectomy	98	32	32.7

(From Ledger, W. J., Reite, A. M., and Headington, J. T.: The surveillance of infection of an inpatient gynecologic service. Am. J. Obstet. Gynecol., *113*:662, 1972.)

highest incidence of postoperative infection when a subcuticular closure was used.[66] Most wound infections are seen four to ten days postoperatively and should be suspected in any febrile postoperative patient who has no evidence of infection in the pelvis or urinary tract on examination.

The clinical evidence of wound infection is an inflamed wound edge or a purulent exudate on a wound dressing. The key to therapy is adequate drainage, which requires opening the wound to the level of the fascia to be sure this layer has remained intact. Results of aerobic and anaerobic cultures of the exudate should be obtained. They may add little to the care of individual patients, but they do provide important microbiologic information if a common source of contamination is suspected when there has been a high frequency of wound infection. A portion of the wound exudate should be Gram stained and examined to determine the predominant microbial forms. Systemic antibiotics are usually not necessary. The exception is in the patient who demonstrates spreading induration and inflammation of the wound edge. Often these infections are caused by a mixture of a coagulase-positive staphylococci and other organisms. For the patient with induration and inflammation of the wound edge, it is important to utilize an antibiotic that is effective against coagulase-positive staphylococci, such as a cephalosporin, to achieve cure. In some instances, the infection is accompanied by thrombosis of vessels that supply the skin, and cure can be achieved only by wide surgical incision of the infected area until normal vascularity is seen.[49] There is increasing evidence that anaerobes can be recovered from infected wounds in gynecologic patients. The role of systemic antibiotics in the treatment of these patients has not been established. The mainstay of care is adequate drainage.

In addition to the care of patients with infections, the physician must be aware of the danger these patients represent to others on the operative service, particularly preoperative patients who can become colonized before elective operation. Women with infected open wounds shed large quantities of bacteria and may be the source of spread to other patients by contact with the medical staff. Some form of isolation is necessary, and the medical staff must wash hands and change gowns before other patients are seen. If a group A beta-hemolytic *Streptococcus,* a coagulase-positive *Straphylococcus,* or *Pseudomonas aeruginosa* is recovered from the wound, isolation should be strictly maintained until culture results from exudate of the open wound are no longer positive. These organisms are easily spread from patient to patient and can be the source of an epidemic of hospital-acquired infection. Most wounds granulate and close by secondary intention, but occasionally a secondary closure can be performed later.

POSTOPERATIVE PELVIC INFECTIONS

Postoperative pelvic infections are common sequelae of hysterectomy. They are not unexpected, for a portion of an abdominal hysterectomy and the entire vaginal hysterectomy are performed in a microbiologically contaminated field—the vagina. The presence of bacterial flora of the vagina and of devitalized tissue and blood products is conducive to the establishment of a soft tissue infection in the pelvis. The frequency of these problems after vaginal hysterectomy has been dramatically reduced by the use of prophylactic antibiotics and the immediate postoperative use of closed suction T-tube drainage. Soft tissue infections take many forms. If the patient has a collection of contaminated material in the vaginal cuff, she usually becomes febrile 48 hours or longer after the operation and complains of a sense of fullness in the lower abdomen. On examination, an infected, often foul-smelling hematoma is readily evacuated and this procedure usually suffices for cure. More frequently, material is obtained by probing the vaginal cuff and there is marked induration of the pelvis on examination. The diagnosis is pelvic cellulitis, and patients are treated with systemic antibiotics. A number of alternative initial antibiotic regimens can be used with equal success. Most commonly, I have employed a combination of clindamycin and an aminoglycoside, usually gentamicin. Alternatively, the second and the third generation cephalosporins or a newer penicillin can be given alone.

SEPTIC PELVIC THROMBOPHLEBITIS AND PELVIC ABSCESS

In patients who remain febrile despite adequate antibiotic coverage, septic pelvic thrombophlebitis, a pelvic abscess, or unrecognized operative damage to a ureter should be considered. Reexamination is indicated, and if no pelvic mass is palpated or found on ultrasonography and the ureters are normal, a tentative clinical diagnosis is septic pelvic thrombophlebitis.[67] This is an uncommon clinical diagnosis in the 1980s, and I believe this is because of greater awareness of anaerobic bacteria and early use of antibiotics that are effective against these organisms[68] when the diagnosis is made clinically. It is wise to obtain results of a pretreatment screening test of clotting time, but a better and more productive measure is the partial thromboplastin time (PTT). A constant infusion of heparin by pump, beginning at 1000 U per hour with increment added on the basis of the PTT, is the preferred method of therapy in postoperative patients who have the potential for serious bleeding from the site of incision. The PTT should be maintained at a level two to two-and-a-half times above normal. This incremental addition of heparin is important, for patients have varying requirements for this agent, which may be related to the discovery that *Bacteroides* produces heparinase in the laboratory.[69] Clinically, patients usually respond dramatically to heparin, becoming afebrile within 36 to 48 hours[70] (Figure 9–4). At arrow 1 the patient whose temperature is shown in Figure 9–4 had a vaginal hysterectomy. At arrow 2 the diagnosis of pelvic cellulitis was made in this patient, who was allergic to penicillin. After she failed to respond to chloramphenicol, heparin was added to the regimen at arrow 3, and her temperature dropped dramatically.

Surgical intervention by inferior vena cava and ovarian vein ligation is reserved for the patient who has continued pulmonary emboli despite adequate anticoagulation. This procedure is rarely performed on our service. If the patient remains febrile despite adequate treatment, this usually indicates the presence of a pelvic abscess that requires operative intervention (Figure 9–5).[70] Many abscesses are

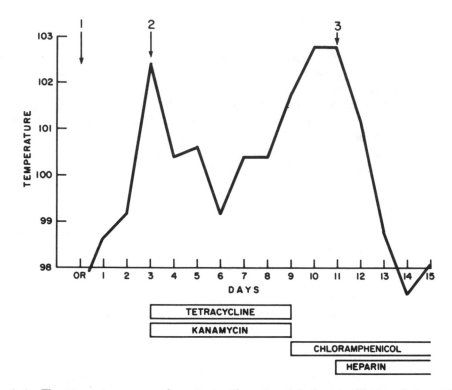

Fig. 9–4. The temperature course of a patient with septic pelvic thrombophlebitis. (Ledger, W. J.: Infections in obstetrics and gynecology: New developments in treatment. Surg. Clin. North Am., *52*:1447, 1972.)

amenable to vaginal drainage, and it is likely that many postoperative adnexal abscesses have been managed this way in the past.[2] Often, the pelvic mass is palpated high in the pelvis, and a laparotomy is indicated for removal of these abscesses.[19]

DRUG FEVER

A noninfectious cause of persistent postoperative fever is reaction to drugs. In gynecologic patients, this should be suspected in the patient with a persistent fever and no clinical evidence of a site of infection. A differential blood count can show an eosinophilia, but this is usually not present. When a trial without antibiotics is carried out, patients almost always are clinically better within 48 hours.[71]

Late Manifestations of Postoperative Infections

Some of the most serious postoperative infections in gynecologic patients are not obvious during their initial hospitalization,[19, 72] and the patients may have no immediate postoperative fever (Figure 9–6),[19] or alternatively they may seemingly have responded rapidly to the initial selection of antibiotics (Figure 9–7).[19] At arrow 1 the patient whose temperature is recorded in Figure 9–7 underwent a vaginal hysterectomy. At arrow 2 sulfisoxizole was prescribed for a suspected urinary tract infection. At arrow 3 the clinical diagnosis of pelvic cellulitis was made, and the patient was treated with intravenous cephalothin. At arrow 4 a

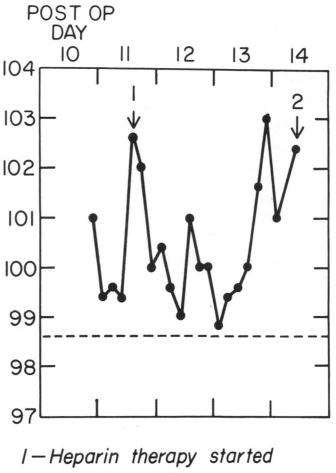

POST OP DAY

1 — Heparin therapy started

2 — Laparotomy — bilateral salpingo — oophorectomy

Fig. 9–5. The failure of the temperature of a patient with a postoperative adnexal abscess to respond to heparin. At arrow 1 heparin therapy was initiated. At arrow 2 a bilateral salpingo-oophorectomy was performed. (Ledger, W. J., and Peterson, E. P.: The use of heparin in the management of pelvic thrombophlebitis. Surg. Gynecol. Obstet., *131*:1115, 1970.)

collection of fluid was drained from the vaginal cuff. After this, this initial hospital course seemed uncomplicated. She was subsequently readmitted with an adnexal abscess. Other factors that may cause a postoperative patient to require read-mission to the hospital are early discharge from the hospital (on the fourth or fifth day following a major operation) and the early use of antibiotics that mask symptoms but do not eradicate the infection. A number of sites of infection can be implicated in these patients. An abdominal wound infection may not become clinically manifest until the patient has left the hospital and been home for a few days. Careful drainage of the wound is needed, but if the fascia is intact the patient can be managed as an outpatient. This discovery of late infection is not

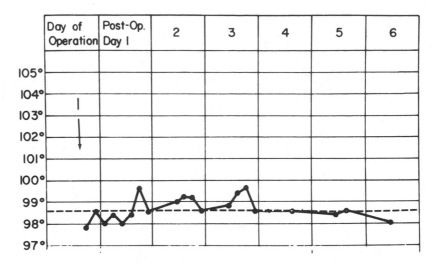

Fig. 9–6. No immediate postoperative febrile morbidity in a patient who later developed an adnexal abscess. (Ledger, W. J., Campbell, C., and Willson, J. R.: Postoperative adnexal infections. Obstet. Gynecol., *31*:83, 1968.)

uncommon. One study of antibiotic prophylaxis in patients undergoing abdominal hysterectomy showed that 19% of the recorded postoperative infections were first diagnosed after discharge from the hospital.[73]

POSTOPERATIVE ADNEXAL ABSCESS

The most serious late postoperative infection complication is the postoperative adnexal abscess. Figure 9–8 documents the time sequence of a series of complications from adnexal abscesses in women patients before prophylactic antibiotics became available.[72] Patients with adnexal abscesses often have a palpable mass high in the pelvis, an indication for immediate removal. However, in the majority of these febrile patients no mass can be palpated and administration of systemic antibiotics can be begun. The frequent isolation of *Bacteroides fragilis* from these sites of infection makes it imperative to use clindamycin, cefoxitin, mezlocillin, or metronidazole. An adnexal abscess is ideally diagnosed by ultrasonography, which can delineate a cystic mass not apparent on pelvic examination. The presence of a mass or the patient's failure to respond to antibiotics, as evidenced by persistent spiking fever, is an indication for laparotomy to remove the abscess.

PELVIC CELLULITIS

Readmission to the hospital for a persistent pelvic infection that is not amenable to operation may be necessary. Patients may have widespread pelvic cellulitis with anaerobic organisms, particularly *Bacteroides fragilis,* and these infections can take a long time to resolve. Sometimes patients have an associated septic pelvic thrombophlebitis that requires heparin therapy for resolution. Occasionally, a diffuse "woody" induration, ligneous cellulitis, is seen. Patients with this condition have widespread pelvic induration and continue to run low grade fevers. They seem to be responsive to adrenal steroids in phamacologic doses.[74] Ligneous cellulitis is infrequently diagnosed; we have not seen it in the past five years at New York Hospital-Cornell Medical Center.

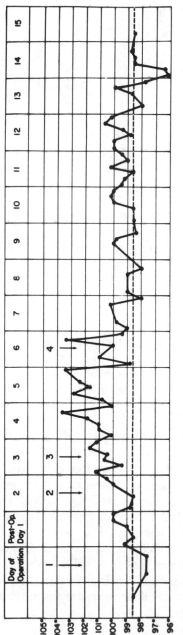
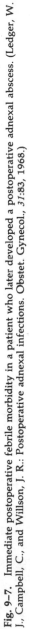

Fig. 9–7.   Immediate postoperative febrile morbidity in a patient who later developed a postoperative adnexal abscess. (Ledger, W. J., Campbell, C., and Willson, J. R.: Postoperative adnexal infections. Obstet. Gynecol., *31*:83, 1968.)

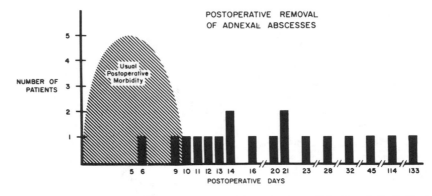

Fig. 9–8. The late onset of postoperative adnexal abscesses. (Ledger, W. J., Campbell, C., Taylor, D., and Willson, J. R.: Adnexal abscess as a late complication of pelvic operations. Surg. Gynecol. Obstet., *129*:973, 1969.)

HEPATITIS

Serum hepatitis may result from injection of contaminated blood and will not become manifest until late in the postoperative period.[75] Most of the attack on this problem has been directed toward prevention, with restricted use of blood and better screening of donors with specific tests to detect carriers of the hepatitis B virus.[32] Despite these measures, blood transfusion will still be needed on occasion, and in some situations hepatitis due to A, B, or nonA–nonB types will occur. Liver function tests should be obtained in patients in whom this diagnosis is suspected.

Another late complication causing persistent fever is "halothane" hepatitis. Frequently, the history of more than one recent induction of anesthesia can be elicited, particularly for the still common conization-hysterectomy sequence. In patients suspected of having this diagnosis, liver function tests should be done.

CYTOMEGALOVIRUS INFECTION

A late complication of hospitalization for gynecologic problems is the development of fever due to cytomegalovirus infection. The patient usually presents several days or weeks after discharge with a spiking fever pattern. Typically, there are no localizing signs of infection and no evidence of a pelvic abscess or an abdominal wound infection on examination. The diagnosis can be confirmed by serial testing of the blood for the presence of antibodies to cytomegalovirus. Although this syndrome has been most frequently seen in patients who have received multiple units of blood, one recent study reported this finding in a patient who had received only one unit of blood during the initial hospitalization.[76] Once the diagnosis is made, the management is expectant. If antibiotics were ordered for this patient at the time of readmission, they can be discontinued.

OSTEOMYELITIS PUBIS

Late developing infections of the symphysis pubis can be seen in women following gynecologic operations. Most frequently they follow suprapubic operations for correction of stress incontinence in which sutures are placed in the symphysis to elevate the urethrovesical junction. Recently, these infections have also been reported in patients following radical gynecologic surgery.[77] In the study, symptoms did not appear until 8 to 17 weeks after the operation. These women present with pubic bone tenderness, avoidance of ambulation, and pain on deduction and abduction. Radiographs often show bone changes. Broad-spectrum antibiotic coverage that is effective against coagulase-positive staphylococci, anaerobes, and gram-negative aerobes should be given for 2 to 4 weeks intravenously, followed by oral antibiotics. In some cases, debridement will be needed for cure.

REFERENCES

1. Ledger, W.J., Reite, A.M., and Headington, J.T.: The surveillance of infection of an inpatient gynecologic service. Am. J. Obstet. Gynecol., *113*:662, 1972.
2. Hall, W.L., Sobel, A.I., Jones, C.P., and Parker, R.J.: Anaerobic postoperative pelvic infections. Obstet. Gynecol., *30*:1, 1967.
3. Ledger, W.J., and Child, M.: The hospital care of patients undergoing hysterectomy. An analysis of 12,026 patients from the Professional Activity Study. Am. J. Obstet. Gynecol., *117*:423, 1973.
4. Eickhoff, T.C., Brachman, P.S., Bennett, J.V., and Brown, J.F.: Surveillance of nosocomial infections in community hospitals: I. Surveillance methods, effectiveness, and initial results. J. Infect. Dis., *120*:305, 1969.
5. Thoburn, R., Fekety, F.R., Jr., Cluff, L.E., and Melvin, V.B.: Infections acquired by hospitalized patients. Arch. Intern. Med., *121*:1, 1968.
6. Pollack, M., Charache, P., Nieman, R.E., Jett, M.P., Reinhardt, J.A., and Hardy, P.H., Jr.: Factors influencing colinisation and antibiotic resistant patterns of gram negative bacteria in hospital patients. Lancet, *2*:668, 1972.
7. Bruce, D.L., and Wingard, D.W.: Anesthesia and the immune response. Anesthesiology, *34*:271, 1971.
8. Green, S.L., and Sarubbi, F.A.: Risk factors associated with postcesarean section Febrile morbidity. Obstet. Gynecol., *49*:686, 1977.
9. Burke, J.F.: The effective period of preventive antibiotic action in experimental incisions and dermal lesions. Surgery, *50*:161, 1961.
10. Cruse, P.: Wound infection surveillance. Rev. Infect. Dis., *3*:734, 1981.
11. Maki, D.G., Alvarado, C.J., Hassemer, C.A., and Zilz, M.A.: Relation of the inanimate hospital environment to endemic nosocomial infection. N. Engl. J. Med., *307*:1562, 1982.
12. Polk, H.C., and Miles, A.A.: Enhancement of bacterial infection by ferric iron: Kinetics, mechanisms, and surgical significance. Surgery, *70*:71, 1971.
13. Bornside, G.H., and Cohn, I.: Hemoglobin as a bacterial virulence enhancing factor in fluids produced in strangulation intestinal obstruction. Am. Surg., *34*:63, 1968.
14. Mead, P.B.: Cervical-vaginal flora of women with invasive cervical cancer. Obstet. Gynecol., *52*:601, 1978.
15. Malinak, L.R., Jeffrey, R.A., Jr., and Dunn, W.J.: Conization-hysterectomy time interval: A clinical and pathologic study. Obstet. Gynecol., *23*:317, 1964.
16. Orr, J.W., Jr., Shingleton, H.M., Hatch, K.D., Mann, W.J., Jr., Austin, J.M., Jr., and Soong, S-J.: Correlation of perioperative morbidity and conization to radical hysterectomy interval. Obstet. Gynecol., *59*:726, 1982.
17. Burkman, R.T., Tonascia, J.A., Atienza, M.F., and King, T.M.: Untreated endocervical gonorrhea and endometritis following elective abortion. Am. J. Obstet. Gynecol., *126*:648, 1976.
18. Curran, J.W., Rendtorff, R.C., Chandler, R.W., Wiser, W.L., and Robinson, H.: Female gonorrhea: Its relation to abnormal uterine bleeding, urinary tract symptoms, and cervicitis. Obstet. Gynecol., *45*:195, 1975.
19. Ledger, W.J., Campbell, C., and Willson, J.R.: Postoperative adnexal infections. Obstet. Gynecol., *31*:83, 1968.
20. Smith, M.R., and Soderstrom, R.: Salpingitis: A frequent response to intrauterine contraception. J. Reprod. Med., *16*:159, 1976.
21. Badra, P.L., Young, J.R., Laros, R.K., Jr., and Peterson, E.P.: Suppurative salpingitis after laparoscopic tubal cauterization. Obstet. Gynecol., *42*:511, 1973.
22. Garibaldi, R.A., Brodine, S., and Matsumiya, S.: Infections among patients in nursing homes. N. Engl. J. Med., *305*:731, 1981.
23. McIntyre, D.M.: An epidemic of *Streptococcus pyogenes* puerperal and postoperative sepsis with an unusual carrier site—the anus. Am. J. Obstet. Gynecol., *101*:308, 1968.
24. Dineen, P., and Drusin, L.: Epidemics of postoperative wound infections associated with hair carriers. Lancet, *2*:1157, 1973.
25. Speers, R., Jr., Bernard, H., O'Grady, F., and Shooter, R.A.: Increased dispersal of skin bacteria into the air after shower-baths. Lancet, *1*:478, 1965.

26. Donowitz, L.G., Marsike, F.J., Hoyt, J.W., and Wenzel, R.P.: *Serratia marcescens* bacteremia from contaminated pressure transducers. J.A.M.A., *242*:1749, 1979.
27. Martone, W.J., Osterman, C.A., Fisher, K.A., and Wenzel, R.P.: *Pseudomonas cepacia:* Implications and control of epidemic nosocomial colonization. Rev. Infect. Dis., *3*:708, 1981.
28. Remington, J.S., and Schimpff, S.C.: Please don't eat the salads. N. Engl. J. Med., *304*:433, 1981.
29. Haley, C.E., Cohen, M.L., Halter, J., and Meyer, R.D.: Nosocomial Legionnaires' disease: A continuing common-source epidemic at Wadsworth Medical Center. Ann. Intern. Med., *90*:583, 1979.
30. Semmelweis, I.P.: Die Aetiologie, der Bergriff und die Prophylaxis des Kindbettfiebers Pest. Vienne-Leipzig, C.A. Hartlebeu's Verlags Expedition, 1961.
31. Mulligan, M.E., Rolfe, R.D., Finegold, S.M., and George, W.L.: Contamination of a hospital environment by *Clostridium difficile.* Curr. Microbiol., *3*:173, 1979.
32. Goldfield, M., Black, H.C., Bill, J., Srihongse, S., and Pizzuti, W.: The consequences of administering blood pretested for HBs Ag by third generation techniques: A progress report. Am. J. Med. Sci., *270*:335, 1975.
33. Drew, W.L., Mintz, L., Miner, R.C., Sands, M., and Ketterer, B.: Prevalence of cytomegalovirus infection in homosexual men. J. Infect. Dis., *143*:188, 1981.
34. Curran, J.W., Lawrence, D.N., Jaffe, H., Kaplan, J.E., Zyla, L.D., Chamberland, M., Weinstein, R., Lui, K-J., Schonberger, L.B., Spira, T.J., Alexander, W.J., Swinger, G., Ammann, A., Solomon, S., Auerbach, D., Mildvan, D., Stoneburner, R., Jason, J.M., Haverkos, H.W., and Evatt, B.L.: Acquired immunodeficiency syndrome (AIDS) associated with transfusions. N. Engl. J. Med., *310*:69, 1984.
35. England, G.T., Randall, H.W., and Graves, W.L.: Impairment of tissue defenses by vasoconstrictors in vaginal hysterectomies. Obstet. Gynecol., *61*:271, 1983.
36. Seropian, R., and Reynolds, B.M.: Wound infections after pre-operative depilatory versus razor preparation. Am. J. Surg., *121*:251, 1971.
37. Morrow, C.P., Hernandez, W.L., Townsend, D.E., and Disaia, P.J.: Pelvic celiotomy in the obese patient. Am. J. Obstet. Gynecol., *127*:335, 1977.
38. Swartz, W.H., and Tanaree, P.: T-tube suction drainage and/or prophylactic antibiotics. Obstet. Gynecol., *47*:665, 1976.
39. Shapiro, M., Munoz, A., Tager, I.B., Schoenbaum, S.C., and Polk, B.F.: Risk factors for infection at the operative site after abdominal or vaginal hysterectomy. N. Engl. J. Med., *307*:1661, 1982.
40. Dicker, R.C., Greenspan, J.R., Strauss, L.T., Cowart, M.R., Scally, M.J., Peterson, H.B., DeStefano, F., Rubin, G.L., and Ory, H.W.: Complications of abdominal and vaginal hysterectomy among women of reproductive age in the United States. Am. J. Obstet. Gynecol., *144*:841, 1982.
41. Richardson, A.C., Lyon, J.B., and Graham, E.E.: Abdominal hysterectomy: Relationship between morbidity and surgical technique. Am. J. Obstet. Gynecol., *115*:953, 1973.
42. Kunin, C.M., and McCormack, R.C.: Prevention of catheter-induced urinary tract infections by sterile closed drainage. N. Engl. J. Med., *274*:1155, 1966.
43. van Nagell, J.R., Jr., Penny, R.M., Jr., and Roddick, J.W., Jr.: Suprapubic bladder drainage following radical hysterectomy. Am. J. Obstet. Gynecol., *113*:849, 1972.
44. Ingram, J.M.: Further experience with suprapubic drainage by trocar catheter. Am. J. Obstet. Gynecol., *121*:885, 1975.
45. Britt, M.R., Garibaldi, R.A., Miller, W.A., Hebertson, R.M., and Burke, J.P.: Antimicrobial prophylaxis for catheter associated bacteriuria. Antimicrob. Agents Chemother., *11*:240, 1977.
46. Sack, R.A.: Epidemic of gram-negative organism septicemia subsequent to elective operation. Am. J. Obstet. Gynecol., *107*:394, 1970.
47. Felts, S.K., Schaffner, W., Melly, M.A., and Koenig, M.G.: Sepsis caused by contaminated intravenous fluids. Ann. Intern. Med., *77*:881, 1972.
48. Ledger, W.J., and Headington, J.T.: Group A beta-hemolytic *Steptococcus*—an important cause of serious infections in obstetrics and gynecology. Obstet. Gynecol., *39*:474, 1972.
49. Baxter, C.R.: Surgical management of soft tissue infections. Surg. Clin. North Am., *52*:1483, 1972.
50. Ledger, W.J., Kriewall, T.J., and Gee, C.: The fever index. A technic for evaluating the clinical response to bacteremia. Obstet. Gynecol., *45*:603, 1975.
51. Goodlin, R.C.: Complications of amnioinfusion with hypertonic saline for midtrimester abortion. Am. J. Obstet. Gynecol., *110*:885, 1971.
52. MacDonald, D., O'Driscoll, M.K., and Geoghegan, F.J.: Intra-amniotic dextrose—a maternal death. J. Obstet. Gynecol. Br. Commonw., *72*:452, 1965.
53. Berger, G.S., Gibson, J.J., Harvey, R.P., Tyler, C.W., Jr., and Pakter, J.: One death and a cluster of febrile complications related to saline abortions. Obstet. Gynecol., *42*:121, 1973.
54. Sabbagha, R.E., and Hayashi, T.T.: Disseminated intravascular coagulation complicating hysterotomy in elderly gravidas. Obstet. Gynecol., *38*:844, 1971.
55. Tietze, C., and Lewit, S.: Legal abortions: Early medical complications. Fam. Plann. Perspect., *3*:6, Oct. 1971.
56. Lowensohn, R.I., and Hibbard, L.T.: Laceration of the ascending branch of the uterine artery: A complication of therapeutic abortion. Am. J. Obstet. Gynecol., *118*:36, 1974.

57. Hamilton, W.K., McDonald, J.S., Fischer, H.W., and Bethards, R.: Post-operative respiratory complications. Anesthesiology, *25*:607, 1964.
58. Pierce, A.K., and Robertson, J.: Pulmonary complications of general surgery. Ann. Rev. Med., *28*:211, 1977.
59. Ledger, W.J., Gee, C., and Lewis, W.P.: Guidelines for antibiotic prophylaxis in gynecology. Am. J. Obstet. Gynecol., *121*:1038, 1975.
60. Swartz, W.H.: Prophylaxis of minor febrile and major infectious morbidity following hysterectomy. Obstet. Gynecol., *54*:284, 1979.
61. Stark, R.P., and Maki, D.G.: Bacteriuria in the catheterized patient. What quantitative level of bacteriuria is relevant? N. Engl. J. Med., *311*:560, 1984.
62. Altemeier, W.A., McDonough, J.J., and Fullen, W.D.: Third day surgical fever. Arch. Surg., *103*:158, 1971.
63. Bentley, D.W., and Lepper, M.H.: Septicemia related to indwelling venous catheter. J.A.M.A., *206*:1749, 1968.
64. Buxton, A.E., Highsmith, A.K., Garner, J.S., West, M., Stamm, W.E., Dixon, R.E., and McGowan, J.E.: Contamination of intravenous infusion fluid: Effects of changing administration sets. Ann. Intern. Med., *90*:764, 1979.
65. Band, J.D., and Maki, D.G.: Safety of changing intravenous delivery systems at longer than 24 hour intervals. Ann. Intern. Med., *91*:173, 1979.
66. Foster, G.E., Hardy, E.G., and Hardcastle, J.D.: Subcuticular suturing after appendectomy. Lancet, *1*:1128, 1977.
67. Ledger, W.J., and Peterson, E.P.: The use of heparin in the management of pelvic thrombophlebitis. Surg. Gynecol. Obstet., *131*:1115, 1970.
68. Ledger, W.J.: Selection of antimicrobial agents for treatment of infections of the female genital tract. Rev. Infect. Dis., *5*:S98, 1983.
69. Gesner, B.M., and Jenkin, C.R.: Production of heparinase by *Bacteroides*. J. Bacteriol., *81*:595, 1961.
70. Ledger, W.J.: Infections in obstetrics and gynecology: New development in treatment. Surg. Clin. North Am., *52*:1447, 1972.
71. Young, E.J., Fainstein, V., and Musher, D.M.: Drug induced fever: Cases seen in the evaluation of unexplained fever in the general hospital population. Rev. Infect. Dis., *4*:69, 1982.
72. Ledger, W.J., Campbell, C., Taylor, D., and Willson, J.R.: Adnexal abscess as a late complication of pelvic operations. Surg. Gynecol. Obstet., *129*:973, 1969.
73. Polk, B.F., Tager, I.B., Shapiro, M., White, B.G., Goldstein, P., and Schoenbaum, S.C.: Randomized clinical trial of perioperative cefazolin in preventing infection after hysterectomy. Lancet, *1*:437, 1980.
74. Campbell, C.: Two unusual uses of steroid hormones in pelvic infections. Clin. Obstet. Gynecol., *12*:247, 1969.
75. Grady, G.F., and Bennett, A.J.E.: Risk of post-transfusion hepatitis in the United States. J.A.M.A., *220*:692, 1972.
76. Rader, D.L., Mucha, P., Jr., Moore, S.B., Farnell, M., Edwon, R., and Smith, T.: Cytomegalovirus infection in noncardiac surgical patients. Surg. Gynecol. Obstet. In press.
77. Hoyme, U.B., Tamimi, H.K., Eschenbach, D.A., Ramsey, P.G., and Figge, P.C.: Osteomyelitis pubis after radical gynecologic operations. Obstet. Gynecol., *63*:47S, 1984.

Chapter 10

MATERNAL INFECTION WITH ADVERSE FETAL AND NEWBORN OUTCOMES

Community-acquired infections during pregnancy causing adverse effects in the newborn are the most varied and intricate of all infectious disease problems facing the obstetrician-gynecologist today. To combat this complex assemblage of syndromes, we must have constant awareness of the impact of both the disease and its treatment on the fetus. The many interactions involved in maternal infections can result in a wide variety of manifestations. Some organisms cause no significant maternal symptoms but have an ill-effect on the fetus that persists after birth. Neither the patient nor the physician may be aware of a problem. Or, the obstetrician may have frequent inquiries from patients about the significance of an ill-defined flulike syndrome some time during pregnancy or have to interpret laboratory data to determine whether maternal antibody has been recently acquired because of the patient's concern about fetal problems. Still other maternal infections with the potential for fetal damage or death can be symptomatic and obvious. In order to delineate these varying clinical presentations, separate segments of this chapter are devoted to all the currently recognized maternal infections that result in an unfavorable fetal outcome. In addition to the importance of recognizing the diverse effects of infection on the fetus during pregnancy, the physician must acknowledge both patients, the mother and the fetus, when contemplating predelivery therapy.

THERAPY WITH ADVERSE FETAL AND NEWBORN EFFECTS

A number of widely used therapeutic regimens in nonpregnant women have the potential of producing ill-effects in the fetus. One major concern is the introduction of a live virus vaccine into a pregnant women, with resulting maternal and fetal viremia. This has been noted in patients receiving the rubella vaccine and represents the physician's failure to ascertain the possibility of pregnancy in the patient.[1] Careful studies of such cases indicate that rubella virus can be recovered from the products of conception. The concern about live virus vaccines in pregnant women is not limited to rubella. Table 10–1 lists the immunization programs available that utilize live viruses and their relative safety for the pregnant woman.[2] In addition, there is the newly developed live rabies virus vaccine as well as the use of killed bacteria and viral immunizations and toxoids used as immunizing agents.[3] At least one study has shown the use of live rabies immu-

Table 10–1. Immunization During Pregnancy

Immunizing Agent	Risk of Disease in Pregnant Female	Risk of Disease in Fetus or Neonate	Type of Immunizing Agent	Risk from Immunizing Agent to Fetus	Indications for Immunization During Pregnancy	Dose Schedule	Comments
Measles	Significant morbidity, low mortality; not altered by pregnancy	Significant increase in abortion rate; may cause malformations	Live attenuated virus vaccine	None confirmed	Contraindicated	Single dose	Vaccination of susceptible women should be part of postpartum care
Mumps	Low morbidity and mortality; not altered by pregnancy	Probable increase rate of abortion in 1st trimester; questionable association of fibroelastosis in neonates	Live attenuated virus vaccine	None confirmed	Contraindicated	Single dose	
Poliomyelitis	No increased disease incidence in pregnancy but may be more severe if it occurs	Anoxic fetal damage reported; 50% mortality in neonatal disease	Live, attenuated virus (OPV) and inactivated virus (IPV) vaccine	None confirmed	Not routinely recommended for adults in U.S., except persons at increased risk of exposure	Primary: 3 doses of IPV at 4–8 week intervals and a 4th dose 6–12 months after the 3rd dose; 2 doses of	Vaccine indicated for susceptible pregnant women traveling in endemic areas or in other high-risk situations

	Risk from disease to mother	Risk to fetus or neonate	Type of vaccine	Risk from vaccine to fetus	Indication during pregnancy	Dose schedule	Comments
						OPV with a 6–8 week interval and a 3rd dose at least 6 weeks later, customarily 8–12 months later; Booster: Every 5 years until 18 years of age for IPV	
Rubella	Low morbidity and mortality; not altered by pregnancy	High rate of abortion and congenital rubella syndrome	Live attenuated virus vaccine	None confirmed	Contraindicated	Single dose	Teratogenicity of vaccine is theoretical, not confirmed to date; vaccination of susceptible women should be part of postpartum care
Yellow fever	Significant morbidity and mortality; not altered by pregnancy	Unknown	Live attenuated virus vaccine	Unknown	Contraindicated except if exposure unavoidable	Single dose	Postponement of travel preferable to vaccination, if possible

(Adapted from The American College of Obstetricians and Gynecologists: Immunization During Pregnancy (ACOG Technical Bulletin 64). Washington, DC, ACOG, 1982.)

nization in a pregnant woman without ill-effects on the fetus.[4] In these days of international jet travel, a number of questions about the safety of various vaccines are directed to the physician, and this table provides a basis for sound advice.

There are other biologic agents with the potential for ill-effects. On occasion physicians have to prescribe systemic antimicrobial agents for pregnant women. Obviously, any decision to use an antibiotic must be tempered by the knowledge of the potential harm of this agent to both the mother and fetus. During pregnancy, there is evidence that high doses of tetracycline are poorly tolerated by the maternal liver, resulting in fatty infiltration, hepatic failure, and sometimes death.[5] In addition to these important maternal considerations, there is the welfare of the fetus to consider. A major area of concern is maternal drug ingestion during the first trimester, when embryogenesis occurs. This is a time when all medications should be avoided if possible. Past use of the drug thalidomide is a tragic case in point of the dangers of exogenous medication at a critical time in pregnancy. This concern for prescribing medication is not limited to the first trimester. A number of effective antimicrobial agents can cause problems in the fetus or newborn without causing maternal difficulty. For example, administration of a dose of tetracycline that is not toxic to the mother has been associated with discoloration of teeth in the newborn.[6] The use of other antibiotics may alter some tests of the maternal-fetal unit. Administration of methenamine mandelate (Mandelamine) to the mother may result in falsely low urinary estriol values,[7] and ampicillin[8] and erythromycin[9] have been demonstrated to be associated with a decrease in estriols because of their reduction of the gastrointestinal microbial flora. When present these bacteria break the conjugation of estriol and permit the reabsorption of unconjugated estriol. When bacteria are absent or present in diminished numbers, increased amounts of conjugated estriol are lost in the bowel. The use of these medications should be acknowledged when test results are interpreted.

Problems of drug toxicity to the newborn can occur, particularly when drugs are administered to the mother just before delivery. The sulfas, particularly long-acting ones, cross the placenta and achieve therapeutic levels in the fetus. If delivery occurs while fetal levels remain high, this drug competes for the same globulin binding site in serum that is utilized by bilirubin, and this can result in higher levels of unbound bilirubin in the newborn.[10] The use of long-acting sulfas should be avoided in the patient near term, but short-acting ones such as sulfi-thoxazole can be used in the antepartum period for uncomplicated lower urinary tract infections. This focus upon the fetus will be examined in the remainder of this chapter.

MATERNAL INFECTIONS PRODUCING ADVERSE FETAL EFFECT

Some viral infections acquired by the mother during pregnancy can produce developmental anomalies in the fetus. The standard for teratogenesis, the rubella virus, was first associated with fetal abnormalities in Gregg's report in 1941.[11] Since then, repeated observations of the offspring of pregnant women who were infected during rubella epidemics have demonstrated microcephaly, deafness, mental retardation, and cardiac malformations. The development of the rubella antibody test to determine host susceptibility and of a vaccine to prevent infection has resulted in the elimination of recurring epidemics of rubella. Despite this, occasional episodes of rubella still occur, for more than 10% of women in the childbearing age group have no antibody to the virus.[12] Another proven viral teratogen is the cytomegalovirus. Malformation of the fetal central nervous system, including microcephaly, polymicrogyria, and microphthalmia[13] and congenital heart disease and deafness[14] have been implicated following maternal cytomegalovirus infections. In addition to rubella and cytomegalovirus, there is evidence that infections with the enteroviruses (including the coxsakie virus) during pregnancy have occasionally been associated with fetal infection and abnormalities of the heart.[15]

STORCH INFECTIONS

The current obstetric preoccupation with improving newborn outcome has resulted in increased emphasis upon maternal infections that can produce newborn disability. To categorize these problems by the organisms involved, I am in agreement with Monif that the acronym STORCH, the German word for stork, is appropriate. In order, S is for syphilis, T for toxoplasmosis, O for other agents, R for rubella, C for cytomegalovirus, and H for herpes. The grouping of these diverse microbiologic agents, which range from viruses to protozoa, is based upon the similarity of the diagnostic and therapeutic dilemmas they cause for physicians. The maternal infections are usually inapparent clinically, the newborns have a wide variety of manifestations at birth from no apparent disease to death from an intrauterine infection, and the surviving infant can have long-term damage with extraordinary costs for the family and society. In utero many of these infants appear to have symmetric intrauterine growth retardation. These infections are not common entities, and Table 10–2 gives an estimate of their frequency.[16, 17]

The clinical presentation for the obstetrician is usually confusing. A minority of women with these problems will have nonspecific symptoms with a febrile illness and occasionally a rash. Most women will have no symptoms of an infection. Some familiarity with laboratory testing procedures is needed to make the correct diagnosis in these patients with vague or absent symptoms, since on laboratory study an asymptomatic pregnant woman may be found to have either a positive antibody screen or a positive culture. A logical sequence of laboratory testing should be followed so that proper advice can be given to the patient. Since these women and their newborns do not have distinct clinical pictures, the subsequent discussion in this chapter will be organized on the basis of specific microbiologic agents.

Table 10–2. Incidence of Maternal, Fetal and Neonatal Infections Caused by Selected Microorganisms

Microorganism	Mother (per 1,000 Pregnancies)	Fetus (per 1,000 Live Births)	Newborns (per 1,000 Live Births)
Cytomegalovirus	40–150	5–25	10–70
Rubella			
Epidemic	20–40	4–30	0
Interepidemic	0.1	0.5	0
Toxoplasma gondii	1.5–6.4	0.8–1	Unknown
Herpes simplex	10–15	Rare	0.1–0.5
Treponema pallidum	0.2	0.1	0
Group B *Streptococcus*	50–250	—	1–4
Escherichia coli	Common	—	1–2

Syphilis

The prototype for asymptomatic maternal infections with an adverse effect upon the fetus is syphilis. This is as true in the 1980's as it was in 1902, when Ballantyne observed that fetal syphilis is the infection that comes to mind when a reference is made to fetal disease.[18] Obstetricians providing prenatal care rarely find a chancre or the rash of secondary syphilis, which is most prominent on the palms of the hands and the soles of the feet. The usual infected pregnant patient is asymptomatic, and the disease is diagnosed because of routine laboratory surveillance. In the maternal host, spirochetes cross the placenta and infect the fetus in utero. In the past, there was a focus upon the 16th week of pregnancy, for the study showed no pathologic evidence of newborn infection before this.[19] However, recent observations have shown that transplacental infection of the fetus with spirochetes can occur before the 16th week of pregnancy.[20] There is a wide range of fetal response to this intrauterine infection. There can be abortion, premature labor and delivery, intrauterine growth retardation, stillbirth, or neonatal death. At birth, however, the signs and symptoms of congenital syphilis may not be apparent; the disease may be suspected by an astute pediatrician by the development in the neonate of lacrimation, nasal discharge, the appearance of mucous patches in the oral cavity, or a costochondritis discovered on roentgen examination. In addition, these infants may have a rash, a bullous skin eruption, and hepatosplenomegaly. If infected at birth, these infants later present with keratosis, notched teeth, nasal malformations, and deafness.

The basis of care for both the mother and the fetus is early accurate diagnosis of syphilis. Rarely, a chancre will be discovered and the diagnosis confirmed by a darkfield examination. The usual diagnosis is made by serologic screening at the first prenatal visit. The universally used test, the reagin test, is nonspecific for syphilis but, despite this, is of great help to the clinician. The test has been standardized, and all clinical laboratories can perform it. Titers can be obtained to aid in the surveillance of the response to therapy. The major shortcoming of the reagin test is the fact that it can be positive in some women who have other infections or systemic diseases such as lupus erythematosus. Because of this, specific syphilis tests such as the Fluorescent Treponemal Antibody Absorption Test (FTA-ABS) should be performed. Although it is not 100% specific, a positive FTA-ABS test should be considered confirmatory for syphilis. This test usually remains positive for life, so it cannot be used as a test for cure.

Although this outline of laboratory testing for syphilis is simple and straightforward, there are a number of difficult areas of interpretation for care. Some antepartum patients may be seen who have a weakly reactive reagin test. These could be patients whose serologic tests remain positive despite adequate past treatment for syphilis, who have produced a biologic false-positive test because of another illness, or who are manifesting the immunologic response of early spirochetal infection. A careful history and review of the medical records is necessary to document past treatment for syphilis. If there has been adequate antibiotic treatment in the past with a significant fall in reagin titer of four tubes' dilution or more posttreatment and no change in the reagin titer during this pregnancy, active syphilis is unlikely. Biologic false-positive results should be considered in the patient with a low reagin titer and a nonreactive FTA-ABS test. Ruling out syphilis in this patient may lead to discovering other problems, for the positive reagin test may herald significant underlying systemic collagen disease with potentially serious problems, and this should be evaluated. Finally, a patient with a high range or rising reagin titer, a positive FTA-ABS test, and no history of antibiotic therapy has syphilis and should receive antibiotic therapy. There are other problems of care. The first negative prenatal reagin screen will be of no aid for the woman who acquires syphilis later in pregnancy. Monif and colleagues reported instances of congenital syphilis in infants of mothers who had a negative serologic test result at the first prenatal visit.[21] On this basis, it has been suggested that a repeat maternal serologic test be done in the third trimester, in addition to the accepted routine of the cord blood serologic study done at birth.[21] Although this represents a large volume of laboratory testing for congenital syphilis, a disease diagnosed in only 331 newborns from over three million deliveries in 1979,[22] the benefits for the few cases thus discovered would be great. If benefit cost analyses and cost-containment pressures preclude screening of all pregnant women, there is a subpopulation at high risk for syphilis who should be reevaluated serologically in the third trimester for the presence of syphilis[23] (see Table 10–3).[24]

The treatment of syphilis in pregnancy is simple if the patient is not allergic to penicillin. The spirochete *Treponema pallidum* is very susceptible to penicillin. Since this antibiotic acts primarily upon the cell wall and the spirochete replicates slowly, approximately every 24 hours, a low level of penicillin should be achieved for an extended time for cure. This therapeutic need is met by the pharmacologic action of benzathene penicillin, which maintains low levels in the bloodstream for longer than a week. The guidelines for therapy are based upon the length of time since acquisition of the disease. If the disease has been present for less than a year, based upon the presence of a chancre, lesions of secondary syphilis, or a documented history of serologic conversion within the past year, the treatment is one dose of intramuscular benzathine penicillin, 2,400,000 U. If the infection was introduced more than a year ago or the time of acquisition is not known, the Centers for Disease Control's recommendation is benzathene penicillin, 2,400,000 U at weekly intervals for three doses, or a total of 7,200,000 U.[25] Although Philipson has demonstrated that equivalent antibiotic dosages produce lower serum levels in pregnant than in nonpregnant women,[26] this regimen seems effective. A test of cure is a fourfold or greater drop in the reagin titer within six months of treatment. The newborn will be surveyed serologically at birth and followed closely after birth to be sure that a positive reagin test on the cord blood is caused

Table 10–3. Pregnant Women at High Risk for Syphilis

1. Unmarried pregnant women
2. Pregnant teenagers
3. Pregnant women with inadequate or no prenatal care
4. Drug abusers
5. Sexually promiscuous pregnant women
6. Pregnant women with ill-defined rashes or ulcerating lesions at such unusual sites as the mouth, anus, or breast (extragenital chancres)
7. Pregnant women who experience preterm delivery
8. Pregnant women with unexplained large placenta
9. Pregnant women with occurrence of unexpected stillbirth or hydrops fetalis
10. Occurrence of symmetric intrauterine growth retardation in the fetus
11. Pregnant women diagnosed as syphilitic but inadequately treated

by the transplacental passage of maternal IgG and not a newborn response to active infection. These reagin titers should diminish and become negative.

The treatment of syphilis for the penicillin-allergic patient is much more complicated. One of the two alternative drugs for use in nonpregnant women is tetracycline; this is not recommended during pregnancy because of both fetal and maternal toxicity. The recommended drug is erythromycin. It is safe for use during pregnancy, but cases of congenital syphilis have been reported when the mother was successfully treated for syphilis.[27] At least one study has shown that very low levels of erythromycin were achieved in fetal tissues when therapeutic doses of the drug were given to women just prior to elective termination of pregnancy.[28] The recommendations for treatment with erythromycin during pregnancy are based upon the clinical determination of acquisition of the disease within the past year, or more than a year ago, or unknown. For less than a year, the regimen is 500 mg orally four times a day for 15 days or a total of 30 g. For more than a year or unknown, the recommendation is 500 mg orally four times a day for 30 days, a total of 60 g.[25] The estolate form is not recommended because of the potential for liver toxicity. These erythromycin recommendations have an aura of unreality, however, for this daily dosage causes so much gastrointestinal distress that few if any asymptomatic pregnant women will complete the treatment course. At delivery, the newborns of these patients should be treated with penicillin as though they have congenital syphilis. This is possible because maternal allergy to penicillin resides chiefly in the IgE fraction and this does not cross the placenta.

Toxoplasmosis

Toxoplasmosis is a disease that is neglected and misunderstood by practicing obstetricians. The damage it causes to the newborn is serious although often insidious. The mother, who acquires the infection during pregnancy, is usually asymptomatic. Although occasionally the infected newborn has obvious manifestations of disease, the usual picture is a normal baby who subsequently develops the serious consequences of infection. These sequelae often require years to develop, and the pediatrician rather than the obstetrician sees the end result. Despite the fact that serologic testing is available and the frequency of occurrence of these infections in pregnant women is greater than either rubella or syphilis infections, the reality of current obstetric practice is that routine antibody testing is done for rubella and syphilis but not for toxoplasmosis. This is tragic, for this disease is amenable to a variety of therapeutic strategies. As advocates for the health of the fetus and the newborn, obstetricians should change their practice patterns in this area. The stimulus for change may come from a better understanding of the disease.

Maternal symptoms of a primary toxoplasmosis infection are difficult to detect. Women with this condition can have lymphadenopathy without fever or fatigue.[29] In less than 10% of cases, patients have lymphadenopathy and atypical lymphocytes in their blood that simulate infectious mononucleosis.[30] With this infrequent and vague clinical picture, it is easy to see that these infections will not be readily diagnosed clinically.

The majority of cases of maternal infection will be diagnosed by testing for antibodies to toxoplasmosis. The test most frequently utilized in the United States is the Sabin-Feldman dye test, which largely reflects the presence of IgG antibody.

The dilemma of the clinician occurs when a positive test is reported from blood obtained at the first prenatal visit. The physician does not know whether this indicates a recent infection during pregnancy or represents an infection that preceded pregnancy. If the titer is very low, the test should be repeated in three weeks. A rising titer is suggestive of a recent infection, while a stable low titer suggests an old infection. Some laboratories do the indirect hemagglutination antibody test (IHA) as their screen instead of the Sabin-Feldman. Since this test takes a longer period of time to become positive than the Sabin-Feldman test, this is not a wise choice. The patient with a high Sabin-Feldman titer presents a difficult problem. Does this represent a fixed high titer from an old infection or is the antibody rise caused by a recent infection? Other tests can help in this differentiation. The indirect hemagglutination (IHA) test can be useful, for positive titers lag several weeks or more behind those of the dye test and tend to remain elevated at higher levels for a longer period of time.[31] In acute maternal infection, this test can be diagnostic if the dye test has already stabilized at a high titer and a rising IHA test is found on serial samples. Positive titers of the complement fixation (CF) test also appear later, and a negative test that becomes positive on subsequent sampling or a CF test with rising titers on serial sampling indicates recent infection. In the event that both of these tests show fixed high titers, blood can be sent to a reference laboratory, either the state or the Centers for Disease Control, for determination of the presence of IgM to toxoplasmosis, indicating a recent infection. The specificity of this test depends upon the antiserum to IgM that has been selected and the willingness of the laboratory to screen for rheumatoid factor, which when present can also give a positive IgM test.[31] If the laboratory has taken steps to avoid these shortcomings, then this test will be extremely helpful.

Acute toxoplasmosis infection of the mother has a wide variety of effects upon the subsequent health of the newborn. A measure of the variation of response of the newborn is noted in Table 10–4.[32, 33] If the mother acquires the infection very early in pregnancy, fewer newborns will be infected but the infections will be more serious. Infection in the newborn can range from clinically inapparent disease to a picture including microcephaly, intracranial calcification, chorioretinitis, hepatosplenomegaly, thrombocytopenia, and anemia. The majority of newborn infants with toxoplasmosis will not be detected by specific clinical findings, although

Table 10–4. Frequency of Adverse Pregnancy Outcomes Among the Offspring of 500 Women Who Acquired *Toxoplasma* Infection During Pregnancy

Outcome	I Number	(%)	II Number	(%)	Trimester When Infection Was Acquired III Number	(%)
1. No infection	109	(86)	173	(71)	52	(41)
2. Congenital toxoplasmosis						
Subclinical	3	(2)	49	(20)	68	(53)
Mild	1	(1)	13	(5)	8	(6)
Severe	7	(6)	6	(2)	0	(0)
3. Stillbirth or perinatal death	6	(5)	5	(2)	0	(0)
Total	126	(100)	246	(100)	128	(100)

Table 10–5. Prevalence of *Toxoplasma* Antibodies in Pregnant Women

NEW YORK		LONDON		PARIS			
				French		NonFrench	
Number	% Positive	Number	% Positive	Number	% Positive	Number	% Positive
4048	32	3169	22	1206	87	293	70

many will be premature or show evidence of symmetric intrauterine growth retardation. The most serious aspect of these inapparent infections is that if they are undetected and untreated, almost all children will develop adverse sequelae, especially neurologic effects, a spectrum including chorioretinitis, lowered intelligence testing, hearing loss, and epilepsy.[34]

The risk of maternal infection varies with the locale and the social habits of the pregnant population. Table 10–5[33] shows the prevalence of toxoplasmosis in three urban centers, New York,[35] London,[36] and Paris.[37] The Paris incidence figures are the highest, indicating the French predilection for the ingestion of uncooked meats. Figure 10–1 shows the relative risk of acquisition of toxoplasmosis in these populations with a varied prior exposure during pregnancy.[38] A high frequency of toxoplasmosis during pregnancy occurs when a population with a low incidence of toxoplasmosis, curve II, moves to an environment in which uncooked meat is widely used. The result, curve III, reflects the experience in Paris among immigrants, especially those from North Africa.

The cornerstone of the treatment of toxoplasmosis is prevention. Obstetricians should require the same screening laboratory tests for toxoplasmosis susceptibility

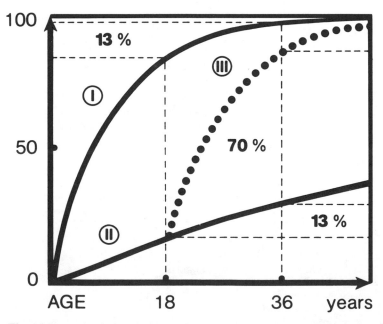

Fig. 10–1. The relative risk of acquiring toxoplasmosis. See text for details. A high frequency of toxoplasmosis occurs when a low incidence population moves to an area in which uncooked meat is served. The result is curve III. (From Desmonts, G., and Couvreur, J.: Toxoplasmosis: Epidemiologic and serologic aspects of perinatal infection. *In* Infections of the Fetus and the Newborn Infant. Progress in Clinical and Biological Research. Edited by S. Krugman and A.A. Gershon. Vol. 3. New York, Alan R. Liss, Inc., 1975.)

in nonpregnant women as now exist for rubella and syphilis in many states as a prerequisite for a marriage certificate. Nonpregnant women with a positive toxoplasmosis test can be advised that they need have no concern about delivering a child infected with *Toxoplasma gondii.* Those nonpregnant women who are seronegative are at risk and should have repeat testing at their first prenatal visit when they become pregnant. If test results are negative, they should be advised to avoid undercooked meats during the pregnancy. In addition, persistent close contact with an infected cat or its litter box can lead to infection. This is particularly true for the owner of a "hunter" cat who has free access to the outdoors, where it can kill and devour infected rodents.

For the woman with serologic evidence of active infection during pregnancy, treatment is still in flux. There is a risk of severe damage to the newborn if the infection occurs in the first trimester. Because of this, many women will elect to have a pregnancy termination. As an alternative to this and for those women who acquire the disease in the second or third trimester, chemotherapy is a possibility. At present, there are a number of chemotherapeutic agents that can be prescribed for toxoplasmosis. Pyrimethamine (Daraprim) is effective against toxoplasmosis. However, it is a folic acid antagonist with teratogenic effects. Although contraindicated during the first trimester of pregnancy, it can be given later with a folic acid supplement and also subsequently to an infected newborn.[39] Sulfonamides are effective, as is spiramycin.[32, 39] Although these drugs can lower the incidence of congenital toxoplasmosis, they do not eliminate it. These drugs have not been approved by the FDA for use in pregnant patients, but the results, which indicate a reduction in incidence, suggest that this will be an accepted mode of therapy in the future.

Other Agents of STORCH

Currently, not all the other agents of the STORCH complex have been defined. Studies by Alford and associates show that the majority of infants born with elevated cord blood IgM levels have not had an intrauterine infection with one of the defined members of the STORCH complex.[40] This section includes a listing of those organisms causing inapparent or mild maternal infections that have an adverse effect upon the fetus or newborn.

GROUP B BETA-HEMOLYTIC *STREPTOCOCCUS*

The group B beta-hemolytic *Streptococcus* is associated with serious problems of infection in the newborn. The newborn disease is classified as early onset when it occurs within the first five days after birth and late onset when it occurs more than a week after delivery. The differentiating features are noted in Table 10–6.[41] The infections can be associated with neonatal sepsis, meningitis, and death. This is a disturbing disease because of the fetal mortality rate. Babies with this syndrome are born to asymptomatic women, with progression from first symptoms to death in hours, despite appropriate antibiotic therapy. The mortality rate in early onset sepsis has been higher than 50% in many series.[42] Alternatively, the newborn may leave the hospital seemingly well, only to be readmitted with meningitis. Although the mortality rate with late onset disease is lower, the residual central nervous system damage is frequent enough to make this a serious clinical problem.

Table 10–6 Clinical Characteristics of Early Onset and Late Onset Disease with Group B Beta-Hemolytic *Streptococcus* in the Newborn

Clinical Characteristics	Early Onset	Late Onset
Mean age at onset	20 hours	24 days
Incidence of prematurity	Increased	Not increased
Obstetric problems	Frequent (60%)	Uncommon
Common manifestations	Septicemia (30–40%)	Meningitis (85%)
	Meningitis (30%)	Bacteremia without focus
	Pneumonia (30–40%)	Bone or joint infection
Serotypes isolated	Ia, Ib, Ic (30%)	III (93%)
	II (30%)	
	III (40% nonmeningeal; 80% meningeal isolates)	
Mortality rate	55%	23%

There are clinical factors that correlate with an increased risk of newborn infections. The premature infant is at greater risk for infection and mortality from the pregnancy in which there is prolonged rupture of membranes.[43] In the absence of maternal fever, fetal tachycardia in labor, at a rate of 160 beats per minute or greater for over 30 minutes, identifies newborns at risk for an infection with this organism.[44] There is also an increased infection rate among newborns who have been subjected to invasive monitoring techniques with the attachment of a fetal scalp electrode during labor.[44] There is a constellation of findings at the time of delivery that should make the physician aware of the possibility of group B beta-hemolytic streptococcal sepsis. The delivery of an unexpectedly limp infant with one and five minute Apgar scores of below five and no prior evidence of fetal heart rate decelerations during labor and a normal cord gas pH at delivery should make the obstetrician highly suspicious of the possibility of group B beta-hemolytic sepsis. These clinical observations support my belief that early onset sepsis is an intrauterine infection and not first acquired during fetal passage through a contaminated birth canal. Despite the recognition of high risk groups, there are two major problems with the assignment of clinical risk factors for group B beta-hemolytic streptococcal infections in the newborn. Although they are at higher risk, the overwhelming majority of patients with these risks factors will not deliver an infant with a group B streptococcal infection. More important, some newborns with fatal group B streptococcal sepsis will have none of the risk factors. For example, early onset group B streptococcal sepsis has been seen in term infants delivered by elective cesarean section in patients with intact membranes.[45]

Group B beta-hemolytic streptococcal infection in the newborn is related to maternal carriage of the organism in the lower genital tract. Many more women are colonized by this organism than have newborns with disease (Table 10–7).[41,46–51] There are some unique aspects of the relationship between maternal colonization by the organism and subsequent newborn disease. Unlike maternal colonization with *Escherichia coli*, which remains constant during pregnancy, the group B *Streptococcus* has a skip factor.[52] Some women who are culture-positive in the first and second trimesters will be culture-negative when labor begins, and in contrast, some women who are culture-negative early in pregnancy will be positive at the

Table 10-7 Attack Rates for Group B Streptococcal Disease in Infants

City	Prevalence of Maternal Genital Colonization per 1,000 Deliveries	Attack Rate per 1,000 for Bacteremic Early Onset Infection	Ratio of Maternal Colonization at Delivery to Neonatal Invasive Disease
Denver	46	2.0	23:1
Houston	225	2.9	78:1
Palm Beach	290	3.4	85:1
Los Angeles	300	3.0	100:1
Birmingham	190	3.7	51:1
Houston	234	2.3	102:1

start of labor. This makes it difficult to assess antepartum antibiotic prophylaxis. Women at risk for transmitting the infection to their infants often have an absence of antibody[53] and are heavily colonized with this organism.[44]

There are other ways in which the newborn can become infected with this organism. Repeated use of intrauterine pressure transducers without adequate cleansing procedures has been associated with contamination by group B beta-hemolytic *Streptococcus*,[54] and nosocomial spread in the nursery has been documented in a few cases.[55]

Understandably, there has been a great deal of interest in techniques of prevention of this disease. Not all the newborns at risk can be identified prior to delivery, and there is awareness that treatment of an infected newborn cannot prevent mortality in every instance of early onset sepsis. One approach has been to screen all pregnant women for this organism and to treat those who are culture-positive with antibiotics. Some investigators have advocated therapy to reduce the incidence of premature rupture of membranes, premature labor, and delivery.[56] The difficulty with this approach is that there is a high failure rate with maternal recolonization after treatment.[57] This can be attributable to carriage of the organism by the male sexual partner[57] or rectal colonization that subsequently results in vaginal colonization.[58] Another alternative management strategy is to identify women at risk in the third trimester and to treat them in labor.[59] This technique has been highly effective in reducing the rate of newborn infections. I favor this approach, although more rapid techniques of microbiologic identification of the group B *Streptococcus* are needed to screen women in labor at the time of admission. An alternative is to treat all newborns at birth, but this will not prevent all serious infections or mortality.[60] One study of the use of penicillin after birth in newborns weighing 2,000 g or less showed no reduction in the death rate from sepsis caused by the group B beta-hemolytic *Streptococcus*.[61] This reinforces the concept that infection occurred in utero and was well established before the first hour of postnatal life. Another preventive measure has been an attempt to immunize mothers against a surface antigen of the group B beta-hemolytic *Streptococcus*.[62] Since there are a variety of serotypes involved with early onset disease and there is concern about immunization effectiveness, this method of control remains under study.

OTHER BACTERIAL SOURCES OF NEWBORN SEPSIS

Early onset sepsis in the newborn can be related to other bacterial pathogens, particularly *Escherichia coli*,[63] *Hemophilus influenzae*,[64] and *Listeria monocytogenes*.[65] All these organisms have many things in common with the group B beta-hemolytic *Streptococcus.* The mother is usually asymptomatic, and problems with newborn infection are more common with premature labor and delivery and premature rupture of the membranes. Both *Escherichia coli,*[63] and *Hemophilus influenzae*[64] infections are related to a specific surface antigen type that has the capability of invasion, particularly of the central nervous system of the newborn. *Listeria monocytogenes* has been associated with a wide range of infectious manifestations in the newborn.[65] Intrauterine infection of the fetus with intact fetal membranes has been proved by the use of transabdominal amniocentesis.[66] After delivery, these infections range from the respiratory to the central nervous system. In view of the poorly defined or absent maternal symptoms, the majority of cases will not be suspected clinically. At present, routine antepartum screening of mothers by culture or antibody surveillance is not done. In the evaluation of women with premature rupture of the membranes, this should be part of the microbiologic screening.

TUBERCULOSIS

This infection is of increasing importance to American obstetricians because of the influx in recent years of immigrants from southeast Asia and the Caribbean with a high incidence of pulmonary tuberculosis. The organism, *Mycobacterium tuberculosis,* produces a syndrome similar to that of the other microbiologic agents of the STORCH group. The mothers are often asymptomatic and are usually diagnosed by chest radiograph examination during pregnancy because their tuberculin skin tests are positive. There is a wide variety of fetal and newborn responses, which range from no apparent disease to generalized sepsis and death.[67] Pregnant women should be tuberculin skin tested, and those with positive results need a chest x-ray examination to rule out active disease. Antitubercular therapy with isoniazid, PAS, and streptomycin can be given if active disease is present. The safety of rifampin and ethambutal for pregnant women has not been established as yet.

CHLAMYDIA

This organism can cause infection problems in the newborn of an asymptomatic woman. The most frequent clinical problem seen is conjunctivitis, which is responsive to local therapy with tetracycline or erythromycin ophthalmic solution. Women whose cultures are positive for *Chlamydia* during pregnancy are particularly prone to having newborns with this problem.[68] Because of concern about this organism as a cause of newborn eye infections, many neonatal services now routinely employ an erythromycin ophthalmic ointment instead of the traditional silver nitrate drops.[69] On occasion, a full-blown pneumonitis is seen, which can be fatal if not recognized and treated with appropriate antibiotics.[70]

NEISSERIA GONORRHOEAE

Neisseria gonorrhoeae has a specific spectrum of disease in the newborn. As in the infections caused by the other members of the STORCH complex, maternal symptoms are usually absent. The most serious problem for the newborn is ophthalmia neonatorum. Although silver nitrate drops have been required treatment for all newborns, recent concern about the irritating effects of these drops, plus awareness of the frequency of *Chlamydia* infection in the newborn, has led to wider use of erythromycin ophthalmic ointments, which are also effective against the gonococcus. A much less frequent newborn problem is gonococcal arthritis. It should be considered in the newborn who presents with septic arthritis one to four weeks after birth. In recent years, scalp abscesses and newborn sepsis with *Neisseria gonorrhoeae* have been reported in the offspring of women who are asymptomatic carriers, and a fetal scalp electrode has been employed in labor.[71] Although an increased frequency of premature labor and premature rupture of membranes has been noted in women whose cultures are positive for *Neisseria gonorrhoeae,*[72] a cause and effect relationship or an improved outcome with antibiotic therapy has not been demonstrated as yet.

OTHER VIRAL AGENTS

There are a wide variety of viral agents with demonstrable effects upon the fetus. The vast majority are seen in pregnant women who have no clinical evidence of serious disease. These include such enteroviruses as the echoviruses and coxsackie A and B viruses, which can have a wide range of fetal response from no apparent infection to clinically apparent infection of the lungs or the central nervous system or both. Coxsakie A and B viruses have been associated in some studies with cardiovascular abnormalities in the newborn.[15]

Hepatitis A, B, and nonA-nonB infections can be acquired by the mother with manifestation of few or no clinical symptoms. There is a wide range of clinical response in the newborn, from no disease to the rare infant who demonstrates jaundice in the nursery.[73] If the mothers are hepatitis antigen–positive, asymptomatic newborns should be treated with the hepatitis B vaccine. Prematurity in the newborn is frequently associated with maternal disease.

Rubella

In the minds of most obstetricians, the rubella virus is the prototype of the STORCH agents. Frequently inapparent maternal infection with this virus leads to a wide range of newborn effects that were documented during the last rubella epidemic in the United States in 1964. There can be serious newborn abnormalities, including cataracts, deafness, cardiac deficiencies, and microcephalus. Many of these infants, exposed early in the pregnancy to the virus, show intrauterine growth retardation, and 10 to 20% die of hepatitis, encephalitis, or myocarditis during the first few months of life.[13] The survivors can continue to carry stigmata of the infection, with hepatosplenomegaly, jaundice, thrombocytopenia, petechiae, ecchymoses, pneumonitis, and radiolucencies of the long bones, persisting for one to six months. Beyond one to six months of age, the children were often smaller than normal and microcephalic, with diminished central nervous system function. These untoward fetal effects were the stimuli for a program of prevention.

In the early 1960's two new bits of knowledge became the basis for the development of a program of prevention of rubella. The first was the discovery of a test to evaluate the presence or absence of antibodies to rubella. This gave obstetricians a tool to define a population of susceptible women and to make the serologic diagnosis of an acute infection during pregnancy. The most important new informational breakthrough was the isolation of the live rubella virus, which subsequently led to the development of a live attenuated rubella vaccine.

There has been controversy associated with the rubella immunization program from the time of the licensing of the vaccine in 1969. When the vaccine first became available, an administrative decision was made to focus on the population age group of one to 14 years.[74] This age group was chosen in order to confer "herd" immunity on a large susceptible population pool that could infect pregnant women. One underlying rationale for this approach was the concern about the frequency of side-effects, particularly arthritis, when a live viral vaccine was given to adult women.[75] Another important consideration was the possibility of the administration of live virus to a pregnant woman.[1] Support for this strategy comes from the observation that there have been no major rubella epidemics in the United States since the introduction of the vaccine in the middle 1960's, the frequency of the newborn rubella syndrome is much lower than before the immunization program, and there is ample evidence that the use of the vaccine in adult women has been accompanied by inadvertent administration to pregnant women (Table 10–8).[1] The Centers for Disease Control states that from 4 to 20% of these products of conception have live virus present, but there have been no reports of congenital rubella syndrome.[1] The critics of the initial decision downgraded the concept of "herd" immunity because a nonimmunized population of women in the childbearing age group would remain, and there was a question as to the length of time of the conferred immunity.[76] Recent outbreaks of rubella in adult women in New York City confirm their prediction about the lack of "herd" immunity. The duration of immunization is still not known. Although the hemagglutinin inhibition (HI) test has declined to nondetectable levels in 10% or more of women eight or more years after initial immunization,[77] the evidence seems strong that they are still immunized in most cases. However, there have been observations of active rubella infection in adults who have been previously immunized, but this has occurred after wild rubella infection.[78] The frequency of infection after immunization is ten times more common than following previous wild virus infection,[78] but the frequency of this in previously immunized pregnant women is not known. Fortunately, this is an extremely rare event.

The obstetrician has a number of evaluations to make about rubella in a patient population. In the nonpregnant woman, the absence of immunity is an indication for vaccine administration if the patient can avoid a pregnancy for at least three months after the immunization has been given. All obstetricians should be aware of the wide variation in the accuracy of tests for rubella immunity that are available through commercial laboratories (Figure 10–2).[79] He or she should be an advocate for the screening and immunization of medical team personnel who have contact with pregnant women in both outpatient and inpatient hospital settings. Out-

Table 10–8.   Live Rubella Vaccine Virus and Virus Administration to Pregnant Women

Prevaccination Immunity Status	Total Cases (%)	Live Births		Spontaneous Abortion and Stillbirth		Induced Abortion		Outcome Unknown	
		No.	%	No.	%	No.	%	No.	%
Susceptible	214	143	(66.8)	6	(2.8)	53	(24.8)	12	(5.6)
Immune	41	37	(90.2)	0	(0)	3	(7.3)	1	(2.4)
Unknown	472	263	(55.7)	20	(4.2)	152	(32.2)	37	(7.8)
Total	727	443	(60.9)	26	(3.6)	208	(28.6)	50	(6.9)

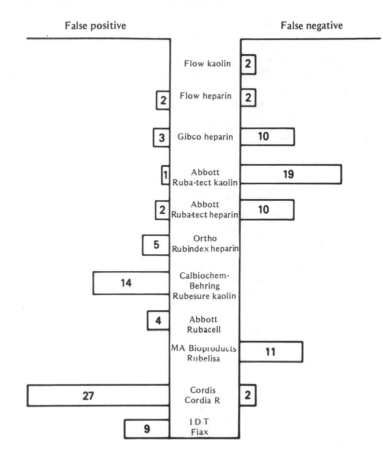

Fig. 10–2. Summary of the number of false-positive and false-negative results obtained with 11 commercial kits. (From Castellano, G.A., Madden, D.L., Hazzard, G.T., Cleghorn, C.S., Vails, D.V., Lay, A.-C., Tzan, N.R., and Sever, J.L.: Evaluations of commercially available diagnostic kits for rubella. J. Infect. Dis., *143*:578, 1981.)

breaks of rubella among hospital personnel place susceptible pregnant women, both hospital workers and patients, at risk for the disease. For patients, rubella antibody screening should be done at the first prenatal visit and those with a high titer should be evaluated for evidence of recent disease. The most specific test for infection is the presence of IgM for rubella. This is available through many commercial laboratories, state laboratories, or the Centers for Disease Control laboratory. During pregnancy, the obstetrician will receive queries from patients about possible exposure to rubella, occasionally because of the occurrence of an undiagnosed flulike illness. If such a patient is known to have a positive HI test, she is immune and not at risk. If no HI antibody is present, she is susceptible and a repeat HI titer in 3 to 4 weeks will give evidence of a recent infection. If there is evidence of active infection in the first 12 weeks of gestation, I would advise termination of the pregnancy. Although gross abnormalities recognized at birth are associated with active rubella infection in the first trimester, later exposure results in persistent viral shedding in some newborns, with the subsequent discovery of hearing defects. The patient should have a choice in this circumstance. For the susceptible woman exposed to rubella who does not elect a pregnancy termination, gamma globulin can be given, although its value in this situation has not been proved. Occasionally, the obstetrician will see a pregnant woman in the first half of pregnancy who has received the live rubella vaccine. Although there is no risk of the fetal rubella syndrome with the vaccine virus, this episode represents fetal exposure to a live virus, and some abnormalities have been reported. If the pregnancy is less than 20 weeks, I would favor termination. For the susceptible woman who has delivered, the postpartum period is an excellent time for immunization. The risk of pregnancy is low, and these women can breast-feed without any fear of damage to their children.

Cytomegalovirus

The next agent of the STORCH complex, the cytomegalovirus, has great importance even though newborn infection is usually not recognized by the obstetrician. There are two aspects to its significance: It is the most frequent microbiologic agent implicated in newborn infections (see Table 10–2), and it can be the source of serious newborn disease[13] that results in death or long-term mental disabilities. The frequency and the severity of these infections are usually underestimated by obstetricians because the majority of infants with this disease have no gross clinical evidence of infection at birth. An added concern for clinicians is the observation that a normal-appearing newborn can go on to develop serious mental disabilities, with hearing loss, which is a hallmark of this syndrome.[80]

Since the first edition of this book there has been a growing volume of knowledge about both the nature of maternal colonization and of fetal and newborn infection caused by the cytomegalovirus. For some time, it has been known that maternal excretion of the virus in the urine or from the cervix occurs more frequently than infection in the fetus or newborn. This asymptomatic maternal shedding of virus is more common in lower socio-economic populations, with increasing frequency in the third trimester, reaching 13.4% in one study of a lower socio-economic black population in the southern United States.[81] The missing link in our information chain is the determination of the susceptibility of the newborn to infections with this virus. In contrast to the frequent maternal excretion of virus, the newborn is less commonly infected, only 1% of all live births.[82] Among infected infants, there is a wide range of response. Five to 10% will have an obvious virulent form of the disease,[13] while another 10% with subclinical congenital infection will develop varying degrees of neurologic and learning disabilities.[80] Although the presence of maternal antibody does not prevent maternal excretion of the virus or subsequent newborn infection, one study documented the occurrence of the most serious newborn infections in women who had a primary cytomegalovirus infection during pregnancy.[83] Even in this high risk group, the newborn risk for infection is not 100%. The authors found that 50% of the infants born after a primary maternal infection were infected,[83] and this was a figure comparable to the 46% reported in a subsequent study.[84] In contrast to this high incidence, only 6% of newborns of mothers with recurrent infections were infected, and their infections were not the most serious types.[83] It is clear that the risk of infection for the newborn, both in frequency and severity, is greater with primary maternal infection.

This new information provides some guidelines for physician care of pregnant women. Since primary infection with the cytomegalovirus usually causes no maternal symptoms, prepregnancy and first trimester screening for the presence of cytomegalovirus antibody should be done whenever possible. If the prenatal blood test shows a high titer, an IgM test can be done to check for recent infection. If this is the case, I would advise termination of the pregnancy because of our present inability to designate the newborn infant who will become infected. If the patient is seronegative at the time of the first prenatal visit, a repeat maternal blood sample should be drawn at the time of delivery. If this is positive, the newborn can be closely screened by the pediatrician. If the child subsequently develops learning defects that are attributed to the "trauma" of delivery, this can be very important information for the obstetrician.

The role of a vaccine for cytomegalovirus is still unclear at this time. The incomplete protection afforded by maternal antibody (i.e., some mothers with antibody excrete virus and deliver infants who are infected) suggests that the vaccine will not provide universal protection. However, the presence of natural antibody seems to provide protection against the most serious infections. Field trials of the vaccine are in progress, but the greatest enthusiasm for the vaccine to date has been in patients receiving multiple blood transfusions, particularly when they are immunosuppressed. Systemic infection due to the cytomegalovirus can occur when blood transfusions are given,[85] and this may be life-threatening in the latter group of patients. A celebrated instance of this syndrome was the readmission to the hospital of Pope John Paul for a febrile illness caused by the cytomegalovirus that resulted from the multiple transfusions required for his initial care after an assassination attempt.

Herpesvirus

There is a huge disparity between the high anxiety level of physicians and lay people about herpes simplex virus and the low risk of newborn infection caused by this virus. Herpes disease has been overpublicized in the popular press, and this is understandable. Genital herpes is linked to sexual activity and its incidence has been rapidly rising, so that forecasters can speculate that everyone in the world will have genital tract herpes by the year 2030. There is also public fascination with an "incurable" disease, particularly when it can cause death or serious life-long morbidity in the newborn. The public's fear of serious newborn infection has been communicated to obstetricians, who often feel the pressures to perform an elective cesarean section in order to avoid this problem. A major factor in the physician's decision of abdominal delivery is that a bad result, an infant with herpes disease, means a lawsuit, and there is a body of opinion that correlates cesarean section with optimal obstetric care. In contrast is the rarity of occurrence of this newborn disease. As noted in Table 10–2, herpes simplex virus has the lowest frequency of newborn infection among the STORCH pathogens and has been estimated to occur once in 7,700 deliveries.[86] There remains this enormous gap between obstetric practice patterns and the rarity of herpes infection in the nursery. On my own obstetric service at the New York Hospital-Cornell Medical Center, in the calendar year 1982 there were 27 cesarean sections performed to avoid newborn infection due to herpes. This works out to 56 cesarean sections per 7500 deliveries. In other words, over 50 cesarean sections were performed to prevent one case of newborn herpes. In that same year, of 3,613 total deliveries there were no infants who had an active infection caused by herpes in the nursery. This discrepancy between obstetric practice and newborn experience requires obstetric knowledge of the basic facts of herpes infections so that appropriate management decisions can be made.

The starting point of understanding is the awareness that the herpesviruses can have a serious impact upon the fetus. Among the newborn infants who develop herpes simplex infections, 50% die, and many survivors suffer permanent neurologic damage.[87] Although intrauterine infection of the fetus occurs rarely,[88] nearly all the fetal infections are acquired during labor and the passage through a birth canal contaminated by herpesvirus. There is difficulty in assessing the risks to each individual newborn. Although the frequency of active maternal genital tract shedding of the virus is not known, one survey found that 4% of a population of pregnant women were culture-positive for the virus during pregnancy.[89] This frequency of 40 in 1000 cases is 300 times more frequent than the occurrence of the rare newborn infection, which is one per 7,500 deliveries. One remarkable example of the lack of correlation between newborn viral exposure and the development of infection was the case report finding of herpesvirus in amniotic fluid obtained by amniocentesis prior to cesarean section, which resulted in the delivery of an unaffected infant.[90] The newborn most at risk for a herpes infection is the child delivered vaginally in a mother with an active herpetic lesion. Even in this high risk situation, only 40% of the newborns are infected.[86] One study showed that the risk of fetal herpes infection in mothers with genital lesions increased with the length of time of ruptured membranes.[91] Cesarean section was not helpful in women whose membranes were ruptured more than four hours.[91] Another aspect of the therapeutic problems with this disease is the realization that 70% of the infants with herpes infection are born to asymptomatic mothers.[92]

Despite this limited basis for understanding, guidelines for the care of pregnant patients can be developed. The highest risk populations are those women with active herpetic lesions found during pregnancy. Women with a history of genital tract herpes need to be instructed by their physicians to be alerted to the clinical progression of the disease (see Chapter 8). They should be able to recognize the prodromal signs in order to alert the obstetrician if they are present when membranes rupture or labor begins. The patient with prodromal symptoms or active genital lesions should make this known to the obstetrician early in labor or when the membranes rupture, so that a cesarean section can be performed before four hours' time of membrane rupture has elapsed. Because the number of patient observations determining the four hour rule is small, I would be willing to do a cesarean section for a patient with genital herpes if the interval of membrane rupture is less than 12 hours. In patients with a history of genital herpes or with an active lesion at some time during pregnancy, culture of the lesion site and of cervical tissue can be used as a guide late in pregnancy if there are no active lesions.[93-95] Viral surveillance of the lesion-free patient depends upon a laboratory equipped to do the cultures and report the results to the physician immediately. A Pap smear of a genital lesion or of a cervical sample is not an acceptable screening technique because there are samples from genital tract sites that will produce positive culture results but in which no giant cells will be seen on the smear. A positive smear from a new perineal lesion in a patient in early labor would be diagnostic for me, but it is impossible to get an expert cytologic reading on a 24-hour basis seven days a week in most hospitals. The major diagnostic aid remains the culture. There is good evidence that asymptomatic mothers who have negative cultures a week or less before delivery can safely have vaginal deliveries.[93-95] The vast majority (92%) of positive cultures become so within four days of incubation in the laboratory.[95] If culture reports are not available or the patient has prodromal signs of a recurrent herpes infection, I believe that cesarean section should be performed. Herpetic lesions at nongenital sites are not an indication for cesarean section, i.e., active "cold" sores in the oral cavity are not a justification for cesarean section. There have been reports of newborn herpetic infection in which the initiation of the infection occurred at the site of application of the scalp electrode during labor.[92] Because of these reports and my concern about asymptomatic maternal carriage of the virus, I do not use a scalp electrode on the fetus of a mother with a history of genital tract herpes infection at any time during pregnancy. There is no uniformity of opinion on this point. In a personal communication, Grossman has stated that he feels that a scalp electrode can be used on the newborn of the culture-negative mother. Following delivery, mothers with genital tract lesions or positive cultures can breast-feed their infants provided that reasonable care is taken to prevent direct contact of the infant with infected surfaces. Most hospitals require isolation techniques for the mother and the baby in the nursery. I prefer a private room for the mother with rooming-in capabilities if possible in order to minimize the mother's feelings of discomfort about the isolation. Despite all these safeguards, the fact that herpes can occur in the newborn of an asymptomatic woman with intact membranes means that this infection cannot be totally prevented by obstetricians.[96] New antiviral agents such as acyclovir may be a treatment option for these infected newborns.

ASYMPTOMATIC MATERNAL INFECTION OR COLONIZATION WITH POSSIBLE EFFECT ON FETAL OUTCOME

Prematurity

When we attempt to relate poor fetal outcome to maternal conditions, we are in a still clouded area of clinical investigation. The major stimulus for this research has been an awareness that the outcome for low birth weight infants is poorer than for those weighing more than 2,500 g. This observation holds whether the differences are the result of prematurity or of intrauterine growth retardation. A number of evaluations of populations of pregnant women have revealed a statistically significant correlation between an inapparent maternal infection and a poorer fetal outcome as measured by fetal weight. Over and over again, there has been a failure in many studies to acknowledge that a cause and effect relationship has not been established. One group of investigators has hypothesized that males are the source of this microbiologic colonization[97] at the time of intercourse. The critical element needed to prove the hypothesis that maternal colonization and poor fetal outcome are related is prospective therapeutic intervention that demonstrates improvement in results. Currently, the National Institutes of Health has funded studies of antibiotic intervention in pregnant women to address this point.

Asymptomatic Bacteriuria

The most striking relationship between inapparent maternal infection and prematurity has been in instances of maternal asymptomatic bacteriuria. This relationship is clear-cut,[98] but it has not been established that antibiotic therapy to rid the mother of these bacteria will have any favorable effect on the prematurity rate. Some studies have shown a lowering of the rate of premature delivery among treated women[99] and others have shown no impact.[100] I personally am skeptical of such a preventive role of antibiotics directed against urinary tract colonization. The most serious urinary tract infection for the pregnant woman is pyelonephritis. One study of women in this highest risk category who were successfully treated during pregnancy showed no increase in the prematurity rate compared with the population at large.[101] It is possible that the common finding of asymptomatic bacteriuria in pregnant women from lower socio-economic classes with a high prematurity rate is only a marker of social class and has no importance by itself as a cause of prematurity.

Mycoplasma

Members of the *Mycoplasma* family, for example *Mycoplasma hominis,* have been found with greater frequency in the lower genital tracts of pregnant women who have a higher incidence of low birth weight infants.[102] In surveys of nonpregnant women, this organism has been recovered more often in sexually active women, particularly those from lower socio-economic classes.[103] However, these same women can also be heavily colonized with *Ureaplasma* or *Chlamydia,* which adds other microbiologic variables to this equation. A great stimulus for serious consideration of the possibility of a direct relationship between these organisms in the mother and pregnancy wastage was provided by Elder and associates, who found the prematurity rate to be lower in pregnant controls who had been treated with tetracycline, an antibiotic with known effectiveness against *Mycoplasma.*[100] This study provided a major incentive for the planning of prospective therapeutic intervention studies to determine the possibility of the benefit of antibiotic treatment of asymptomatic pregnant women. There is still considerable controversy about these observations. Is the significant factor in prematurity colonization of the mother with one or all of these organisms or is it related to actual invasion and infection? One recent study of a large number of women showed no correlation between the isolation of either *Mycoplasma hominis* or *Ureaplasma urealyticum* from the lower genital tract and an increased incidence of prematurity.[104]

Chlamydia

There has been a recent parallel interest in the relationship of maternal genital tract colonization with *Chlamydia* and identification of a population that has a higher incidence of prematurity.[105] Again, this observation was not confirmed in a recent study of genital tract colonization.[104] A small subgroup of colonized women, those with IgM antibodies to *Chlamydia* in their serum indicative of recent systemic infection, had a significant risk of delivering prematures.[104] Clearly, more studies are needed before obstetricians embark upon a large-scale surveillance program of *Chlamydia* colonization of the lower genital tract and treatment of pregnant women.

SYMPTOMATIC MATERNAL INFECTION WITH POSSIBLE ADVERSE FETAL OUTCOME

Primary Site Not the Genital Tract

There have been many studies relating symptomatic systemic maternal infection to a poor fetal outcome. Viral infections such as hepatitis[106] or bacterial infections including pyelonephritis[107] or pneumonia[108] have been associated with an increased incidence of premature labor and a higher perinatal mortality rate. In some of these cases, it is possible that either maternal fever or systemic release of viral or bacterial products is a factor in the initiation of premature labor. Added to the stress of premature labor is the increased risk to the fetus caused by the elevated temperature of the mother. All of these components add up to a poorer fetal outcome.

This clear-cut relationship between maternal infection and a poorer fetal outcome has been modified by some recent observations. This is particularly true in the case of bacterial infections such as pyelonephritis[101] and bacterial pneumonia,[109] in which the prematurity rate has been much lower than in previous studies and the perinatal mortality rate very close to that seen on the obstetric service in general.

I think these better clinical results reflect improvement in physician understanding of infection with resultant modifications of maternal care. Obstetricians now have a wider range of antibiotics with which to treat patients with these bacterial infections. Physicians are more aware of the importance of intravenous fluid hydration to achieve proper fluid balance, and they employ antipyretic agents to achieve a more favorable intrauterine environment for the fetus. Add to this increased fund of obstetric care knowledge the tremendous advances that have taken place in the neonatal nursery, with more efficient resuscitation at birth and better survival in the nursery. All of these have combined to improve the outlook of the babies of the mothers with these systemic infections.

Obstetricians should be aggressive in the care of these patients. In addition to the concern for appropriate antibiotic selection if a bacterial infection is suspected, more than the usual intravenous hydration should be ordered. This should not be standard maintenance therapy; sufficient volumes of fluids should be given (with close monitoring of serum electrolytes and urine output) to replace the huge insensible fluid loss associated with an elevated maternal temperature and vomiting in some instances. Many of these women will require 6 L or more of fluid in the first 24 hours. In addition, acetaminophen (Tylenol) should be used with a normal loading dose and then a half-dose given every two hours instead of a full dose every four hours in an attempt to avoid recurrent elevations of maternal temperature because of the short half-life of this medication. Concomitant with this maternal care, there should be frequent monitoring of the fetal condition with such biophysical parameters as the fetal heart rate.

Primary varicella (chickenpox) infection in the adult produces an easily recognizable clinical syndrome that can have profound fetal and newborn effects. It differs from the entities in the STORCH complex because these mothers have identifiable systemic disease, with the appearance of skin vesicles and occasionally life-threatening pneumonia. For the fetus, the risks vary with the timing of the infection. Early pregnancy exposure can produce a wide variety of untoward fetal effects, including cataracts and microphthalmus. The range goes from effects indistinguishable from some of those produced by the STORCH pathogens to a pathognomonic clinical picture with skin scarring and limb hypoplasia.[110] These adverse fetal outcomes are not preventable and the mother should be aware of these possibilities and offered the opportunity for a pregnancy termination if the systemic varicella infection is noted in the first 20 weeks of gestation. Maternal infection late in pregnancy is an acute problem that demands obstetric and pediatric decision making. If the maternal infection occurs 5 to 20 days before delivery, disease is frequently seen in the newborn, but this is usually not serious, presumably because of the protection conferred by transplacental passage of maternal antibody. However, these newborns are a potential source of this viral infection for all susceptible personnel and babies, and strict isolation techniques should be employed. If maternal infection is confirmed in the interval from four days before delivery to two days postpartum, the infant can have serious systemic disease with a 30% mortality rate.[111] These high risk infants should receive varicella-zoster immunoglobulin (VZIG) as soon as possible after birth. This is available through regional laboratories. The physician can locate the site of the nearest center by contacting the Centers for Disease Control.

Primary Site of Maternal Infection—The Genital Tract

In the mother with premature rupture of the membranes, there is a potential risk of infection of the newborn. Indeed, the therapeutic algorithm in this situation in the minds of most physicians weighs the risk of infection for the newborn against the risk of prematurity. There have been a number of important observations made about these risks for the fetus. It is clear that the possibility of fetal infection is greater the longer the time of membrane rupture (see Figure 10–3)[112] and is more frequent with premature babies (see Figure 10–4).[112] These observations on increased fetal and newborn risks of infection were dovetailed in many minds with findings noted in Figure 10–5[113] that documented a higher perinatal mortality rate with increasing time intervals of membrane rupture. The inexorable conclusion was obviously that a prolonged length of time of membrane rupture is equated with a heightened risk of newborn infection and a higher perinatal mortality rate. To combat this, aggressive obstetric intervention to achieve delivery and shorten the time interval of membrane rupture should result in improved perinatal mortality rates. However, this represents flawed reasoning based upon

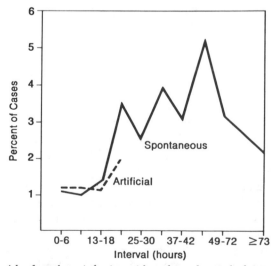

Fig. 10–3. Increasing risk of newborn infection with prolonged period of time of membrane rupture. (Reprinted with permission from the American College of Obstetricians and Gynecologists. From Shubeck, F., Benson, R.C., Clark, W.W., Jr., Berendes, H., Weiss, W., and Deutschberger, J.: Fetal hazard after rupture of membranes. Obstet. Gynecol., *28*:22, 1966.)

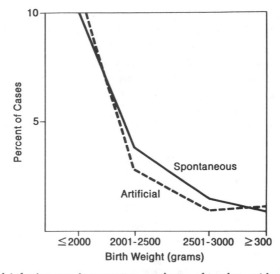

Fig. 10–4. Increased infection rate in premature newborns of mothers with premature rupture of membranes. (Reprinted with permission from the American College of Obstetricians and Gynecologists. From Shubeck, F., Benson, R.C., Clark, W.W., Jr., Berendes, H., Weiss, W., and Deutschberger, J.: Fetal hazard after rupture of membranes. Obstet. Gynecol., *28*:22, 1966.)

the assumption that the observed relationships are cause and effect ones. Review Figure 10–3 again. Although the risk of newborn infection increases with the length of time of membrane rupture, the risk of infection for any individual newborn is quite small, less than 10%. Evaluate Figure 10–5 again. Although the perinatal death rate increases with prolonged membrane rupture, this only reflects the biologic reality that far fewer women with spontaneous rupture of membranes before 36 weeks of gestation will go into spontaneous labor within 24 hours than women in whom this event occurs at term. Figure 10–5 reflects the biologic reality that the infants born after the longest time intervals of membrane rupture are

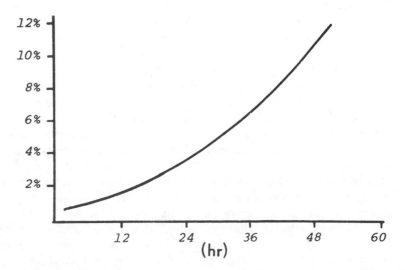

Fig. 10–5. Increasing perinatal mortality with increasing length of time of membrane rupture. (From Gunn, G.C., Mishell, D.R., Jr., and Morton, D.G.: Premature rupture of membranes. Am. J. Obstet. Gynecol., *106*:469, 1970.)

usually the most premature. The most telling arguments against this obstetric obsession with time are the recent observations that the majority of the deaths of these infants can be related to prematurity and not to infection.[114, 115] Active intervention to secure an even more immature fetus than would have occurred naturally cannot be expected to improve newborn outcome. Even in the highest risk situation, in which the mother develops chorioamnionitis with an elevated temperature and a tender uterus, the newborn infection rate is only 1 to 6%.[116] These observations should influence obstetric management of the pregnant patient with premature rupture of the membranes.

The pathophysiology of premature rupture of the membranes has significance for the clinician. There are a few women with premature rupture of the membranes in whom the bacterial colonization of the amniotic fluid precedes the clinical event of membrane rupture. This has been best documented by the finding of elevated IgM immunoglobulin levels in a subgroup of infants born of mothers with premature rupture of the membranes.[117] These women are at higher risk for having a newborn with infection in the nursery. Rather than regard the whole population of women with premature rupture of the membranes as at equal risk for newborn infection that increases with the length of time of membrane rupture, our focus should be to attempt to identify the subgroup of women who are at higher risk for fetal infection from the beginning.

The first priority of physician care for the patient with suspected premature rupture of membranes is diagnosis. In these women with a history of sudden loss of fluid per the vagina, the initial examination should be performed efficiently so that repeated vaginal manipulation will not be necessary. A sterile speculum examination should be performed, and if a pool of fluid is present, the diagnosis is obvious. The fluid should be aspirated for pulmonary maturity studies if the fetus is less than 36 weeks' gestation. The lecithin-sphingomyelin ratio from such fluid does not correlate well with fluid obtained transabdominally, but the presence of phosphatidylglycerol does seem to be an important marker suggesting pulmonary maturity.[118] If no pooling is present in the vagina, the posterior fornix of the vagina should be sampled for pH, and a smear obtained for microscopic examination. An alkaline pH and ferning seen on the smear confirm the diagnosis. Other studies need to be done. A culture of the fluid or of the surface of the cervix if no fluid is present should be obtained to determine the presence of such important pathogens for the newborn as the group B beta-hemolytic streptococci, *Escherichia coli, Hemophilus influenzae, Listeria monocytogenes,* and *Neisseria gonorrhoeae,* and cultures should be done for the herpesvirus. Routine blood studies should be obtained in these women, although the value of the white blood cell count and sedimentation rate in predicting subsequent infection has not been proved. A few years ago, there was a surge of interest in the C-reactive protein test because it allegedly identified all pregnant women with a subsequent risk of developing an infection.[119] This observation was not confirmed by subsequent study,[120] however, and thus probably represents an inappropriate decision in the original study to include those patients with a pathologic diagnosis of chorioamnionitis alone who had no clinical evidence of infection. This pathologic diagnosis of chorioamnionitis is made far more frequently than that of clinical infection (Table 10–9).[121]

The most controversial aspect of diagnostic care in these women is the use of amniocentesis to evaluate the presence of bacterial contamination as well as to

Table 10–9. Correlation of Histologic Inflammation in 1,536 Consecutive Placentas with Fetal Outcome

	Vasculitis and Chorionitis (%)	Neither (%)
Stillbirths	2	2
Neonatal morbidity	25	15
Neonatal infection	5	Less than 1
Neonatal deaths	5	2
Normal course	73	84

more accurately assess pulmonary maturity. There is legitimate concern because this is an invasive procedure, and it is not possible to obtain fluid in 100% of the candidates for this approach. The initial reports for this transabdominal approach were enthusiastic, since the presence of bacteria in the amniotic fluid obtained this way identified a high risk population.[122] This enthusiasm has persisted in two subsequent reports[123, 124] in which the ability to obtain amniotic fluid was high (51%[123] and 68.8%[124]) and the findings were helpful in management. Despite this enthusiasm, this procedure has not been accepted on most services. Many physicians have found the difficulty in obtaining fluid to be the rule rather than the exception, and therefore management for the majority of these patients proceeds without the benefit of an amniotic fluid analysis. When the responsible physicians become accustomed to management without amniocentesis, there is less inclination to perform this invasive procedure in the next case. I adhere to the following guidelines in the initial care of these women. In the patient with premature rupture of the membranes before 36 weeks' gestation of the fetus, an ultrasonographic examination is performed. If there is a pocket of fluid that can be safely obtained, amniocentesis is performed. The finding of bacteria in the microscopic examination of an unspun specimen correlates well with high risk for the fetus. If no pocket is present, no intervention is employed.

The major controversies in the care of women with premature rupture of the membranes involve active obstetric intervention. One camp of physicians advocates the use of steroids to hasten lung maturity in less than 32 weeks' gestation and then achieve delivery after a 24 to 48 hour interval.[125] The rationale for this approach is that it reduces the risk of infection for the newborn, and there is evidence from older studies that only 7.6% of the women with premature rupture of membranes and a premature infant in utero will carry the pregnancy a week or more.[126] The argument is advanced that since so few of these infants gain any significant time in utero, the obstetrician is better served by active intervention to lower the risk of infection in the newborn. For the patient who is 36 weeks pregnant or more, the concern about prematurity is gone and early intervention is indicated, because older studies showed an increase in the perinatal mortality rates when the interval between membrane rupture and delivery exceeds 48 hours.[126] I do not support the view of active obstetric intervention in these women. In a carefully controlled prospective study of the use of steroids in women with premature rupture of the membranes,[127] there was no benefit for the infants who were subsequently delivered. I favor no intervention, and more recent studies have shown that 20 to 46% of women whose infants have achieved a week or more in utero after premature rupture of the membranes.[128-131] On the obstetric service at the New York Hospital-Cornell Medical Center where there are a high number of maternal transfers, nearly 19% of the women gain a week or more before delivery.[132] There are important therapeutic decisions to make in these women. Although daily white blood cell counts are usually obtained, there is no evidence that this is predictive for infection in these women. In at least one study, the only correlation with an elevated white blood cell count was the spontaneous onset of labor with 24 hours of that observation.[114] Tocolytic agents should not be used in these women because uterine activity can be the response to a developing chorioamnionitis. The one exception to this is the instance in which uterine activity occurs after amniocentesis and the fluid shows no evidence of bacterial contamination. For me, one of the highest risk groups for infection are women with premature rupture of the membranes who have a cerclage in place. The cerclage should be removed immediately and the pregnancy terminated at that point, without waiting for clinical signs of infection. Although the conservative approach gains added time in utero and results in the delivery of larger babies, in the total population of women with premature rupture of the membranes the newborn results have not been as good as they are for equivalent-sized infants whose mothers did not undergo premature rupture. There is a higher incidence of fetal abnormalities in this group, and we have seen infants with hypoplastic lungs after prolonged periods in utero with little or no amniotic fluid.[132]

The role of antibiotics for the fetus is of women with premature rupture of membranes is still controversial. There are points of agreement. There is no enthusiasm for the use of prophylactic antibiotics in all patients in the antepartum period. However, there are many individuals in whom antibiotics will be employed. These include those patients in whom a potential pathogen for the fetus has been recovered on initial screening of the lower genital tract. Although I would begin the therapy immediately if *Neisseria gonorrhoeae* were recovered, I have withheld therapy until the onset of labor with an organism such as the group B *Streptococcus.* Many physicians will begin treatment as soon as this culture report is available. The role of the routine use of intrapartum antibiotics for all patients with a history of premature rupture of the membranes has not been established by a comparative prospective study. One study was enthusiastic in its support of the routine use of antibiotics in these patients in labor.[133] I remain selective in my prescription of antibiotics. If any known pathogen has been isolated at the time of admission, if the fetus develops tachycardia during labor (i.e, a pulse rate of 160 beats/minute or greater for one half-hour or more), or if the mother becomes febrile, I do begin systemic antibiotics. Since the most commonly involved organisms in newborn sepsis are the group B beta-hemolytic streptococci or *Escherichia coli,* either ampicillin or cefoxitin could be prescribed. Cefoxitin provides better coverage of *Escherichia coli.* If the patient is allergic to penicillin or cephalosporins or both, I usually prescribe clindamycin and gentamicin in combination. If *Hemophilus influenzae* is a frequent source of newborn infection on your service, then ampicillin, cefamandole, or cefotoxime would be a good choice.

A subgroup of women with premature labor and intact membranes can have unsuspected intraamniotic fluid contamination with an increased risk of subsequent newborn infection. One study by Bobitt and Ledger[134] showed a number of women with premature labor who subsequently delivered premature babies who had heavy bacterial contamination of the amniotic fluid. Another later study demonstrated that bacterial products are substrates for the production of pros-taglandins, which will initiate labor.[135] This led to investigations of the use of amniocentesis in the care of women with premature labor to rule out the presence of bacterial contamination of the amniotic fluid. Since the recovery of bacteria in this situation was so infrequent in one study in 1981,[136] these investigators felt that amniocentesis should not be a routine diagnostic procedure in these women. I tend to agree with this philosophy in general. Since bed rest and hydration will cure 50% of the women with a diagnosis of premature labor, the routine use of an invasive diagnostic procedure that has associated morbidity does not seem prudent. However, currently on the obstetric service of the New York Hospital-Cornell Medical Center amniocentesis is attempted if a pocket of fluid is visualized on ultrasound examination, at which point a second course of intravenous tocolysis is planned. In the population of women with asymptomatic bacterial contami-nation of the amniotic fluid and premature labor, subsequent infection of the newborn is a rare event that occurs in less than 5%.

Despite all our preventive measures, the obstetrician will have to care for pregnant women with a clinical diagnosis of chorioamnionitis. There has been some confusion about fetal and newborn risks in this population. Earlier studies demonstrated a high perinatal mortality rate in this population[137] and many ser-vices imposed strict time rules, i.e., the woman with chorioamnionitis had to be delivered within eight hours of diagnosis in order to lower these risks. This reasoning was flawed, for in many of these women chorioamnionitis develops after an intrauterine death occurs, and many of these newborn deaths are related to prematurity. This etiology will not be modified favorably by time limits on labor. In fact, one careful review of chorioamnionitis patients found that diagnosed newborn infections occurred in only 1 to 6% of the cases.[116] As a result, the current standard of care in these women is to employ antibiotics in labor, either ampicillin or cefoxitin alone or a combination of clindamycin and gentamicin, and to only intervene by cesarean section for such obstetric indications as failure to progress or "fetal distress." The failure to progress has been noted to appear with some frequency in this population[138] (Figure 10–6). This individual management has resulted in a vaginal delivery in the majority of patients, and perinatal mortality rates have been similar to those of the population at large.[139, 140] Despite these findings, the obstetrician should not be cavalier about the risks to the fetus in this population. One recent study of women with chorioamnionitis who delivered premature infants showed a higher than expected perinatal mortality rate.[115] This increased death rate was not caused by sepsis, and it is possible that the increased maternal temperature adds to the stress for these premature babies.

NEWBORN INFECTIONS ASSOCIATED WITH THE USE OF A FETAL SCALP ELECTRODE

Fetal infections can result from the use of a fetal scalp electrode or scalp sampling for pH during labor. Most of these infections are not serious, and there is a variation in the estimate of frequency of this condition from 0.34/1,000[141] to 4.7% of all deliveries.[142] Serious life-threatening infections have been reported, including osteomyelitis of the skull,[143] sepsis and death,[144] and herpes infection of the scalp.[92] To date, there have been no techniques of application that have totally eliminated this problem, although a higher scalp infection rate was reported with one barbed

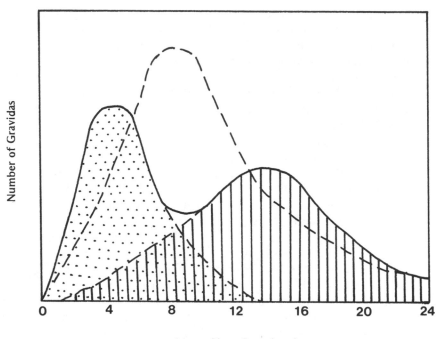

Fig. 10–6. The lack of uniformity of a labor pattern in women with chorioamnionitis. Instead of the idealized figure demonstrated by the dotted lines, there are two distinct populations, with the population on the right characterized by a prolonged labor. (From Friedman, E.A.: Obstetric infection in labor. *In* Obstetric and Perinatal Infections. Edited by D. Charles and M. Finland. Philadelphia, Lea & Febiger, 1973.)

electrode that is no longer being sold in this country.[142] The treatment of infants with this problem is usually simple and straightforward. Simple local drainage usually suffices, but cultures for anaerobic organisms should be obtained because of the high frequency of anaerobic involvement in these infections. If there is any evidence of a spreading infection, systemic antibiotics should be prescribed and wide excision of the infection site may be necessary for a cure.

REFERENCES

1. Rubella vaccination during pregnancy—United States 1971–1981. M.M.W.R., *31*:477, 1982.
2. Immunization during pregnancy. ACOG Tech. Bull., *64*:1, 1982.
3. Amstey, M.S.: Nonviral vaccine in pregnancy. Infect. Dis. Letters for OB/GYN, *5*:55, 1983.
4. Varner, M.W., McGuinness, G.A., and Galask, R.P.: Rabies vaccination in pregnancy. Am J. Obstet. Gynecol., *143*:717, 1982.
5. Schultz, J.C., Adamson, J.S., Jr., Workman, W.W., and Norman, T.D.: Fatal liver disease after intravenous administration of tetracycline in high dosage. N. Engl. J. Med., *269*:999, 1963.
6. LeBlanc, A.L., and Perry, J.E.: Transfer of tetracycline across the human placenta. Tex. Rep. Biol. Med., *25*:541, 1967.
7. Greene, J.W., Jr., and Touchstone, J.C.: Urinary estriol as an index of placental function. Am. J. Obstet. Gynecol., *85*:1, 1963.
8. Boehm, F.H., DiPietro, D.L., and Goss, D.A.: The effect of ampicillin administration on urinary estriol and serum estradiol in the normal pregnant patient. Am. J. Obstet. Gynecol., *119*:98, 1974.
9. Gallagher, J.C., Ismail, M.A., and Aladjem, S.: Reduced urinary estriol levels, with erythromycin therapy. Obstet. Gynecol., *56*:381, 1980.
10. Lucey, J.F., and Driscoll, T.J.: Hazards to newborn infants of administration of long-acting sulfonamides to pregnant women. Pediatrics, *24*:498, 1959.

11. Gregg, N. McA.: Congenital cataract following German measles in the mother. Trans. Aust. Coll. Ophthalmol., *3*:35, 1941.
12. Center for Disease Control: Current status of rubella in the United States, 1969–1979. J. Infect. Dis., *142*:776, 1980.
13. Kibrick, S.: Viral infections of the fetus and newborn. Perspect. Virol., *2*:140, 1961.
14. McCracken, G.H., Jr., Shinefield, H.R., Cobb, K., Rausen, A.R., Dische, M.R., and Eichenwald, H.F.: Congenital cytomegalic inclusion disease. Am. J. Dis. Child., *117*:522, 1969.
15. Brown, G.C., and Karunas, R.S.: Relationship of congenital anomalies and maternal infection with selected enteroviruses. Am. J. Epidemiol, *95*:207, 1972.
16. Alford, C.A., and Pass, R.F.: Epidemiology of chronic congenital and perinatal infections of man. Clin. Perinatol., *8*:397, 1981.
17. Klein, J.O., Remington, J.S., and Marcy, S.M.: Current concepts of infection of the fetus and newborn infant. *In* Infectious Diseases of the Fetus and Newborn. Edited by J.S. Remington and J.O. Klein. 2nd ed., Philadelphia, W.B. Saunders, 1983.
18. Ballantyne, J.W.: Manual of Antenatal Pathology and Hygeine. Edinburgh, William Green & Son, 1902.
19. Dippel, A.L.: The relationship of congenital syphilis to abortion and miscarriage, and the mechanism of intrauterine protection. Am. J. Obstet. Gynecol., *47*:369, 1944.
20. Harter, C.A., and Benirschke, K.: Fetal syphilis in the first trimester. Am. J. Obstet. Gynecol., *124*:705, 1976.
21. Monif, G.R.G., Williams, B.R., Jr., Shulman, S.T., and Baer, H.: The problem of maternal syphilis after serologic surveillance during pregnancy. Am. J. Obstet. Gynecol., *117*:268, 1973.
22. Centers for Disease Control: Annual summary 1979: Reported morbidity and mortality in the U.S. M.M.W.R., *28*:83, 1980.
23. Stray-Pederson, B.: Economic evaluation of maternal screening to prevent congenital syphilis. Sex. Trans. Dis., *10*:167, 1983.
24. Ingall, D., and Musker, D.: Syphilis. *In* Infectious Diseases of the Fetus and Newborn. Edited by J.S. Remington and J.O. Klein. 2nd ed., Philadelphia, W.B. Saunders, 1983.
25. Centers for Disease Control: Syphilis—CDC recommended treatment schedules. M.M.W.R., *25*:101, 1976.
26. Philipson, A.: Pharmacokinetics of antibiotics in the pregnant woman. *In* Antibiotics in Obstetrics and Gynecology. Edited by W.J. Ledger. Boston. Martinus Nijhoff, 1982.
27. Fenton, L.J., and Light, I.J.: Congenital syphilis after maternal treatment with erythromycin. Obstet. Gynecol., *47*:493, 1976.
28. Philipson, A., Sabath, L.D., and Charles, D.: Transplacental passage of erythromycin and clindamycin, N. Engl. J. Med., *288*:1219, 1973.
29. Remington, J.S.: Toxoplasmosis in the adult. Bull. N.Y. Acad. Med., *50*:211, 1974.
30. Remington, J.S., Barnett, C.G., Meikel, M., and Lunde, M.N.: Toxoplasmosis and infectious mononucleosis. Arch. Intern. Med., *110*:744, 1962.
31. Welch, P.C., Masur, H., Jones, T.C., and Remington, J.S.: Serologic diagnosis of acute lymphodenopathic toxoplasmosis. J. Infect. Dis., *142*:256, 1980.
32. Desmonts, G., and Couvreur, J.: Congenital toxoplasmosis: A prospective study of the offspring of 542 women with acquired toxoplasmosis during pregnancy. Perinatal Medicine Sixth European Congress. Edited by O. Thalhammer, K. Baumgarten, and A. Pollok. Stuttgart, Thieme, 1979.
33. Remington, J.S., and Desmonts, G.: Toxoplasmosis. *In* Infectious Diseases of the Fetus and Newborn Infant. Edited by J.S. Remington and J.O. Klein. 2nd ed., Philadelphia, W.B. Saunders, 1983.
34. Wilson, C.B., Remington, J.S., Stagno, S., and Reynolds, D.W.: Development of adverse sequelae in children born with subclinical congenital *Toxoplasma* infection. Pediatrics, *66*:767, 1980.
35. Kimball, A.C., Kean, B.H., and Fuchs, F.: Congenital toxoplasmosis: A prospective study of 4,048 obstetric patients. Am. J. Obstet. Gynecol., *111*:211, 1971.
36. Ruoss, C.F., and Bourne, G.L.: Toxoplasmosis in pregnancy. J. Obstet. Gynecol. Br. Commonw., *79*:1115, 1972.
37. Desmonts, G., Couvreur, J., and Ben Roclid, M.S.: Le toxoplasme, à la mère et l'enfant. Arch. Fr. Pediatr., *22*:1183, 1965.
38. Desmonts, G., and Couvreur, J.: Toxoplasmosis: Epidemiologic and serologic aspects of perinatal infection. *In* Infections of the Fetus and the Newborn Infant. Progress in Clinical and Biological Research. Edited by S. Krugman and A.A. Gershon. Vol. 3. New York, Alan R. Liss, Inc., 1975.
39. Thalhammer, D.: Prevention of congenital toxoplasmosis. Neuropaediatrie, *4*:233, 1973.
40. Alford, C.A., Jr., Foft, J.W., Blankenship, W.J., Cassady, G., and Benton, J.W., Jr.: Subclinical central nervous system disease of neonates: A prospective study of infants born with increased levels of IgM. J. Pediatr., *75*:1167, 1969.
41. Baker, C.J., and Edwards, M.S.: Group B streptococcal infections. *In* Infectious Diseases of the Fetus and Newborn Infant. Edited by J.S. Remington and J.O. Klein. 2nd ed., Philadelphia, W.B. Saunders, 1983.

42. McCracken, G.H., Jr.: Group B streptococci: The new challenge in neonatal infections. J. Pediatr., *82*:703, 1973.
43. Baker, C.J.: Early onset group B streptococcal disease. J. Pediatr., *93*:124, 1978.
44. Bobitt, J.R., and Ledger, W.J.: Obstetric observations in 11 cases of neonatal sepsis due to the group B beta hemolytic streptococcus. Obstet. Gynecol., *47*:439, 1976.
45. Eickhoff, T.C., Klein, J.O., Daly, A.K., Ingall, D., and Finland, M.: Neonatal sepsis and other infections due to group B beta-hemolytic streptococci. N. Engl. J. Med., *271*:1221, 1964.
46. Francoisi, R.A., Knostman, J.D., and Zimmerman, R.A.: Group B streptococcal neonatal and infant infections. J. Pediatr., *82*:707, 1973.
47. Baker, C.J., and Barrett, F.F.: Transmission of group B streptococci among parturient women and their neonates. J. Pediatr., *83*:919, 1973.
48. Aber, R.C., Allen, N., Howell, J.T., Wilkenson, H.W., and Facklam, R.R.: Nosocomial transmission of group B streptococci. Pediatrics, *58*:346, 1976.
49. Anthony, B.F., and Okada, D.M.: The emergence of group B streptococci in infections of the newborn infant. Ann. Rev. Med., *28*:355, 1977.
50. Pass, M.A., Gray, B.M., Khare, S., and Dillon, H.C., Jr.: Prospective studies of group B streptococcal infections in infants. J. Pediatr. *95*:437, 1979.
51. Baker, C.J.: Group B streptococcal infections in neonates. Pediatr. Rev., *64*:5, 1979.
52. Lewin, E.B., and Amstey, M.S.: Natural history of group B streptococcus colonization and its therapy during pregnancy. Am. J. Obstet. Gynecol., *139*:512, 1981.
53. Baker, C.J., and Kasper, D.L.: Correlation of maternal antibody deficiency with susceptibility to neonatal group B streptococcal infection. N. Engl. J. Med., *294*:753, 1976.
54. Davis, J.P., Gutman, L.T., Higgins, M.V., Katz, S.L., Welt, S.I., and Wilfert, C.M.: Nasal colonization of infants with group B *Streptococcus* associated with intrauterine pressure transducers. J. Infect. Dis., *138*:804, 1978.
55. Winterbauer, R.H., Fortuine, R., and Eickhoff, T.C.: Unusual occurrence of neonatal meningitis due to Group B beta hemolytic streptococci. Pediatrics, *38*:661, 1966.
56. Regan, J.A., Chao, S., and James, L.S.: Premature rupture of membranes, preterm delivery, and group B streptococcal colonization of mothers. Am. J. Obstet. Gynecol., *141*:184, 1981.
57. Gardner, S.E., Yow, M.D., Leeds, L.J., Thompson, P.K., Mason, E.O., Jr., and Clark, D.J.: Failure of penicillin to eradicate group B streptococcal colonization in the pregnant woman: A couple study. Am. J. Obstet. Gynecol., *135*:1062, 1979.
58. Anthony, B.F., Eisenstadt, R., Carter, J., Kim, K.S., and Hobel, C.J.: Genital and intestinal carriage of group B streptococci during pregnancy. J. Infect. Dis., *143*:761, 1981.
59. Boyer, K.M., Gadzala, C.A., Kelly, P.D., and Gotoff, S.P.: Selective intrapartum chemoprophylaxis of neonatal group B streptococcal early-onset disease. III. Interruption of mother to infant transmission. J. Infect. Dis., *148*:810, 1983.
60. Siegel, J.D., McCracken, G.H., Jr., Threlkeld, N., Depasse, B.M., and Rosenfeld, C.R.: Single dose penicillin prophylaxis of neonatal group B streptococcal disease: Conclusion of a 41 month controlled trial. Lancet, *1*:1426, 1982.
61. Pyati, S.P., Pildes, R.S., Jacobs, N.M., Ramamurthy, R.S., Yeh, T.F., Raval, D.S., Lilein, L.D., Amma, P., and Metzger, W.I.: Penicillin in infants weighing two kilograms or less with early onset group B streptococcal disease. N. Engl. J. Med., *308*:1383, 1983.
62. Baker, C.J.: Summary of the workshop on perinatal infections due to group B *Streptococcus.* J. Infect. Dis., *136*:137, 1977.
63. McCracken, G.H., Jr., Sarff, L.D., Glode, M.P., Mize, S.G., Schiffer, M.S., Robbins, J.B., Gotschlich, E.C., Orskov, I., and Orskov, F.: Relation between *Escherichia coli* k1 capsular polysaccharide antigen and clinical outcome in neonatal meningitis. Lancet, *2*:246, 1974.
64. Wallace, R.J., Jr., Baker, C.J., Quinones, F.J., Hollis, D.G., Weaver, R.E., and Wiss, K.: Nontypable *Haemophilus influenzae* (biotype 4) as a neonatal, maternal, and genital pathogen. Rev. Inf. Dis., *5*:123, 1983.
65. Zervoudakis, I.A., and Cederqvist, L.L.: Effect of *Listeria monocytogenes* septicemia during pregnancy on the offspring. Am. J. Obstet. Gynecol., *129*:465, 1977.
66. Petrilli, E.S., D'Ablaing, G., and Ledger, W.J.: *Listeria monocytogenes* chorioamnionitis: Diagnosis by transabdominal amniocentesis. Obstet. Gynecol., *55*:5S, 1980.
67. Niles, R.A.: Puerperal tuberculosis with death of infant. Am. J. Obstet. Gynecol., *144*:131, 1982.
68. Schachter, J., Grossman, M., Holt, J., Sweet, R., and Spector, S.: Infection with *Chlamydia trachomatis:* Involvement of multiple anatomic sites in neonates. J. Infect. Dis. *139*:232, 1979.
69. Hammerschlag, M.R., Chandler, J.W., Alexander, E.R., English, M., Chiang, W.T., Koutsky, L., Eschenbach, D.A., and Smith, J.R.: Erythromycin ointment for ocular prophylaxis of neonatal chlamydial infection. J.A.M.A. *244*:2291, 1980.
70. Arth, C., VonSchmidt, B., Grossman, M., and Schachter, J.: Chlamydial pneumonitis. J. Pediatr., *93*:447, 1978.
71. Thadepalli, H., Rambhatla, K., Maidman, J.E., Arce, J.J., and Davidson, E.C., Jr.: Gonococcal sepsis secondary to fetal monitoring. Am. J. Obstet. Gynecol., *126*:510, 1976.

72. Handsfield, H.H., Hodson, W.A., and Holmes, K.K.: Neonatal gonococcal infection. I. Orogastric contamination with *Neisseria gonorrhoeae*. J.A.M.A., *225*:697, 1973.
73. Fawaz, K.A., Grady, G.F., Kaplan, M.M., and Gellis, S.S.: Repetitive maternal-fetal transmission of fatal hepatitis B. N. Engl. J. Med., *293*:1357, 1975.
74. Horstmann, D.M.: Rubella: The challenge of its control. J. Infect. Dis., *123*:640, 1971.
75. Thompson, G.R., Ferreyra, A., and Brackett, R.G.: Acute arthritis complicating rubella vaccination. Arthritis Rheum., *14*:19, 1971.
76. Schoenbaum, S.C., Hyde, J.N., Jr., Bartoshesky, L., and Crampton, K.: Benefit-cost analysis of rubella vaccination policy. N. Engl. J. Med., *294*:306, 1976.
77. Schiff, G.M., Rauh, J.L., Young, B., Trimble, S., Rotte, T., and Schiff, B.E.: Rubella-vaccinated students: Follow up in a public school system. J.A.M.A. *240*:2635, 1978.
78. Horstmann, D.M., Liebhaber, H., LeBouvier, G.L., Rosenberg, D.A., and Halstead, S.B.: Rubella: reinfection of vaccinated and naturally immune persons exposed in an epidemic. N. Engl. J. Med., *283*:771, 1970.
79. Castellano, G.A., Madden, D.L., Hazzard, G.T., Cleghorn, C.S., Vails, D.V., Ley, A.-C., Tzan, N.R., and Sever, J.L.: Evaluations of commercially available diagnostic kits for rubella. J. Infect. Dis., *143*:578, 1981.
80. Reynolds, D.W., Stagno, S., Stubbs, K.G., Dahle, A.J., Livingston, M.M., Saxon, S.S., and Alford, C.A.: Inapparent congenital cytomegalovirus infection with elevated cord IgM levels. N. Engl. J. Med., *290*:291, 1974.
81. Reynolds, D.W., Stagno, S., Hosty, T., Tiller, M., and Alford, C.A., Jr.: Maternal cytomegalovirus excretion and perinatal infection. N. Engl. J. Med., *289*:1, 1973.
82. Stagno, S., Pass, R.F., and Alford, C.A.: Perinatal infections and maldevelopment. Birth Defects, *17*:31, 1981.
83. Stagno, S., Pass, R.F., Dworsky, M.E., Henderson, R.E., Moore, E.G., Walton, P.D., and Alford, C.A.: Congenital cytomegalovirus infection. N. Engl. J. Med., *306*:945, 1982.
84. Hunter, K., Stagno, S., Capps, E., and Smith, R.J.: Prenatal screening of pregnant women for infections caused by cytomegalovirus, Epstein-Barr virus, herpesvirus, rubella, and *Toxoplasma gondii*. Am. J. Obstet. Gynecol., *145*:269, 1983.
85. Monif, G.R.G., Daicoff, G.I., and Flory, L.L.: Blood as a potential vehicle for the cytomegaloviruses. Am. J. Obstet. Gynecol., *126*:445, 1976.
86. Nahmias, A.J., Alford, C.A., and Korones, S.B.: Infection of the new-born with herpes virus hominis. Adv. Pediatr. *17*:185, 1970.
87. Nahmias, A.J., Visintine, A.M., Reimer, C.B., Del Buono, I., Shore, S.L., and Starr, S.E.: Herpes simplex virus of the fetus and newborn. *In* Infections of the Fetus and Newborn Infant. Edited by S. Krugman and A. Gershon. New York, Alan R. Liss, Inc., 1975.
88. Mitchell, J.E., and McCall, F.C.: Transplacental infection by herpes simplex virus. Am. J. Dis. Child., *106*:207, 1964.
89. Scher, J., Bottone, E., Desmond, E., and Simons, W.: The incidence and outcome of asymptomatic herpes simplex genitalis in an obstetric population. Am. J. Obstet. Gynecol., *144*:906, 1982.
90. Zervoudakis, I.A., Silverman, F., Senterfit, L.B., Strongin, M.J., Read, S., and Cederqvist, L.L.: Herpes simplex virus in the amniotic fluid of an unaffected fetus. Obstet. Gynecol., *55*:16S, 1980.
91. Amstey, M.S., and Monif, G.R.G.: Genital herpes virus infection in pregnancy. Obstet. Gynecol., *44*:394, 1974.
92. Whitley, R.J., Nahmias, A.J., Visintine, A.M., Fleming, C.L., and Alford, C.A.: The natural history of herpes simplex virus infection of mother and newborn. Pediatrics, *66*:489, 1980.
93. Grossman, J.H., III, Wallen, W.C., and Sever, J.L.: Management of genital herpes simplex virus infection during pregnancy. Obstet. Gynecol., *58*:1, 1981.
94. Boehm, F.H., Estes, W., Wright, P.F., and Growdon, J.F. Jr.: Management of genital herpes simplex virus infection occurring during pregnancy. Am. J. Obstet. Gynecol., *141*:735, 1981.
95. Harger, J.H., Pazin, G.J., Armstrong, J.A., Breinig, M.C., and Ho, M.: Characteristics and management of pregnancy in women with genital herpes simplex virus infection. Am. J. Obstet. Gynecol., *145*:784, 1983.
96. Hain, J., Doshi, N., and Harger, J.H.: Ascending transcervical herpes simplex infection with intact fetal membranes. Obstet. Gynecol., *56*:106, 1980.
97. Naeye, R.L.: Coitus and associated amniotic fluid infections. N. Engl. J. Med., *301*:1198, 1979.
98. Norden, C.W., and Kass, E.H.: Bacteriuria of pregnancy—a critical appraisal. Ann. Rev. Med., *19*:431, 1968.
99. Kass, E.H.: The significance of bacteriuria. J. Infect. Dis., *138*:546, 1978.
100. Elder, H.A., Santamarina, B.A.G., Smith, S., and Kass, E.H.: The natural history of asymptomatic bacteriuria during pregnancy. The effect of tetracycline on the clinical course and the outcome of pregnancy. Am. J. Obstet. Gynecol., *111*:441, 1971.
101. Gilstrap, L.C., Leveno, K.J., Cunningham, F.G., Whalley, P.J., and Roark, M.L.: Renal infection and pregnancy outcome. Am. J. Obstet. Gynecol., *141*:709, 1981.

102. DiMusto, J.C., Bohjalian, O., and Millar, M.: *Mycoplasma hominis* type I infection and pregnancy. Obstet. Gynecol., *41*:33, 1973.
103. McCormack, W.M., Rosner, B., and Lee, Y.-H.: Colonization with genital mycoplasmas in women. Am. J. Epidemiol., *97*:240, 1973.
104. Harrison, H.R., Alexander, E.R., Weinstein, L., Lewis, M., Nash, M., and Sim, D.A.: Cervical *Chlamydia trachomatis* and mycoplasmal infections in pregnancy. J.A.M.A., *250*:1721, 1983.
105. Martin, D.H., Koutsky, L., Eschenbach, D.A., Daling, J.R., Alexander, E.R., Benedetti, J.K., and Holmes, K.K.: Prematurity and perinatal mortality in pregnancies complicated by maternal *Chlamydia trachomatis* infections. J.A.M.A., *247*:1585, 1982.
106. Heiber, J.P., Dalton, D., Shorey, J., and Combes, B.: Hepatitis and pregnancy. J. Pediatr., *91*:545, 1977.
107. Kass, E.H., and Zinner, S.H.: Bacteriuria and pyelonephritis in pregnancy. *In* Obstetric and Perinatal Infections. Edited by D. Charles and M. Finland. Philadelphia, Lea & Febiger, 1973.
108. Oxorn, H.: The changing aspects of pneumonia complicating pregnancy. Am. J. Obstet. Gynecol., *70*:1057, 1955.
109. Benedetti, T.J., Valle, R., and Ledger, W.J.: Antepartum pneumonia in pregnancy. Am. J. Obstet. Gynecol., *144*:413, 1982.
110. Srabstein, J.C., Morris, N., Larke, R.P.B., deSa, D.J., Castelino, B.B., and Sum, E.: Is there a congenital varicella syndrome? J. Pediatr., *84*:239, 1974.
111. Raine, D.N.: Varicella infection contracted in utero: Sex incidence and incubation period. Am. J. Obstet. Gynecol., *94*:1144, 1966.
112. Shubeck, F., Benson, R.C., Clark, W.W., Jr., Berendes, H., Weiss, W., and Deutschberger, J.: Fetal hazard after rupture of membranes. Obstet. Gynecol., *28*:22, 1966.
113. Gunn, G.C., Mishell, D.R., Jr., and Morton, D.G.: Premature rupture of the fetal membranes. Am. J. Obstet. Gynecol., *106*:469, 1970.
114. Schreiber, J., and Benedetti, T.: Conservative management of preterm premature rupture of the fetal membranes in a low socioeconomic population. Am. J. Obstet. Gynecol., *136*:92, 1980.
115. Garite, T.J., and Freeman, R.K.: Chorioamnionitis in the preterm gestation. Obstet. Gynecol., *59*:539, 1982.
116. Siegel, J.D., and McCracken, G.H., Jr.: Sepsis neonatorum. N. Engl. J. Med., *304*:642, 1981.
117. Cederqvist, L.L., Zervoudakis, I.A., Ewool, L.C., and Litwin, S.D.: The relationship between prematurely ruptured membranes and fetal immunoglobulin production. Am. J. Obstet. Gynecol., *134*:784, 1979.
118. Stedman, C.M., Crawford, S., Staten, E., and Cherney, W.B.: Management of preterm premature rupture of membranes: Assessing amniotic fluid in the vagina for phosphatidyl glycerol. Am. J. Obstet. Gynecol., *140*:34, 1981.
119. Evans, M.I., Hajj, S.N., Devoe, L.D., Angerman, N.S., and Moawad, A.H.: C-reactive protein as a predictor of infectious morbidity with premature rupture of the membranes. Am. J. Obstet. Gynecol., *138*:648, 1980.
120. Farb, H.F., Arnesen, M., Geistler, P., and Knox, G.E.: C-reactive protein with premature rupture of membranes and premature labor. Obstet. Gynecol., *62*:49, 1983.
121. Benirshke, K.: Routes and types of infection in the fetus and the newborn. Am. J. Dis. Child., *99*:714, 1960.
122. Platt, L.D., Schmidt, P.L., Manning, F.A., and Ledger, W.J.: Amniocentesis can influence the management of patients with premature rupture of the membranes. Soc. Gyn. Inv., San Diego, 1979, Abstract 9, p. 7.
123. Garite, T.J., Freeman, R.K., Linzey, E.M., and Braly, P.: The use of amniocentesis in patients with premature rupture of membranes. Obstet. Gynecol., *54*:226, 1979.
124. Cotton, D.B., Hill, L.M., Strassner, H.T., Platt, L.D., and Ledger, W.J.: Use of amniocentesis in preterm gestation with ruptured membranes. Obstet. Gynecol., *63*:38, 1984.
125. Mead, P.B., and Clapp, J.F. III: The use of betamethasone and timed delivery in management of premature rupture of the membranes in the pre-term pregnancy. J. Reprod. Med., *19*:3, 1977.
126. Guilbeau, F.: Editorial comment. Obstet. Gynecol. Surv., *10*:14, 1955.
127. Garite, T.J., Freeman, R.K., Linzey, E.M., Braly, P.S., and Dorchester, W.L.: Prospective randomized study of corticosteroids in the management of premature rupture of the membranes and the premature gestation. Am. J. Obstet. Gynecol., *141*:508, 1981.
128. Christensen, K.K., Christensen, P., Ingemarsson, I., Mardh, P.A., Nordenfelt, E., Ripa, T., Solum, T., and Svenningsen, N.: A study of complications in preterm deliveries after prolonged premature rupture of the membranes. Obstet. Gynecol., *48*:670, 1976.
129. Fayez, J.A., Hasan, A.A., Jonas, H.S., and Miller, G.L.: Management of premature rupture of the membranes. Obstet. Gynecol., *52*:17, 1978.
130. Kappy, K.A., Cetrulo, C.L., Knuppel, R.A., Ingardia, C.J., Sbarra, A.J., Scerbo, J.C., and Mitchell, G.W.: Premature rupture of the membranes: A conservative approach. Am. J. Obstet. Gynecol., *134*:655, 1979.

131. Taylor, J., and Garite, T.J.: Premature rupture of membranes before fetal viability. Obstet. Gynecol., *46*:615, 1984.
132. Druzin, M., Toth, M., and Ledger, W.J.: Nointervention in premature rupture of the amniotic membranes: A study of the natural history. Surg. Gynecol. Obstet. (In press).
133. Haesslein, H.C., and Goodlin, R.C.: Delivery of the tiny newborn. Am. J. Obstet. Gynecol., *134*:192, 1979.
134. Bobitt, J.R., and Ledger, W.J.: Amniotic fluid analysis: Its role in maternal and neonatal infection. Obstet. Gynecol., *51*:56, 1978.
135. Bejar, R., Curbelo, V., Davis, C., and Gluck, L.: Premature labor. II. Bacterial sources of phospholipase. Obstet. Gynecol., *57*:479, 1981.
136. Wallace, R.L., and Herrick, C.N.: Amniocentesis in the evaluation of premature labor. Obstet. Gynecol., *57*:483, 1981.
137. Clark, D.M., and Anderson, G.V.: Perinatal mortality and amnionitis in a general hospital population. Obstet. Gynecol., *31*:714, 1968.
138. Friedman, F.A.: Obstetric infection in labor. *In* Obstetric and Perinatal Infections. Edited by D. Charles and M. Finland. Philadelphia, Lea & Febiger, 1973.
139. Koh, K.S., Chan, F.H., Monfared, A.H., Ledger, W.J., and Paul, R.H.: The changing perinatal and maternal outcome in chorioamnionitis. Obstet. Gynecol., *53*:730, 1979.
140. Gibbs, R.S., Castillo, M.S., and Rodgers, P.J.: Management of acute chorioamnionitis. Am. J. Obstet. Gynecol., *136*:709, 1980.
141. Cordero, L., Jr., and Hon, E.H.: Scalp abscess: A rare complication of fetal monitoring. J. Ped., *78*:533, 1971.
142. Okada, D.M., and Chow, A.W.: Neonatal scalp abscess following intrapartum fetal monitoring: Prospective comparison of two spiral electrodes. Am. J. Obstet. Gynecol., *127*:875, 1977.
143. Overturf, G.D., and Balfour, G.: Osteomyelitis and sepsis: Severe complication of fetal monitoring. Pediatrics, *55*:244, 1975.
144. Turbeville, D.F., Heath, R.E., Jr., Bowen, F.W., Jr., and Killam, A.P.: Complications of fetal scalp electrodes: A case report. Am. J. Obstet. Gynecol., *122*:530, 1975.

Chapter 11
COMMUNITY-ACQUIRED OBSTETRIC INFECTIONS

The type and severity of community-acquired infections in women can be unfavorably influenced by pregnancy. These modifications in response are caused by a number of factors. There is an altered immunologic state during pregnancy. Although these changes enable the pregnant woman to successfully maintain a foreign protein graft—the placenta and fetus—they can be a hindrance when the maternal host is exposed to new viral or bacterial pathogens during pregnancy. This added risk factor can be particularly damaging when it is compounded by poor host response to infection in an undernourished pregnant population. Because of this, the risk of infection during pregnancy, and particularly for serious complications, is increased among those in lower socio-economic groups. There may be no measurable clinical significance of these changes in the pregnant host response for most clinicians. The widespread use of vaccines has eliminated some serious systemic viral infections, while the availability of safe and effective antibiotics has markedly reduced serious maternal outcomes in many bacterial infections. In addition to these systemic factors, local changes can influence the nature of maternal infections. The expansion of the urinary collecting system and the slowed transit time of urine create an environment in which the prolonged presence of urine in the collecting system increases the potential for bacterial proliferation and subsequent infection. The uterus undergoes marked changes in pregnancy and is susceptible to infection, particularly when invasive techniques have been employed to terminate the pregnancy.

There are many inherent difficulties in the laboratory evaluation of the pregnant patient with an infection. Commonly employed blood tests have different parameters during pregnancy. The white cell count is elevated with some shift to the left, i.e., there is an increase in the number of immature white blood cells, and the sedimentation rate is elevated. Physical changes during pregnancy can be confusing to the uninformed, such as consultants in internal medicine or general surgery. For example, the site of the most acute pain in the pregnant woman with appendicitis is usually the midquadrant rather than the lower quadrant. There are other changes in normal pregnant women that must be acknowledged. A dilated urinary collecting system is normal during pregnancy and not evidence in itself of urinary tract disease.

SYSTEMIC VIRAL INFECTIONS

Some serious systemic viral infections have been eliminated from obstetric practice. Prior to the development of effective vaccines and the attempt to establish a universal program of immunization, both smallpox and poliomyelitis had adverse effects upon pregnant women. Smallpox during pregnancy was associated with an increased mortality rate,[1] and poliomyelitis produced higher rates of both paralysis and mortality.[2] Fortunately, smallpox has been eradicated worldwide, and poliomyelitis is rarely seen except for a few scattered outbreaks among non-immunized patients.

Influenza remains a serious problem for the pregnant patient. This concern is of more than historical interest. In the preantibiotic era, the influenza pandemic of 1918 caused by a new strain of virus was accompanied by a higher mortality rate in pregnant than nonpregnant women.[3] This concern about the potential for a pandemic with a new strain of "flu" virus led to the rapid production and utilization of a swine flu vaccine. Fortunately, a swine flu pandemic never materialized. The cause of death in many of these women in the past was a secondary pulmonary infection, frequently attributable to the coagulase-positive *Staphylococcus*.[4] Antibiotics have not eliminated mortality in this clinical situation, but the availability of a large number of safe and effective antistaphylococcal antibiotics has increased the therapeutic options for physicians and enhanced the chances for successful therapy. There is some consensus on prevention. Routine vaccination before the "flu" season is not recommended for every pregnant woman, but it should be given to any antepartum patient with serious underlying pulmonary or cardiac disease. If a new strain of influenza virus is recognized, there will be considerable discussion again about the widespread use of a vaccine in pregnant women, weighing the concern for a possible pandemic against the potential side-effects of the vaccine.

There are still widely divergent views about the impact of primary varicella infections on pregnant women. Occasionally, these women can develop a varicella pneumonia, with rapid progression to respiratory distress and death.[5] In one recent evaluation of this problem, pregnant women were not found to be more at risk for serious complications than nonpregnant women.[6] Any pregnant woman with primary varicella runs the potential risk of developing pneumonitis. Patients should be advised of this and if they have any respiratory symptoms, they should be admitted to the hospital immediately for respiratory supportive care. Although the pneumonitis is viral, antibiotics should be employed to cover the possibility of a superimposed coagulase-positive *Staphylococcus* pneumonia.

Hepatitis has become a much more frequent consideration for the obstetrician in the 1980's. The influx of Asian and Caribbean refugees, who have a high frequency of both hepatitis B and nonA-nonB, has increased the size of the population pool of pregnant women who either have active disease or have been exposed to it in the past. In this same time interval, there has been a burgeoning of medical information on hepatitis. For the physician, this has meant a proliferation of new tests, particularly for the presence of either hepatitis B antigen or antibody in the bloodstream. Figure 11-1 is a schematic view of the sequence of appearance of these abnormal blood test findings in a patient with hepatitis.[7] There is controversy about the significance of hepatitis during pregnancy. The usual view in the United States is that the outcome does not vary from that of

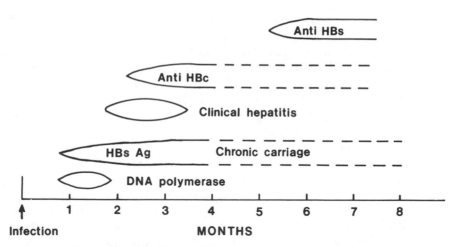

Fig. 11–1. The sequence of clinical findings and laboratory testing with hepatitis B virus infection. (From Greenman, R.L.: Viral hepatitis. Gastroenterology, A Weekly Update. *1*:15, 1979.)

a nonpregnant population.[8] This has not been true in studies of Middle Eastern women, in whom the mortality rate has been considerably higher.[9] This probably represents increased host susceptibility because of malnutrition. Pregnant patients with hepatitis or who are carriers of the hepatitis antigen represent a threat to susceptible medical personnel who care for them. Precautions are necessary, with hand washing and appropriate care when hypodermic needles are used and disposed of. Hepatitis B vaccine is available. Although there are concerns about the population pool that has been the source of the vaccine in which there are homosexuals, to date there have been no problems with an increased incidence of AIDS in people receiving the vaccine. For the physician who deals with a high risk population, this vaccine is probably a good option. If an inadvertent needle stick occurs on the ward or in the operating room in susceptible medical personnel caring for the patient, hepatitis B–specific gamma globulin should be given.

OTHER MATERNAL INFECTIONS DURING PREGNANCY

Vaginitis

The most common symptom of vaginal infection for pregnant women is an irritating vaginal discharge. Although the vast majority of patients with these symptoms have *Candida albicans* vaginitis, other problems including *Trichomonas vaginalis* vaginitis, nonspecific vaginitis, and lower genital tract infection with *Neisseria gonorrhoeae* or herpes simplex genitalis can be present.

There is often a major gap between the pregnant patient's concern and the physician's emphasis on care. The patient may be deeply troubled by a series of frequently unstated questions. Is this discharge a danger to her baby? Is it the result of intercourse that should have been avoided? Has her male sexual partner infected her with organisms acquired through an extramarital affair? Will the medical treatment harm the baby? Too frequently the physician regards the discharge as an unimportant minor complaint or a normal symptom of pregnancy and not a serious problem and certainly as unworthy of any measured consideration. This gap between patient concern and physician performance can easily be bridged.

The first step in physician care of these women is to make an accurate diagnosis of the problem. This requires a careful examination of the lower genital tract, and an immediate microscopic examination of vaginal secretions with saline and potassium hydroxide solutions. Adequate prenatal care requires this capability. In these women, a culture should be carried out for *Neisseria gonorrhoeae*. *Candida* cultures should be obtained if there is a question on the microscopic examination, and cultures for herpes simplex should be obtained if the history is suggestive or local perineal or cervical lesions are seen.

There are several important aspects of treatment for these women. I believe the most important first step is to immediately tell the patient the most likely diagnosis based upon the microscopic examination, e.g., *Candida albicans* vaginitis or *Trichomonas vaginalis* vaginitis. In outlining therapy, the physician should actively address obvious maternal concerns. *Candida* from the lower genital tract is such a rare invader of the upper genital tract that such events are published as case reports in the literature.[10] For women with a yeast vaginitis, the most serious concern should be that the infant will acquire the organism during its passage during labor and will have thrush in the nursery. This is easily treated. For *Trichomonas* infections, there is no evidence to support any direct untoward fetal or newborn effects. It is possible that a *Trichomonas vaginalis* vaginitis increases the risk of premature rupture of the membranes and premature labor, but this relationship has not been established. There should be discussion with patients about therapy during pregnancy before any medications are prescribed. All medication should be avoided in the first trimester of pregnancy. After this, because of the concern about the possible impact of any systemic maternal infections on the fetus, physicians should limit therapy to local medications if possible. It is fortunate that the most common vaginal infection in pregnant women is *Candida* vaginitis. Many theories have been advanced to explain this relationship, including changes in vaginal glycogen content secondary to the hormonal alterations of pregnancy or vaginal contamination from the commonly encountered glycosuria of pregnancy. Although these events usually represent physiologic changes of pregnancy, it is wise to do a carbohydrate metabolic screen in the patient to be certain that she does not have an elevated blood glucose level. When prescribing local medications, both the physician and the patient should be aware that the vagina is an efficient absorbing surface, and systemic levels may be achieved with some local preparations. For those women with *Candida* vaginitis, ancillary care can be important. Vulvar itching and scratching can lead to vulvar macerations and increased pruritus, creating a vicious cycle. Ancillary care to promote vulvar healing includes instructions to the patient to avoid the local use of soap, which is a tissue irritant, and to wear underclothes made of cotton rather than synthetic materials, so that surface moisture has a chance to evaporate. Patient care is more difficult with a *Trichomonas* vaginitis. Both patients and physicians are concerned about the use of metronidazole during pregnancy because of its oncogenic effects in animals. I frequently treat the symptoms of these patients with a local preparation, and in the late second or early third trimester suggest oral therapy with metronidazole for the patient and her male sexual partner. The patient should be aware that this therapy is not approved by the FDA, and she may wish to forego it until after delivery. If herpes simplex is isolated, the patient should be advised and surveillance started so that decisions about delivery can be made. If *Neisseria gonorrhoeae* is isolated, both partners should be treated with penicillin. After a specific diagnosis has been made and the treatment prescribed, the physician must be willing to spend some time answering the patient's questions. Patients may be worried about the safety of intercourse during pregnancy or about spousal infidelity, and they should be able to voice these concerns to their physicians and get a sympathetic response.

URINARY TRACT INFECTIONS

The urinary tract is another frequent and not unexpected site of infection in pregnant women. Asymptomatic bacteriuria occurs in from 5 to 10% of pregnant women, and there are changes in urinary tract functioning that increase the susceptibility to infection during pregnancy. These include the dilatation of the urinary collecting system, an increase in the amount of residual urine, and a slower urine transit time from kidney to bladder, related in part to the decreased ureteral peristalsis of pregnancy. With this background, urinary tract infections occur with great frequency, and the most serious sequela, pyelonephritis, is more common in pregnant than nonpregnant women.

The starting point in the care of the pregnant patient with a urinary tract infection is prevention. The value of this approach has been clearly demonstrated. Many studies,[11, 12] have demonstrated a subsequent increased incidence of pyelonephritis among pregnant women who had asymptomatic bacteriuria at the time of their first screening examination in pregnancy. Figure 11–2 shows the decrease in the incidence of pyelonephritis when a screening examination was done early and therapy was given to eradicate the bacteriuria.[13] I prefer the use of nitrofurantoin for 10 days. The nitrofurans are an effective family of antimicrobials, and they are so well absorbed that they have little impact on the flora of the gas-

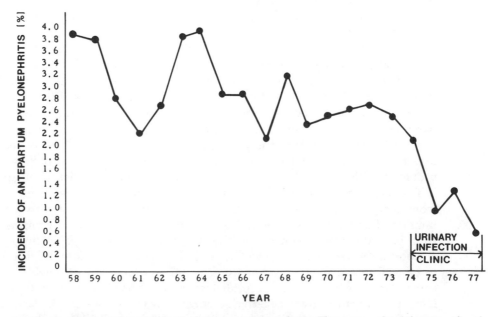

Fig. 11–2. The annual incidence of antepartum pyelonephritis. There was a sharp decrease after the establishment of a urinary infection clinic. (From Harris, R.E.: The treatment of urinary tract infection during pregnancy. *In* Antibiotics in Obstetrics and Gynecology. Edited by W. J. Ledger. Boston, Martinus Nijhoff, 1982.)

trointestinal tract, so that subsequent infection with resistant flora is not a problem. This is not the only available approach. Harris has shown equivalent results with ampicillin, the cephalosporins, or the sulfas.[13] Although single dose therapy has been effective in the elimination of asymptomatic bacteriuria in nonpregnant patients,[14] it has not proved so in a pregnant population.[15] Repeat urine cultures should be obtained after treatment to be sure the bacteriuria has been eliminated.

Pregnant patients with acute dysuria will be seen by physicians. They need to be examined for evidence of vaginitis and to have lower genital tract cultures done for *Neisseria gonorrhoeae* and *Chlamydia trachomatis*. The vast majority of these women with dysuria have cystitis. Recent work by Stamm and colleagues has demonstrated that a colony count of less than 10^5 *Escherichia coli* has significance in these women.[16] They should be treated with either nitrofurantoin or a sulfa drug. Alternatively, equivalent therapeutic results have been obtained with ampicillin or cephalexin. The treatment course should be for at least seven days.

Pyelonephritis

Patients with pyelonephritis are still seen on the obstetric service. There are some important standards of care. The diagnosis is usually not in doubt. These patients are febrile, sometimes septic, with costovertebral angle pain, and have white blood cells and bacteria present in the microscopic examination of an unspun urine specimen. Although urinary tract stones are occasionally present, they are infrequent enough for the clinician to limit the diagnostic workup for renal calculi to those patients who fail to respond to the initial choice of antibiotics. All these patients should be admitted to the hospital. In addition to the systemic administration of antibiotics, hospitalization enables the physician to ensure appropriate hydration for these often dehydrated patients.

A logical starting place for the therapy of pyelonephritis is the choice of the proper antibiotic for the bacteria involved in the infection. Prior to the culture report, physicians have to play the odds of the most likely isolates. In pyelonephritis, about 90% will be gram-negative aerobes, with *Escherichia coli* being the most common. If gram-positive cocci are seen on Gram stain, the group B beta-hemolytic *Streptococcus,* the enterococcus, and the coagulase-positive *Staphylococcus* can be involved. In those young women who are usually free of renal stones, pyelonephritis is invariably caused by a single organism. When dealing with this type of infection problem, the physician and the patient are best served by the prescription of a single antibiotic. This is usually effective, and if there are any problems with a patient reaction to the drug, the cause is quickly apparent.

The selection of the initial antibiotic for the treatment of pyelonephritis varies from hospital to hospital. This depends upon clinical experience with the various families of antibiotics and the clinical microbiologic data on the organisms isolated from patients with pyelonephritis. Most physicians favor a penicillin or a cephalosporin. Obstetricians have had a lot of experience with these drugs, they seem to be well tolerated by pregnant women, and an oral form is available. There are some attractive aspects to the cephalosporins. In many hospitals, they cover a large number of the gram-negative aerobes in the laboratory, particularly *Klebsiella,* and they are more effective against the coagulase-positive *Staphylococcus*. In one study by Cunningham and associates, cephalothin seemed superior to ampicillin.[17] On the other hand, the cephalosporins have not been uniformly superior in the treatment of urinary tract infections,[18] and they are not effective against enterococci. Local experience with the organisms isolated in pyelonephritis will help to guide these choices. Patients with pyelonephritis will be seen who are allergic to penicillin and the cephalosporins. These are difficult treatment problems. Some of the frequently used alternative antibiotics have little appeal to me. Chloramphenicol can be prescribed, but there is always concern about the possibility of the patient's developing aplastic anemia.[19] The aminoglycosides are another alternative, but they require close monitoring of the serum levels in this clinical situation. Standard doses can result in toxic levels of these drugs if given to a pregnant woman with the marked reduction in creatinine clearance that is seen in some patients with acute pyelonephritis.[20] Alternatively, in the young woman with excellent renal function, standard dosing regimens can result in less than optimal serum levels.[21] No matter which antibiotic is given initially, a repeat urine culture should be obtained after 48 hours of therapy. A positive bacterial growth of 10^3 colonies or more of organisms resistant to the antibiotic initially prescribed is an indication to switch the antibiotic to one effective in vitro against the causative organisms.

The choice of antibiotic is not the sole focus of care in these women. Fluid balance is very important. When admitted to the hospital, many of these patients are dehydrated from the insensible fluid loss caused by hyperpyrexia, a limited oral intake because of nausea, and the fluid losses associated with vomiting. Blood electrolyte levels should be obtained at the time of admission, and appropriate fluid replacement prescribed, with close monitoring or urinary output. The strategy for intravenous fluid replacement should be sufficient hydration to ensure a minimum hourly urinary production of 60 to 100 ml. A small percentage of patients with pyelonephritis are acutely ill, with septic shock. In most of these cases, patients respond to appropriate antibiotics and fluid replacement, although steroids have been necessary on occasion.

BACTERIAL PNEUMONIA

An infrequent infection of the pregnant patient is bacterial pneumonia. Although some of these women can be seriously ill, the outlook for these patients has changed considerably. In the preantibiotic era, there was a poor prognosis for pregnant women with pneumococcal pneumonia, for they had a higher mortality rate than nonpregnant women.[22] Articles published in the 1950's and the 1960's showed improved results with antibiotics in patients with bacterial pneumonia, but there was still a substantial maternal mortality rate.[23, 24] Since the 1950's, there has been a wider spectrum of antibiotics available for care, and there is better understanding of fluid and electrolyte balance as well as greatly improved respiratory care with ventilatory support. In this setting, no deaths were reported in a recent study of 28 women with bacterial pneumonias in pregnancy.[25] Although the pneumococcus is the most common bacterial pathogen in community-acquired pneumonias, other microbiologic agents can be involved. A Gram stain of a carefully obtained sputum sample usually confirms the diagnosis of pneumococcal pneumonia by the presence of gram-positive diplococci. In recent years, there has been an increasing awareness of the importance of both *Mycoplasma* organisms and *Legionella pneumophilia* disease in nonlobar pneumonia. In women with an atypical pneumonia, erythromycin is a good initial choice of antibiotic because it effectively covers both of these agents.

PULMONARY TUBERCULOSIS

There have been wide swings in physician concern about pulmonary tuberculosis in pregnancy. In urban hospitals caring for the poor in the immediate post
World War II era, there was a focus upon pulmonary tuberculosis, and chest
roentgen examinations were performed in all antepartum patients. The low positive
yields and the awareness of the dangers of radiation exposure led to modification
of this policy on most services to skin testing and x-rays only for those who had
positive skin tests. There was not the same concern shown for the patient who
failed to get a skin test as for the woman who did not receive a Pap smear. In
the last five years, this relaxed attitude about tuberculosis has been modified. The
massive influx of Caribbean and Far Eastern refugees into many urban centers in
this country has been accompanied by an upswing in the number of cases of
active pulmonary tuberculosis. On these services, a new emphasis has been placed
on this disease. Skin testing has become universal, and subsequent chest films
are closely reviewed to detect women with active pulmonary tuberculosis. There
has been controversy about the care of pregnant women who have positive skin
test results and normal chest x-rays. In an attempt to avoid exposure of the fetus
to isoniazid (INH) and paraaminosalicylic acid (PAS), one strategy was to avoid
therapy during pregnancy and plan to treat the mother after delivery. The problem
with this was that many urban poor patients did not or would not avail themselves
of care and did not return to the medical care system when they were pregnant
again. In my opinion, a recent tuberculin converter should be started on prophylaxis with INH after the first trimester of pregnancy and should receive supplemental pyridoxine (vitamin B_6). In women with positive or suspicious findings
on x-rays, sputum samples should be obtained for acid–fast bacterial cultures. In
pregnant women with active pulmonary tuberculosis, the physician has many
therapeutic options. Unless the patient is seriously ill or plans to terminate the
pregnancy, therapy should be withheld in the first trimester. After this time
interval, there are a number of acceptable and effective drugs. In addition to the
standbys of INH, PAS, and streptomycin, ethambutol is available and in use.
Obstetricians usually do not have extensive experience with this disease. It is
important to plan therapy on the basis of the standard of care in the community
established by physicians who have experience with the antibiotic susceptibilities
of the acid-fast bacteria in that area.

SYSTEMIC FUNGAL INFECTIONS

Although uncommon, systemic fungal infections can occur in pregnancy. The
most frequent cause is *Coccidioides immitis,* and this is frequently seen in California.[26]
Those infections are serious and can present as a pneumonia or meningitis or
both. Prior to the introduction of amphotericin B into clinical practice, all these
patients died. In seriously ill patients, the diagnosis can be suspected in those
with a positive skin test and a positive culture. The treatment is amphotericin B,
and this has resulted in clinical cures.

Serious infections caused by *Cryptococcus neoformans* also can be seen in pregnant
women. Unlike coccidioidomycosis, this problem is not limited to California but
can be seen in the Midwest and the southern United States as well. Patients
usually initially have a lung infection, followed by dissemination to the brain and
its meninges.[27] They present with central nervous system symptoms and a stiff

neck. In addition to standard cultures, an India ink preparation may reveal encapsulated organisms. Treatment is with systemic amphotericin B and flucytosine in combination.

BACTERIAL MENINGITIS

Bacterial meningitis is an uncommon infection during pregnancy. Patients present with central nervous system alterations and have a stiff neck as well. The spinal tap is diagnostic, and cultures will guide subsequent antibiotic therapy. Central nervous system infections are difficult to treat because of the inability to deliver effective levels of antibiotics to the site of infection. In addition to identifying the organism and knowing its susceptibility to antibiotics, the physician must be aware of the pharmacokinetics of the agent. For example, clindamycin would be a poor choice for any central nervous system infection because it penetrates the central nervous system in such low levels. In addition to these pharmacologic concerns, there are microbiologic considerations. In recent years, there has been the appearance of ampicillin-resistant *Hemophilus influenzae* strains.[28] This organism can be a differential diagnostic concern in a pregnant teenager with meningitis. In this situation, chloramphenicol is probably the drug of choice, although the second and third generation cephalosporins are also under study.

INTRAABDOMINAL INFECTIONS

Primary Bacterial Peritonitis

A rare infection during pregnancy is primary bacterial peritonitis. These sick febrile patients present with abdominal pain and ileus. Primary bacterial peritonitis in nonpregnant women usually occurs secondary to an upper respiratory infection with the pneumococcus, with an associated bacteremia and then intraabdominal infection. Occasionally, the group A beta-hemolytic *Streptococcus* is involved. This is more commonly seen in postsplenectomy patients or those with sickle cell disease. During pregnancy, primary peritonitis has been reported to occur secondary to upper genital tract infection with *Neisseria gonorrhoeae*[29] and in a patient with sickle cell disease.[30] This diagnosis should be considered in pregnant patients with diffuse abdominal pain and no localizing signs. Nasopharyngeal and endocervical cultures for *Neisseria gonorrhoeae* should be performed. Positive culture results and a rapid clinical response to penicillin or a cephalosporin should confirm this diagnosis. If in doubt, paracentesis can be performed. Gram staining of a smear of the peritoneal fluid should indicate the appropriate diagnosis and the likely organisms. In addition to the proper selection of antibiotics, intravenous fluid administration is important in these patients. Peritoneal infection can result in massive accumulation of fluid in the third space, so that large volumes of fluid may be necessary to assure an adequate urinary output.

Cholecystitis

Cholecystitis is a more common problem during pregnancy. This diagnosis should be suspected in women who have right upper quadrant discomfort and intolerance to fatty foods. Fortunately, the development of ultrasonography has eliminated the routine use of x-ray examination to make the diagnosis of associated stone formation. If confirmed, the primary therapy is surgical, but antibiotics will be necessary as well. In urban centers with large Mexican-American populations, another important differential diganosis is amebic abscess of the liver. These patients are usually thought to have cholecystitis, but an ultrasonographic examination often will demonstrate a liver abscess.[31] This is an important differential diagnosis to make, for the treatment is medical, with metronidazole, instead of the surgical approach for cholecystitis. This is a good example of successful medical therapy for an abscess in which surgery is rarely needed.

Parasitic Diseases

A more common problem for the clinician in the 1980's is the pregnant patient who presents with intestinal parasites. Each year, millions of Americans travel to foreign areas that have poor environmental hygiene, and in recent years the United States had an influx of 262,602 refugees from Indochina, and 125,000 Cubans plus a large number of Haitians.[32] Parasitic gastrointestinal infections are prevalent in these populations.

There are two major clinical considerations in the pregnant patient with a parasitic gastrointestinal disease. Does the infection pose any threat to the mother, and are the medications safe during pregnancy? A disease in point is giardiasis. The symptoms of nausea, vomiting, and diarrhea can result in an undernourished dehydrated pregnant patient who requires hospital admission for intravenous rehydration.[33] The standard antiparasitic drugs, quinacrine hydrochloride, metronidazole, or furazolidone, are all absorbed from the gastrointestinal tract and have toxicities. As an alternative, paromomycin, an oral, poorly absorbed aminoglycoside, is a potentially less toxic agent for the pregnant patient.

The evaluation of the patient with diarrhea should follow a common course. There should be inquiries about recent foreign travel or the use of broad-spectrum antibiotics. For example, if ampicillin has been given for a urinary tract or an upper respiratory infection, it is possible that the patient has pseudomembranous enterocolitis caused by *Clostridium difficile*. Anaerobic stool culture and a test for *C. difficile* toxin should be done. In those patients with no history of recent antibiotic ingestion, a stool sample should be obtained for examination for ova and parasites. It is important for the physician to know the capabilities of the laboratories to do these studies and to direct the specimen to the laboratory best suited to do these tests.

After the diagnosis has been made, the clinician must make an appropriate therapeutic decision. Table 11–1 details the drugs available through the Centers for Disease Control and commercially for the various parasitic infections.[32] The

Table 11–1. Drugs Available from the Centers for Disease Control.*

Infection	Drug
Onchocerciasis	Suramin
Dracunculiasis	Niridazole
Leishmaniasis	Pentostam
Central nervous system trypanosomiasis	Melarsoprol (Mel B)
Early infection with *Trypanosoma rhodesiense*	Suramin
Early infection with *T. gambiense*	Pentamidine
Chagas' disease	Nifurtimox
Amebiasis	Dehydroemetine, (Furamide)
Malaria	Parenteral quinine

* Parasitic Disease Drug Service, Centers for Disease Control, Atlanta, GA 30333 (404) 452–4174.

decision about the use of these agents during pregnancy should be made after consultation with local public health physicians, experts at a medical center, or the Parasitic Drugs Service at the Centers for Disease Control in Atlanta, Georgia (404–452–4174).

Appendicitis

Appendicitis can be a serious problem for the pregnant woman. Alterations in anatomy modify the presenting symptoms and both the location and the severity of peritoneal signs, so that the disease is more likely to progress to abscess formation and rupture than it is in nonpregnant women.[34] The primary treatment is surgical, but antibiotics to cover anaerobes and gram-negative aerobes are indicated as well. Premature labor can be seen with the peritoneal irritation, and this creates a therapeutic dilemma because of the tachycardia associated with many of the tocolytic agents. In this clinical situation, I favor the use of magnesium sulfate in the first round of therapy to inhibit uterine activity.

OTHER LOCALIZED INFECTIONS SEEN IN PREGNANT WOMEN

Infectious Arthritis

An uncommon infection in pregnant women is infectious arthritis. This is rarely seen, but when it does occur, the most common causative organism is *Neisseria gonorrhoeae*.[35] It is interesting that this organism can be involved in these joint infections without causing pelvic symptoms. In the evaluation of these patients, it is important to obtain an endocervical culture for *Neisseria gonorrhoeae* as well as a similar culture from fluid aspirated from the involved joint site. If this diagnosis is suspected or confirmed by culture, a number of treatment regimens are recommended. These include 10,000,000 U of penicillin G intravenously per day until improvement occurs, followed by amoxicillin or ampicillin, four times a day for at least seven days. Alternatively, only oral penicillins can be given. One dose of amoxicillin 3.0 g or ampicillin 3.5 g, each with probenecid 1.0 g, followed by amoxicillin 500 mg or ampicillin 500 mg by mouth four times a day for at least seven days. If there is concern about penicillin-resistant *Neisseria gonorrhoeae*, cefoxitin 1.0 g or cefotaxime, 500 mg, should be given intravenously four times a day for at least seven days. In the penicillin-allergic patient, erythromycin, 500 mg by mouth, can be given four times a day for at least seven days.[36]

Herpes Zoster Infections

Another uncommon problem during pregnancy is herpes zoster infection.[37] This occurs in patients with a previous history of varicella. The unilateral segmental distribution of the lesions suggests the diagnosis, which can be confirmed by abrasion of the vesicles followed by viral culture. A positive culture confirms the diagnosis, and local symptomatic therapy can be utilized. Systemic drugs should be avoided, and the lesions will disappear with time. There is no concern with fetal infection as there is with a primary varicella infection.

PELVIC INFECTIONS

Salpingitis

Salpingitis can occur in the first trimester of pregnancy. This is uncommon,[38] but is should be considered in every woman who has pelvic and lower abdominal pain in the first trimester of pregnancy. In these patients, an endocervical culture for *Neisseria gonorrhoeae* should be performed and appropriate antibiotics prescribed. It is appropriate to admit those patients in whom this diagnosis is suspected to the hospital for inpatient care.

Infected Abortion

The lack of historical perspective often limits the younger obstetrician-gynecologist's view of current clinical problems. The most striking change in the character of urban gynecologic services in the past 15 years has been the tremendous reduction in the number of women admitted to the hospital with infected abortions. One common response of our specialty is to look for cause and effect relationships. One tenet has been that the availability of pregnancy termination on demand has decreased the numbers of patients with community-acquired infected abortions. However, there are other factors. Santamarina and Smith at the Baton City Hospital noted a reduction in the number of women who had infected abortions before pregnancy termination was freely available.[39] In addition, gynecologists serving the urban poor in New Orleans who had limited access to local pregnancy termination services noted a similar downward trend in the number of women with infected abortions.[40] These trends have to be attributable in part to the more readily available methods of contraception, including oral contraceptives and intrauterine devices.

The sudden appearance of a seeming epidemic of cases of endotoxic shock seen in patients in the late 1950's and the early 1960's is difficult to understand. Following the description by Studdiford and Douglas of this syndrome in 1958,[41] clinicians became increasingly aware of this entity, and it was a major cause of maternal death from infection. A review of the obstetric literature of the 1930's and the 1940's reveals no emphasis on this condition. The current diminished incidence of serious infection from abortions may be part of the ebb and flow of serious problems with infections. Despite the reduced number of cases seen, the patient with an infected abortion can still present difficult therapeutic problems for the clinician.

The diagnosis of an infected abortion should be suspected in every febrile woman who is diagnosed as having a pregnancy loss. In the majority of instances, the cervical os is open, with evidence of the passage of products of conception, and the diagnosis can be made of an incomplete septic abortion.

A number of parameters should be assessed in these patients to see if they are at high risk for a serious infection. High spiking fevers or the presence of hypotension dictates close observation, particularly of the urinary output. The white blood cell count should be assessed, for leukopenia can be present with septic shock. In these women the length of gestation is important, for pregnancies beyond 12 weeks are associated with the most serious infections. The pelvic examination is also important beyond the evaluation of uterine size. Neuwirth and Friedman found that patients who had evidence of infection beyond the uterus had the most serious infections.[42]

In those patients at high risk for serious infection, radiographs of the abdomen should be obtained, both in the supine and upright positions. These films will demonstrate the presence of intraperitoneal or myometrial gas. Either condition should dictate operative intervention in order to assess the extent of uterine

Table 11–2. Treatment Results in Patients with Infected Abortions

Total number of patients	247	
Cure	240	97%
Failure (required other antibiotics)	5	2%
Failure (pelvic abscess)	2	1%

damage as well as any damage to the bowel, which would cause continued peritoneal contamination.

A rare laboratory finding is the presence of myometrial gas, which is layered (the "onion skin" effect). This finding is synonymous with extensive necrosis of uterine tissue and a *Clostridium perfringens* infection, indications for laparotomy and removal of the infected pelvic organ.

The microbiologic evaluation of the patient with an infected abortion is a straightforward matter. Aerobic cultures of endocervical specimens should be obtained to determine the presence of such important pathogens as *Neisseria gonorrhoeae,* the group A beta-hemolytic streptococci, and *Escherichia coli.* Anaerobic cultures of the endocervix are not evaluated. Blood cultures also should be obtained, and there should be a high yield of both positive cultures and anaerobic organisms.[43]

The treatment of these patients is straightforward. Almost any antibiotic or combination of antibiotics will be effective when combined with curettage (Table 11–2).[44–47] In addition, the febrile response of these patients as measured by the fever index, is better than in any other community-acquired infections.[48] There are patients who will require specific antibiotic coverage for *Bacteroides fragilis.* Figure 11–3 documents a patient in whom *Bacteroides fragilis* was recovered from both the endocervix and the bloodstream.[49] At arrow 1, blood cultures were performed, with *Bacteroides* and enterococci recovered; at arrow 2, dilatation and curettage were performed. At arrow 3, curettage was performed again, and another blood culture

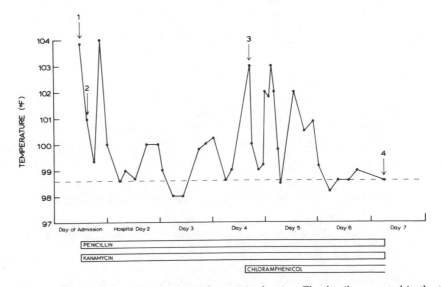

Fig. 11–3. The hospital course of a patient with a septic abortion. The details are noted in the text. (From Ledger, W.J.: Anaerobic infections. Am. J. Obstet. Gynecol., *123*:111, 1975.)

was positive for *Bacteroides*. Chloramphenicol was added to the therapy. At arrow 4, the patient was discharged from the hospital.

Steroids are rarely necessary for the treatment of the patient with an infected abortion. If septic shock is present I believe they are indicated,[50] but they represent supportive care. Operative intervention should not be delayed if indicated.

Operative removal of the pelvic organs is rarely necessary. In the patient with a *Clostridium perfringens* infection or septic shock, laparotomy and hysterectomy may be indicated, but this is rarely necessary.

INFECTIONS OF THE AMNIOTIC FLUID AND UTERUS

Infections of the amniotic fluid and the uterus occur infrequently in pregnant women. A number of investigators have shown the presence of a number of antibacterial substances in amniotic fluid.[51-54] This is fortunate, for it has enabled obstetricians to do a diagnostic amniocentesis knowing that the risk of infection is quite low, as little as 1 per 1,000 in one recent survey.[55] Most problems with amniotic or uterine infections follow a pattern of ruptured membranes; the subsequent development of clinical evidence of infection with septic shock is a rare phenomenon.

There have been misguided therapeutic strategies in the care of women with premature rupture of the membranes. The observation that the greater length of time of membrane rupture was associated with a higher incidence of maternal infection led to many therapeutic interventions to induce labor in order to prevent infection. This ignored the huge increase in maternal infection that occurred when a cesarean section was required[56] and the fact that many inductions of labor failed, necessitating cesarean section.[57] The outcome on many services was a higher maternal infection rate than if no intervention was done. To avoid this, my approach has been not to interfere before a pregnancy of 36 weeks' gestation and to let labor begin spontaneously. In the woman beyond 36 weeks, we still induce labor because the fetus is mature, but at least one study has had good results when no intervention was employed in this population.[58] Unless these women are febrile or require a cesarean section, antibiotics are not required. If the patient becomes febrile and has symptoms of chorioamnionitis, rapid delivery is necessary and systemic antibiotics are indicated. I prefer cefoxitin, but ampicillin can be employed in this situation. Some patients with chorioamnionitis have poor progress in labor[59] and may require a cesarean section for failure to progress. With better knowledge of the significance of anaerobic bacteria, cesarean sections can be done successfully in these women. An extraperitoneal cesarean section[60] or a cesarean hysterectomy is an option,[61] but these are usually not necessary.

REFERENCES

1. Immunization during pregnancy. ACOG Tech. Bull., *64*:1, 1980.
2. Siegel, M., and Goldberg, M.: Incidence of poliomyelitis in pregnancy. N. Engl. J. Med., *253*:841, 1955.
3. Harris, J.W.: Influenza occurring in pregnant women. J.A.M.A., *72*:978, 1919.
4. Freeman, D.W., and Barno, A.: Death from Asian influenza associated with pregnancy. Am. J. Obstet. Gynecol., *78*:1172, 1959.
5. Harris, R.E., and Rhoades, E.R.: Varicella pneumonia complicating pregnancy: Report of a case and review of literature. Obstet. Gynecol., *25*:734, 1965.
6. Amstey, M.S.: Varicella in pregnancy. J. Reprod. Med., *21*:89, 1978.
7. Greenman, R.L.: Viral hepatitis. Gastroenterology, A weekly update. *1*:15, 1979.
8. Davidson, C.S.: Hepatic disease and pregnancy. J. Reprod. Med., *10*:107, 1973.

9. Gelpi, A.P.: Fatal hepatitis in Saudi Arabian women. Am. J. Gastroenterol, *53*:41, 1970.
10. Dixon, B.L., and Houston, C.S.: Fatal neonatal pulmonary candidiasis. Radiology, *129*:132, 1978.
11. Harris, R.E., and Gilstrap, L.C., III: Prevention of recurrent pyelonephritis during pregnancy. Obstet. Gynecol., *44*:637, 1974.
12. Harris, R.E.: The significance of eradication of bacteriuria during pregnancy. Obstet. Gynecol., *53*:71, 1979.
13. Harris, R.E.: The treatment of urinary tract infections during pregnancy. *In* Antibiotics in Obstetrics and Gynecology. Edited by W.J. Ledger. Boston, Martinus Nijhoff, 1982.
14. Gruneberg, R.N., and Brumfitt, W.: Single dose treatment of acute urinary tract infection: A controlled trial. Br. Med. J., *3*:649, 1967.
15. Williams, J.D., Brumfitt, W., Leigh, D., and Percival, A.: Eradication of bacteriuria in pregnancy by a short course of chemotherapy. Lancet, *1*:831, 1965.
16. Stamm, W.E., Counts, G.W., Running, K.R., Fihn, S., Turck, M., and Holmes, K.K.: Diagnosis of coliform infection in acutely dysuric women. N. Engl. J. Med., *307*:463, 1982.
17. Cunningham, F.G., Morris, G.B., and Mickal, A.: Acute pyelonephritis of pregnancy: A clinical review. Obstet. Gynecol., *42*:112, 1973.
18. Sheehan, G., Harding, G.K.M., and Ronald, A.R.: Advances in the treatment of urinary tract infection. Am. J. Med., *76, 5A*:141, 1984.
19. Best, W.R.: Chloramphenicol associated blood dyscrasias. J.A.M.A. *201*:181, 1967.
20. Whalley, P.J., Cunningham, F.G., and Martin, F.G.: Transient renal dysfunction associated with acute pyelonephritis of pregnancy. Obstet. Gynecol., *46*:174, 1975.
21. Bernard, B., Garcia-Cazares, S.J., Ballard, C.A., Thrupp, L.D., Mathies, A.W., and Wehrle, P.F.: Tobramycin: Maternal-fetal pharmacology. Antimicrob. Agents Chemother., *11*:688, 1977.
22. Finland, M., and Dublin, T.D.: Pneumococcal pneumonias complicating pregnancy and the puerperium. J.A.M.A. *112*:1027, 1939.
23. Oxorn, H.: The changing aspects of pneumonia complicating pregnancy. Am. J. Obstet. Gynecol., *70*:1057, 1955.
24. Hopwood, H.G.: Pneumonia in pregnancy. Obstet. Gynecol., *25*:875, 1965.
25. Benedetti, T.J., Valle, R., and Ledger, W.J.: Antepartum pneumonia in pregnancy. Am. J. Obstet. Gynecol., *144*:413. 1982.
26. McCoy, M.J., Ellenberg, J.F., and Killam, A.P.: Coccidioidomycosis complicating pregnancy. Am. J. Obstet. Gynecol., *137*:739, 1980.
27. Stafford, C.R., Fisher, J.F., Fadel, H.E., Espinel-Ingroff, A.V., Shadomy, S., and Hamby, M.: Cryptococcal meningitis in pregnancy. Obstet. Gynecol., *62*:35S, 1983.
28. Lerman, S.J., Brunken, J.M., and Bollinger, M.: Prevalence of ampicillin-resistant strains of *Hemophilus influenzae* causing systemic infection. Antimicrob. Agents Chemother., *18*:474, 1980.
29. Browne, M.K., and Cassie, R.: Spontaneous bacterial peritonitis during pregnancy. Br. J. Obstet. Gynaecol., *88*:1158, 1981.
30. Stauffer, R.A., Wygal, J., and Lavery, J.P.: Spontaneous bacterial peritonitis in pregnancy. Am. J. Obstet. Gynecol., *144*:104, 1982.
31. Wagner, V.P., Smale, L.E., and Lischke, J.H.: Amebic abscess of the liver and spleen in pregnancy and the puerperium. Obstet. Gynecol., *45*:562, 1975.
32. Most, H.: Treatment of parasitic infections of travelers and immigrants. N. Engl. J. Med., *310*:298, 1984.
33. Kreutner, A.K., Del Bene, V.E., and Amstey, M.S.: Giardiasis in pregnancy. Am. J. Obstet. Gynecol., *140*:895, 1981.
34. Reed, C., and Killackey, M.: The acute surgical abdomen in pregnancy. Infect. Surg., *1*:26 (Nov.-Dec.), 1982.
35. Taylor, H.A., Bradford, S.A., and Patterson, S.P.: Gonococcal arthritis in pregnancy. Obstet. Gynecol., *27*:776, 1966.
36. Centers for Disease Control: Sexually transmitted diseases. Treatment guidelines 1982. M.M.W.R. supplement, *31*:335, 1982.
37. Eyal, A., Friedman, M., Peretz, B.A., and Paldi, E.: Pregnancy complicated by herpes zoster. J. Reprod. Med., *28*:600, 1983.
38. Acosta, A.A., Mabray, C.R., and Kaufman, R.H.: Intrauterine pregnancy and coexistent pelvic inflammatory disease. Obstet. Gynecol., *37*:282, 1971.
39. Santamarina, B.A., and Smith, S.A.: Septic abortion and septic shock. Clin. Obstet. Gynecol., *13*:291, 1970.
40. Mickal, A.: Personal communication, 1977.
41. Studdiford, W.E., and Douglas, G.W.: Placental bacteremia: A significant finding in septic abortion accompanied by vascular collapse. Am. J. Obstet. Gynecol., *71*:842, 1956.
42. Neuwirth, R.S., and Friedman, E.A.: Septic abortion. Am. J. Obstet. Gynecol., *85*:24, 1963.
43. Rotheram, E.A., and Schick, S.J.: Nonclostridial anaerobic bacteria in septic abortion. Am. J. Med., *46*:80, 1969.

44. Ostergard, D. R.: Comparison of two antibiotic regimens in the treatment of septic abortion. Obstet. Gynecol., *36*:473, 1970.
45. Josey, W.E., and Farrar, W.E., Jr.: Cephaloridine in septic abortion. Comparison with a conventional combined antibiotic regimen in a conservative program of management. Am. J. Obstet. Gynecol., *106*:237, 1970.
46. Dahm, C.H., Jr., Ostapowicz, F., and Cavanagh, D.: Use of cephalothin in septic abortion. Obstet. Gynecol., *41*:693, 1973.
47. Chow, A.W., Marshall, J.R., and Guze, L.B.: A double-blind comparison of clindamycin with penicillin plus chloramphenicol in treatment of septic abortion. J. Infect. Dis., *135*:S35, 1977.
48. Ledger, W.J., Kriewall, T.J., and Gee, C.: The fever index: A technic for evaluating the clinical response to bacteremia. Obstet. Gynecol., *45*:603, 1975.
49. Ledger, W.J.: Anaerobic infections. Am. J. Obstet. Gynecol., *123*:111, 1975.
50. Schumer, W.: Steroids in the treatment of clinical septic shock. Ann. Surg., *184*:333, 1976.
51. Galask, R.P., and Snyder, I.S.: Bacterial inhibition by amniotic fluid. Am. J. Obstet. Gynecol., *102*:949, 1968.
52. Larsen, B., Snyder, I.S., and Galask, R.P.: Bacterial growth inhibition by amniotic fluid. II. Reversal of amniotic fluid bacterial growth inhibitor by addition of a chemically defined medium. Am. J. Obstet. *119*:497, 1974.
53. Schlievert, P., Johnson, W. and Galask, R.P.: Bacterial growth inhibition by amniotic fluid VI. Evidence for a zinc-peptide antibacterial system. Am. J. Obstet. Gynecol., *125*:906, 1976.
54. Blanco, J.D., Gibbs, R.S., Krebs, L.F., and Castaneda, Y.S.: The association between the absence of amniotic fluid bacterial inhibitory activity and intra-amniotic infection. Am. J. Obstet. Gynecol., *143*:749, 1982.
55. Golbus, M.S., Loughman, W.D., Epstein, C.J., Halbasch, G., Stephens, J.D., and Hall, B.D.: Prenatal genetic diagnosis in 3000 amniocenteses. N. Engl. J. Med., *300*:157, 1979.
56. Sweet, R.L., and Ledger, W.J.: Puerperal infectious morbidity: A two year review. Am. J. Obstet. Gynecol., *117*:1049, 1973.
57. Kappy, K.A., Cetrulo, C.L., Knuppel, R.A., Ingardia, C.J., Sbarra, A.J., Scerbo, J.C., and Mitchell, G.W.: Premature rupture of the membranes: A conservative approach. Am. J. Obstet. Gynecol., *134*:655, 1979.
58. Kappy, K.A., Cetrulo, C.L., Knuppel, R.A., Ingardia, C.J., Sbarra, A.J., Scerbo, J.C., and Mitchell, G.W.: Premature rupture of the membranes at term. J. Reprod. Med., *27*:29, 1982.
59. Friedman, E.A.: Obstetric infection in labor. *In* Obstetric and Perinatal Infections. Edited by D. Charles and M. Finland. Philadelphia, Lea & Febiger, 1973.
60. Perkins, R.P.: Merits of extraperitoneal cesarean section: A continuing experience. J. Reprod. Med., *19*:154, 1977.
61. Ledger, W.J.: Postoperative pelvic infections. Clin. Obstet. Gynecol., *12*:265, 1969.

Chapter 12
HOSPITAL-ACQUIRED OBSTETRIC INFECTIONS

CHANGES IN OBSTETRIC PRACTICE

No discussion of hospital-acquired obstetric infections can be divorced from the background of recent dramatic changes in practice patterns. There has been a major medical emphasis upon improvement of newborn outcome. One gross measure of these practice endeavors has been a steady nationwide reduction in the perinatal mortality rates in this country in the past 20 years. The importance of factors outside the control of medicine is reflected by a rise in perinatal mortality rates in 1982 in states such as Michigan, which were severely affected by the economic recession.

Physician interventions, which have contributed to this reduction in perinatal mortality rates, have taken many forms in the first half of pregnancy. Pregnancy termination by physicians is readily available across the United States. This is reflected by the statistics for 1980; in that year 1,297,606 of these procedures were performed.[1] Combined with the wide-spread prescription of effective family planning methods such as oral contraceptives, this service has decreased the number of unwed teenagers with unwanted pregnancies from the population pool of pregnant patients. This is an important development, because in the past this group has contributed heavily to perinatal mortality figures. Other physician interventions in the first half of pregnancy have improved both perinatal survival figures and the quality of the newborns delivered. New diagnostic techniques, including amniocentesis for chromosomal analysis and alpha-fetoprotein determinations in serum and amniotic fluid, in concert with ultrasonographic examination of the fetus with increasingly sophisticated equipment, have resulted in termination of pregnancies that in the past would have been carried to term. With our present diagnostic technology, this means that most of these terminations are now done after the 16th week of pregnancy. This will change, for new techniques will result in earlier intervention. These diagnostic efforts in the first 20 weeks of pregnancy will be expanded in the future. Since infants born with a defect such as Down's syndrome require a lifetime of care, there is increasing interest in prenatal genetic analysis of all pregnant women. Fortunately, new methods of obtaining fetal tissue by villous biopsy permit these diagnostic attempts to be carried out earlier than amniocentesis.[2] This in turn means that termination can be achieved earlier in the pregnancy with fewer problems.

The physician's concern for the fetus has also revolutionized obstetric practice.

Biophysical monitoring of the fetus has become a standard of care, and in situations in which there is concern about fetal health, invasive techniques with the continuous utilization of a fetal scalp electrode and an intrauterine pressure catheter are frequently employed. This, in conjunction with analysis of fetal scalp blood pH by direct puncture, permits more accurate diagnosis of fetal distress. Other obstetric practices also have changed. A premium has been placed upon atraumatic deliveries. Most fetuses with breech presentation will be delivered by cesarean section, and any clinical questions about the adequacy of the pelvis for an easy vaginal delivery will result in cesarean section for failure to progress, which is the most common cause of primary cesarean section on obstetric services in the United States.[3] Improvements in neonatal survival have modified obstetric decision making, for we now see intervention by cesarean section for the fetus estimated to weigh more than 700 g. These small fetuses would have been written off in the past and no intervention planned because of the lack of survival in the nursery. The result of this primary concern for the fetus has been a steep reduction in the number of midforceps deliveries and a marked increase in the number of cesarean sections being performed in the United States.

These obstetric advances, reflected by reduced perinatal mortality figures, have been achieved at a cost. This cost is an increasing rate of infection in mothers. In the first half of pregnancy, all terminations carry the risk of postprocedure pelvic infection, and this increases with advancing gestational age. Beyond 16 weeks, serious infections can result from hypertonic saline or urea infusion with prostaglandins,[4] the use of prostaglandins,[5] or dilatation and evacuation.[6] Any future diagnostic advances that reduce the number of these late terminations will have a beneficial effect on the frequency and severity of infections. In the latter half of pregnancy, a number of studies indicate that the maternal risk for infection is markedly increased when a cesarean section is performed, particularly when the woman is in labor. An increased number of women develop postpartum uterine infections[7] with associated bacteremia,[8] and the severity of the infection as measured by the fever index is greater as well.[9] The reality of current obstetric practice in the United States is that more frequent and more serious maternal infections are being and will continue to be seen because of the necessity to perform pregnancy terminations beyond the 16th week of pregnancy and the markedly increased cesarean section rate.

This problem of increased risk of maternal infection will not be eliminated by a return to old practice patterns. The benefits to the family unit of improved fetal mortality and morbidity figures have become a standard of medical care. This will continue. Advances in our understanding of the bacteriology and treatment of pelvic infection have made it possible to do interventions such as transperitoneal cesarean section in the presence of chorioamnionitis. Although maternal infection must be treated in every case in this situation, death from sepsis is now a rare event. There are social influences that will not permit disregard of abnormalities of the fetus. The delivery of a damaged baby is no longer acceptable. A baby with Down's syndrome becomes a lifetime burden for the family and society. If this is preventable with our current technology, steps will be taken to make prenatal diagnosis available to all pregnant women and not just those over the age of 35. In obstetrics, there is increased physician sensitivity to the possibility of malpractice litigation. In many instances, there has been too much attention paid to the mode of delivery when assessing the cause of a poor infant outcome. For example, studies have shown the safety of vaginal delivery of the fetus with breech presentation in selected cases,[10] and it has been observed that infants delivered by cesarean section without labor who presented as a breech have a higher incidence of subsequent learning disabilities than similarly delivered infants who had a vertex presentation.[11] Despite this, all too often subsequent learning or behavioral disability in the child who presented as a breech will be attributed to a vaginal delivery. Unfortunately, optimal medical care for the fetus has been equated with cesarean section in lay minds. Physicians are acutely aware of this, and it is another factor contributing to the high cesarean section rate in the United States.

PREVENTION OF INFECTION

Soft Tissue Infections—Genital Tract and Abdominal Wounds

The genital tract or the adominal wound of a recently pregnant patient is susceptible to bacterial infection. In the preantibiotic era, there was a major focus on the introduction of organisms such as the group A beta-hemolytic *Streptococcus* into the genital tract with resulting postpartum infection. Past admonitions about the use of rectal examinations to monitor cervical dilation during labor reflected this concern. Today, it is obvious from the microbiologic surveys of patients with postpartum endomyometritis[12] and those with associated bacteremia[8, 13] that this organism is rarely isolated and that the organisms isolated from the primary site of infection and from the bloodstream are residents of the vagina of normal pregnant women.[14] There is a simple clinical equation that expresses the conditions for a clinical infection. If the number or virulence of the bacteria introduced during labor or at the time of delivery, plus the extent of the soft tissue damage and the amount of foreign material left in place, exceeds the abilities of the host's local and systemic mechanisms to eliminate the organisms, an infection will result. Any attempt to evolve methods of prevention is directed toward shifting the balance of this equation in favor of the host.

It is difficult to delineate the risk factors in maternal soft tissue infection. One major problem has been a persisting physician preoccupation with time. Classic obstetric teaching has been that infection is more likely to occur when labor or the length of time of membrane rupture exceeds a certain number of hours or if an internal uterine pressure catheter is in place for a prolonged period of time. This focus ignores the individual patient variation in response to these stresses and the large differences noted among institutions when some risk factors are assessed. These major variances from hospital to hospital make it difficult to get enthusiastic about multifactoral analysis of risk factors in order to accurately weigh the importance of each factor. This analysis assesses the clinical reality at a particular institution but is not an accurate assessment for another institution in which different results have been obtained. It is more likely that a multiplicity of risk factors can tip the equation toward infection. To date, we have not recognized all of the factors, and we have been unable to accurately assess the significance of every factor that has been analyzed.

There are circumstances that result in greater risk for maternal infection. In pregnancy terminations, more frequent and more serious infections occur in women who are more than 16 weeks pregnant when compared to those earlier in their pregnancy.[4-6] Serious life-threatening infections have occurred in women over the age of 35 who have had hysterotomies;[15] for this reason, this procedure has been abandoned by most American obstetricians. Further, both the frequency[7] and the severity[9] of pelvic soft tissue infections are greater when cesarean section is performed compared with vaginal delivery. There are obviously other factors in these observed differences. The difficult midforceps delivery, with extensive soft tissue trauma and subsequent serious pelvic infection, has nearly been eliminated from modern obstetrics. In addition, many cesarean sections are performed in women with long labors or massive third trimester bleeding in whom a higher rate and greater severity of postoperative infection would be expected. The risk for cesarean section is not limited to morbidity, for the mortality rate from sepsis is higher than with a vaginal delivery.[16] Another factor in the soft tissue infection rate is the social class of the mother. A higher rate of infection is seen among women with lower socio-economic status, particularly when a cesarean section is performed.[12, 17, 18] Whether this is due to differences in medical care available to these women, variations in the bacterial flora of the lower genital tract, or differences in host defense mechanisms is not known at the present time. These risk factors are uniformly associated with a greater risk of infection, although the mechanisms are poorly understood at present.

There have been many confusing analyses of risk factors for soft tissue infection in recently pregnant women. The confusion stems from the variety of responses noted in different institutions.

The length of labor has not been a uniform factor in predicting subsequent infection. Many studies from a wide variety of investigation sites have documented an increased rate of infection with increasing length of time of labor.[19-23] The correlation was strong in two studies from Scandinavia in which there were no indigent patients.[22, 23] In contrast, a number of similarly well-done studies have shown no correlation with increased infection rates and prolonged labor.[24-27] Because of this diversity in response, I am no longer a firm advocate of intervening early to prevent long labors and presumably to automatically reduce the risk of infection. This is particularly true on a service where many patients are indigent. I still believe it is good obstetric practice to attempt to safely limit the length of labor when there is deviation from normal cervical dilatation patterns, but there is no evidence that this strategy will reduce the risk of subsequent infection for patients treated in this manner.

When analyzing the factor of physician examination of the woman in labor, there is no uniformity in the postpartum response. Traditional obstetric teaching focuses upon the importance of careful examination technique, and one recent study cited fewer vaginal examinations and increased utilization of the rectal route as a control measure to reduce the incidence of infection.[28] At least one study from the 1950's showed no difference in the maternal infection rate when routine vaginal examination replaced the rectal exam.[29] Some obstetricians have equated an increasing number of vaginal examinations with a higher infection rate.[21, 22] This view is not uniformly held. Two studies showed no correlation between an increased number of examinations and more infections.[19, 27] Both of these studies were multifactoral analyses. In the study that correlated prolonged labor with an increased infection rate[19] and another study that showed no increased risk with a prolonged labor,[27] no heightened risk of infection with increased numbers of vaginal examinations was found. Unnecessary internal examinations should not be performed in a woman in labor, but there is no universal evidence that a diminished number of examinations decreases the subsequent infection rate in all women.

There is no uniformity of opinion about the impact of the length of time of membrane rupture upon the rate and severity of infection. In recent reviews, the same studies that correlated long labors with an increased infection rate also showed an increased rate of infection with a prolonged period of membrane rupture.[19-23] In contrast, the studies that showed no correlation of infection rate with the length of labor also found no correlation with the length of time of membrane rupture.[24-27] There are other interesting observations. One of the studies[23] that found an increased number of infections with prolonged rupture of membranes also found an increased infection rate with labor and intact membranes. This observation confirms previous studies that have shown bacterial contamination of the amniotic fluid during labor in the presence of intact membranes.[30-32] In addition, prospective evaluations of two treatment regimens in an indigent population who developed postpartum endomyometritis after cesarean section showed no correlation between the length of time of membrane rupture and the severity of the infection as measured by the fever index (Figure 12–1).[33]

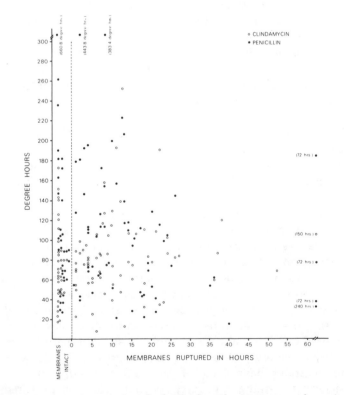

Fig. 12–1. Lack of correlation between length of time of membrane rupture and severity of postpartum infection. (From DiZerega, G., Yonekura, L., Roy, S., Nakamura, R.M., and Ledger, W.J.: A comparison of clindamycin-gentamicin and penicillin-gentamicin in the treatment of post-cesarean endomyometritis. Am. J. Obstet. Gynecol., *134*:238, 1979.)

These diverse results make it difficult to categorize this risk factor in an individual patient. Present obstetric care should avoid decision delays in the patient in labor with ruptured membranes, but early intervention will not diminish the risk of infection in every patient.

There is also no agreement on the risk of the use of an internal pressure catheter and the subsequent development of infection. The use of an indwelling foreign object in a microbiologically contaminated area seems to be a perfect setting for infection. Some reports have shown an increase in infection rate when catheters are used,[18, 26] while others[19, 21, 22, 27] found no correlation. It is again of interest that both of the studies showing an increased infection rate[18, 26] found this with a middle class population and not with an indigent population. There is also lack of correlation between the length of time of the invasive monitoring techniques and a higher incidence of infection. One study showed an increased infection rate when monitoring exceeded eight hours,[34] while two others showed no correlation.[24, 25] These conflicting results do not lend credence to the concept that the intrauterine catheter invariably increases the risk of infection. If a patient requires intravenous oxytocin (Pitocin) or it is difficult to accurately time the relationship of fetal heart rate decelerations with uterine contractions, an internal pressure catheter should be used.

There has been obstetric concern about the risk of infection from manipulations at the time of delivery. Opinions are divided as to the safety of routine exploration of the uterine cavity after vaginal delivery. However, one controlled prospective study found no increase in maternal infection rate when manual removal of the placenta was done in every case.[36] The use of local forms of anesthesia prior to vaginal delivery, such as pudendal or pericervical block anesthesia, can be associated with extensive and serious soft tissue pelvic infections.[37] The use of the vertical incision in cesarean section has been implicated in more serious postpartum infections,[16, 38] while one controlled study found no increase in the infection rate.[39] With these varied results, it is impossible to formulate rules about the best surgical choice of uterine incision.

There have been a wide variety of opinions about other patient factors that might increase the risk of infection. Two studies found a correlation between obesity and an increased postpartum infection rate,[20, 23] while two others could not confirm this.[21, 25] Anemia was also correlated as a factor in infection,[20, 23] but a number of other studies could not confirm this.[21, 22, 25, 40] The use of general anesthesia has also been cited as a contributing factor,[20, 27] but a larger number of articles showed no correlation.[21, 25, 40] This diversity of patient response from one center to another does not support the view that there are risk factors that have uniform weight for all patients on all services.

There are a number of possible explanations for the varied results obtained in evaluating risk factors. Infections with multiple etiologies can make it difficult to pinpoint the individual components of risk. Alternatively, it is possible that we have been looking at the wrong risk factors. Why do women of lower socioeconomic status have a higher rate of infection? Is it the less skilled care of physicians in training, a different bacterial flora, or impaired local and systemic host immunologic responses related to nutrition? I favor the latter and hope to be able to confirm this hypothesis in the future. In addition, much more detailed microbiologic analysis is needed. It is possible that specific species of bacteria, alone or in combination, are more virulent than others and increase the risk of infection in individual patients.

Antibiotic prophylaxis has been widely used in obstetric patients. Guidelines for the use of prophylactic antibiotics in pregnancy termination and delivery are provided in Chapter 7.

Patients developing a postpartum infection can be a source of nosocomial spread of infection to other patients on the service. There are a number of organisms that are easily spread from one patient to another. These include the group A beta-hemolytic *Streptococcus,* the coagulase-positive *Staphylococcus,* and *Clostridium difficile.* Fortunately, the recovery of these organisms is rare. There are specific clinical situations in which these bacteria can be suspected. In the postabortion or postpartum patient with a high temperature elevation, the absence of any localizing clinical signs, and an overwhelming number of gram-positive cocci on the smear of the exudate from the uterus, the presence of group A beta-hemolytic *Streptococcus* should be suspected. An abdominal wound abscess in which gram-positive cocci are seen on microscopic examination of the exudate should raise suspicion of the coagulase-positive *Staphylococcus.* Diarrhea developing in a patient after antibiotic therapy is suggestive of pseudomembranous enterocolitis caused by *Clostridium difficile.* If the clinician is suspicious of the presence of these organisms, or they have been confirmed by microbiologic study, these patients should be isolated in order to encourage care in medical staff contact with the patient and handwashing before any other patients are seen. This will dramatically reduce the problems of nosocomial spread of infection.

Urinary Tract

The urinary tract is particularly vulnerable to infection in the postpartum period. Changes produced in the urinary tract by pregnancy result in dilatation of the urinary collecting system, a slowing of ureteral peristalsis and of the transit of urine from kidney to bladder, and an increase in the volume of residual urine. Labor and delivery create additional stresses for the urinary tract. The base of the bladder is traumatized during normal labor, as evidenced by the common finding of red and white blood cells in the urine at the time of delivery or in the immediate postpartum period. As the fetal head enters the pelvis, the bladder becomes a nonpelvic organ and often is overdistended. Lapides has suggested that the overdistended bladder has a decreased arterial blood supply and thus is much more susceptible to bacterial infection.[41] The woman in labor frequently has difficulty voiding in bed. Vaginal delivery may produce trauma to the base of the bladder and urethra as well as perineal discomfort from the episiotomy incision and its subsequent repair.

Besides local factors, most patients receive intravenous fluids during labor and delivery. This fluid load, combined with the normal postdelivery mobilization of extracellular fluid, results in a postpartum diuresis that presents large quantities of urine to the traumatized bladder in the patient who has perineal discomfort. Some forms of modern anesthesia, particularly long-acting regional anesthesia, can have residual effects on the bladder, and they have been related to difficulty in voiding with subsequent urinary tract infection.[42] Frequently, urethral catheterization is necessary during labor or just before delivery, and this maneuver carries with it a small but significant risk of bacterial contamination of the bladder and subsequent infection. The bladder of a postpartum patient is larger than that of a nonpregnant patient, with a large capacity of residual urine, which increases the risk for a postpartum urinary tract infection.[43] With all these events concentrated around the time of delivery, it is little wonder that the urinary tract is a common site of postpartum infection.

Prevention of a postpartum urinary tract infection includes measures to prevent overdistention and to decrease the use of transurethral catheterization of the bladder. Medical personnel should direct their efforts toward the prevention of overdistention of the bladder during labor. All patients should be evaluated regularly for an overdistended bladder and encouraged to void. A narrow view of obstetric problems focused on the urinary tract dictates that long-acting regional anesthesia, such as continuous caudal or continuous epidural, should be avoided so that the overdistention-urethral catheterization cycle in the postpartum bladder can be avoided. There are many obstetric patients in labor for whom continuous regional anesthesia is indicated, but it should be employed with full recognition of its potential for postpartum urinary tract problems. Unless the patient has an overdistended bladder at the time of delivery, or a forceps rotation is planned, urethral catheterization is not necessary as a routine obstetric procedure. However, catheterization should not be banned, for an overdistended bladder at the time of delivery or immediately postpartum poses more of a risk to the long-term health of the patient's urinary tract than a single catheterization followed by spontaneous voiding, because patients with an overdistended bladder can have difficulty voiding postpartum. Awareness of the vulnerability of the urinary tract to infection should aid in the prevention of at least some postpartum urinary tract problems.

Respiratory Tract

The pregnant patient is particularly vulnerable to the complication of postoperative aspiration pneumonia. Nausea and vomiting can be complications, either during induction or at the termination of general inhalation anesthesia, and it must be guarded against to prevent aspiration of gastric contents. The risk for this complication is greater in pregnant patients, for they usually have a greater volume of gastric contents at the time of induction of anesthesia because of decreased gastrointestinal activity. Gastric emptying time is delayed and more gastric secretions are present than in nonpregnant patients. It is not uncommon for the woman in labor who is made ready for cesarean section to have several hundred milliliters of acid gastric contents present when anesthesia is induced, despite having had nothing by mouth for many hours. Awareness of these risk factors permits the utilization of preventive measures in the patient at risk.

A number of techniques decrease the incidence of aspiration pneumonia. The high risk of all pregnant women for this condition should be recognized, and patients receiving intravenous ethanol to prevent premature labor and delivery are even more at risk because of the stimulating action of alcohol on the stomach.[44] Besides careful use of a cuffed endotracheal tube, which should not be removed until the patient is fully conscious, the prophylactic administration of antacids to these patients prior to the induction of anesthesia has been associated with a lower incidence of complications from aspiration pneumonia; this is because of the relationship of the acidity of gastric contents to the acute inflammatory reaction in the lungs.[45] Perhaps the greatest deterrent to pulmonary complications in obstetric patients is the 24-hour availability of anesthesia and medical personnel skilled in the management of pregnant women. This standard should be the goal of every obstetrics service.

DIAGNOSIS AND TREATMENT

Despite an awareness of risk factors and the use of preventive measures, postoperative and postpartum infections do occur. The remainder of this chapter will be devoted to the evaluation and treatment of women with puerperal infections. The format will be a discussion of the postdelivery patient when first presenting to the physician. Figure 12–2 documents the timing of the first elevation of temperature in postpartum women.[42] Too often, the task of evaluation is relegated to the most junior house officer, or the physician orders the patient placed on systemic antibiotics by telephone at night without benefit of physical examination or prior culture. These events are unfortunate, for the time before administration of antibiotics is the best time to evaluate the extent of the infection, to obtain cultures, or to establish operative drainage; these will help avoid the use of systemic antibiotics. The key to the care of patients is an awareness of the possible sites of infection.

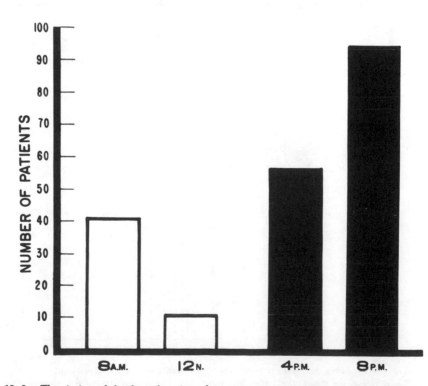

Fig. 12–2. The timing of the first elevation of temperature in postpartum women. (Reprinted with permission from the American College of Obstetricians and Gynecologists. From Ledger, W.J., Reite, A.M., and Headington, J.T.: A system for infectious disease surveillance on the obstetric service. Obstet. Gynecol., *37*:769, 1971.)

Predelivery Infection

A number of pregnant patients with hospital-acquired infections have their first symptoms prior to delivery. These infections can be serious and require careful diagnostic techniques and a careful physical examination. For patients who are undergoing termination of pregnancy after 16 weeks, instillation of hypertonic glucose[46] and hypertonic saline[47] has been associated with a serious uterine infection and associated bacteremia. This is a diagnostic consideration in these women, and after performing blood cultures the patient should be placed on a combination of antibiotics such as clindamycin and gentamicin, particularly since anaerobes[8] and the coagulase-positive *Staphylococcus*[12] have been recovered in these infections. The cornerstone of care remains rapid evacuation of the uterus. Fortunately, the prognosis for cure in these patients is excellent, as noted in Figure 12–3,[9] in which the patients presented had the best results of any of the women with hospital-acquired infections. There are some diagnostic difficulties in the evaluation of a febrile patient undergoing pregnancy termination. Some women who receive prostaglandins for this purpose will have a febrile response,[48] and attempts to differentiate this response from the response to an intrauterine infection are impossible on clinical and laboratory grounds. The uterus can be tender upon examination, and patients usually have a leukocytosis. Blood cultures should be done and antibiotic coverage employed until delivery is accomplished. In pregnancies beyond 20 weeks, fever during labor can be a late sign of chorioamnionitis. It is often a late sign because oral temperatures are less accurate than rectal

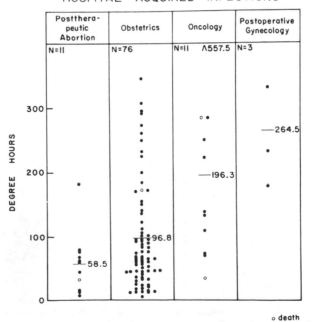

Fig. 12–3. Fever indices in patients with bacteremia secondary to a hospital-acquired infection. The bar indicates the mean fever index for each group. The lowest fevers occur in women with an infection following pregnancy termination. (Reprinted with permission from the American College of Obstetricians and Gynecologists. From Ledger, W.J., Kriewall, T.H., and Gee, C.: The fever index: A technique for evaluating the clinical response to bacteremia. Obstet. Gynecol., *45*:603, 1975.)

temperature owing to the hyperventilation associated with normal labor.[49, 50] When patients are found to be febrile, it can be difficult to pinpoint the site of infection. If an intrauterine catheter is in place, a portion of amniotic fluid can be withdrawn and examined after Gram staining, and another portion can be sent for culture. A microscopic examination is diagnostic only if no white blood cells or bacteria are found. This suggests the site of infection is elsewhere. However, bacteria and white cells are usually present in the patient in labor who has no clinical evidence of infection (Figure 12–4).[51] Amniotic fluid and blood cultures should be obtained. If delivery is imminent, antibiotics can be withheld until after delivery so that the newborn evaluation will not be confused by the presence of antibiotics. If it is necessary for the patient to go through labor, then I favor giving a cephalosporin such as cefoxitin, for it provides good coverage of the group B streptococci and

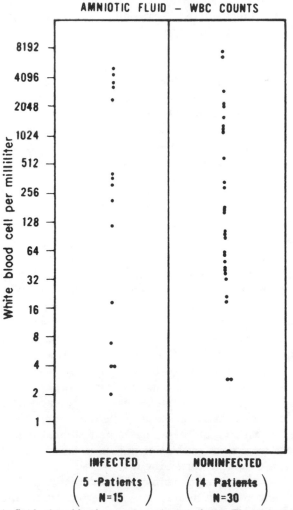

Fig. 12–4. Amniotic fluid white blood count in patients in labor. The group of 15 patients on the left developed infections, while the 30 patients on the right had no infections. (Reprinted with permission from the American College of Obstetricians and Gynecologists. From Bobitt, J.R., and Ledger, W.J.: Amniotic fluid analysis. Its role in maternal and neonatal infection. Obstet. Gynecol., *51*:56, 1978.)

Escherichia coli, the two most common bacterial pathogens for the newborn. I have little concern about the seriousness of the subsequent maternal infection unless a cesarean section is needed. If this is the case, I favor the use of clindamycin and gentamicin as treatment for these patients postpartum. Finally, a rare and serious condition may be noted prior to delivery—malignant hyperthermia from general anesthesia.[52] Early signs are tachycardia followed by a rapid rise in temperature. If suspected, the general anesthesia should be stopped immediately and therapeutic efforts begun to lower the patient's temperature.

Onset of Fever Within 48 Hours of Delivery

The differential diagnosis of the postpartum patient with early onset of sepsis should include the possibility of an exogenous source of infection, such as a contaminated intravenous infusion. The logical sequence and subsequent therapy have been detailed in the discussion of early onset postoperative infections in gynecologic patients in Chapter 9.

ASPIRATION PNEUMONIA

A serious and still common cause of an early febrile response in a postpartum patient is aspiration pneumonia. This condition should be suspected in any patient with onset of fever within 12 hours of delivery who demonstrates some respiratory distress. She will usually have a low arterial pO_2, and frequently abnormal changes in the lungs are noted on chest radiographs. Early diagnosis is a critical factor in management, for the initiation of the pulmonic changes noted with this syndrome seems to be related to the acid pH of the gastric contents. The goal of therapy is to recognize the aspiration immediately and to suction the tracheobronchial tree to minimize the volume of the gastric secretions and their subsequent effect on the pulmonary system. The fact that aspiration was not noted in the operating room does not rule out this differential diagnosis, because regurgitation and aspiration of gastric contents can occur on the entry to or in the recovery room before the patient regains full consciousness after general anesthesia. Established aspiration pneumonia is not likely to yield to aggressive lavage or bronchial suction.

The goal of treatment is to improve ventilatory status, which can usually be accomplished by the use of 100% oxygen by positive pressure, the systemic use of pharmacologic amounts of adrenocortical steroids, and the administration of systemic antibiotics. The first maneuver is free of controversy. One hundred percent oxygen administered by a positive-pressure breathing apparatus usually results in an elevation in the patient's arterial pO_2. The other regimens are open to question. Animal experiments have not demonstrated any benefit from the administration of massive doses of steroids,[53] but there is faith in the anti-inflammatory activity of these agents and clinical belief that patients appear to improve. The use of antibiotics is just as controversial. In animal experiments sterile gastric fluid produced the widespread reactive changes of aspiration pneumonia.[54] However, this experimental model ignores the fact that the gastric contents traverse the mouth and carry its bacterial flora into a respiratory tract that is damaged by the acid gastric content and susceptible to the establishment of a pulmonary infection by contamining bacteria. The plausibility of this bacterial involvement was confirmed by Bartlett and associates, who recovered anaerobic bacteria in 93% of nonobstetric patients with aspiration pneumonia,[55] but these serious infections were seen in nonhospitalized patients who were alcohol or drug abusers with poor dental hygiene. Despite this, I use antibiotics in such hospitalized patients. Since most of the anaerobes recovered in patients with aspiration pneumonia are sensitive to penicillin, this agent remains my first choice. In a few instances, *Bacteroides fragilis* has been recovered in patients with aspiration pneumonia.[56] In the patient whose septic infection persists despite administration of penicillin, consideration should be given to using clindamycin.

BACTEREMIA

A common cause of the early postpartum febrile response in women is bacteremia, with the uterus as the primary site of infection. High risk women include those who have undergone cesarean section.[8] These patients, who have early onset of fever, are frequently misdiagnosed and treated inappropriately. In the early stage of infection, localizing signs of a uterine infection may be minimal. Many physicians include only urinary tract infections in their differential diagnosis and diagnose pyelonephritis on the basis of red and white blood cells seen in a urine specimen of a postpartum patient with sudden onset of fever. Having made this diagnosis, they treat the patient appropriately for a urinary tract infection with a single antibiotic that concentrates in the urine and is effective against gramnegative aerobes. Figure 12–5 graphically portrays this diagnostic confusion in a patient who had an uncomplicated vaginal delivery at arrow 1.[57] At arrow 2 she became febrile, and the original diagnosis was pyelonephritis. Urine culture subsequently produced no growth. However, the blood and endometrial cultures grew the gram-negative aerobic rod, *Klebsiella.* The patient had endomyometritis. Even though material from the endometrial cavity obtained prior to antibiotic therapy had only intermediate susceptibility to ampicillin, the patient became afebrile at arrow 3 and remained so for the remainder of her hospitalization.

Fortunately for the obstetrician-gynecologist, most patients have intact host defense mechanisms and recover from bacteremia. In two separate studies of bacteremia in postpartum patients, a wide variety of microorganisms was recovered.[8, 13] The most commonly recovered bacteria include group B beta-hemolytic streptococci, enterococci, *Escherichia coli, Bacteroides,* and anaerobic cocci. Bacteremia in postpartum patients does not identify a population at risk for serious infection, for in one study these women's infections were no more serious than those without a bacteremia.[13] A major factor in the severity of infection is the route of delivery. Those patients who delivered by cesarean section had more serious infections than those who delivered vaginally[9] (Figure 12–6). The frequency with which certain bacteria are isolated should be acknowledged in the antibiotic coverage of these patients. Minimum coverage of the postcesarean patient usually includes clindamycin and an aminoglycoside, or alternatively one of the newer cephalosporins or penicillins alone. In patients who have delivered vaginally, single agent therapy is appropriate.

URINARY TRACT

An infrequent source of an early febrile response in the postpartum patient is the urinary tract. The development of pyelonephritis de novo in the immediate postpartum period is not a common event. Most patients in whom the urinary tract is the source of the early postpartum rise of temperature have a history of urinary tract difficulties during pregnancy, and many have had unexplained low

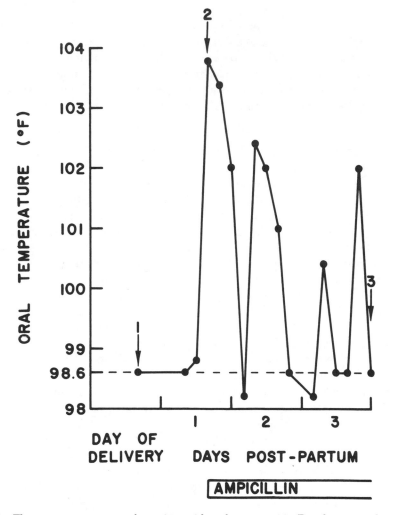

Fig. 12–5. The postpartum course of a patient with endomyometritis. Details are noted in the text. (From Ledger, W.J.: Anaerobic infections. *In* Communicable and Infectious Diseases. Edited by F.H. Top, Sr., and P.F. Wehrle. 8th ed., St. Louis, C.V. Mosby Co., 1976.)

grade fever during labor. These facts suggest that the patients had an infection incubating in the urinary tract during pregnancy, and that pyelonephritis became clinically evident only after delivery. These patients often have costovertebral angle pain on minimal palpation and usually have bacteriuria on microscopic examination of urine and a positive urine culture. In such women, single antibiotic coverage against gram-negative aerobes is appropriate because it usually suffices for cure. Agents such as ampicillin or a cephalosporin can be utilized unless the patient has been exposed to these antibiotics during pregnancy, in which case an aminoglycoside is a good alternative agent. If flank pain develops suddenly postpartum following cesarean section or a difficult repair of a sulcus laceration, an intravenous pyelogram or an ultrasonogram should be obtained to demonstrate the absence of any ureteral compromise.

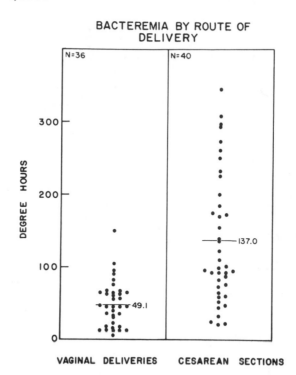

BACTEREMIA BY ROUTE OF DELIVERY

Fig. 12–6. The fever indices of patients who developed an endomyometritis following vaginal or cesarean section delivery. (Reprinted with permission from the American College of Obstetricians and Gynecologists. From Ledger, W.J., Kriewall, T.H., and Gee, C.: The fever index: A technique for evaluating the clinical response to bacteremia. Obstet. Gynecol., *43*:603, 1975.)

ENDOMYOMETRITIS AND BACTEREMIA FROM GROUP A AND GROUP B
BETA-HEMOLYTIC *STREPTOCOCCUS*

One cause of early onset fever in a postpartum patient is endomyometritis caused by group A or B beta-hemolytic *Streptococcus*. Although uncommon, it should be considered because of the severity of the infection and the potential for spread to other patients. This condition can present a confusing diagnostic picture in the individual patient, because the rapid tissue invasion and spread of these organisms occur without the usual clinical signs of infection. The patients are obviously septic, have high temperatures, and appear acutely ill.[58, 59] However, attempts to delineate the primary site of infection by physical examination may be frustrating for the clinician. Although there frequently is some tenderness on pelvic examination, both induration and the purulent uterine discharge usually associated with uterine infection are absent. Instead, there is minimal diffuse pelvic tenderness and grossly clear cervical discharge, which is seen to be filled with gram-positive cocci when a smear has been Gram stained and viewed under the microscope. The patients are critically ill, particularly when group A *Streptococcus* is isolated, and treatment should not be delayed until the final laboratory identification of the organism is made. Patients should be placed on high doses of penicillin or clindamycin if they are allergic to penicillin. Despite the great susceptibility of these bacteria to these antibiotics in the laboratory, patients may require more than 24 hours to become afebrile (Figure 12–7).[58] The patient whose temperature response to antibiotics is shown in Figure 12–7 had a spontaneous

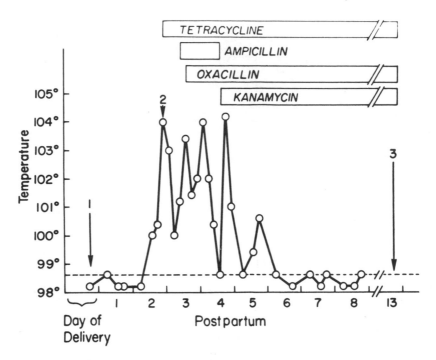

Fig. 12–7. The temperature response of a patient with a postpartum endomyometritis due to group A beta-hemolytic *Steptococcus.* Details are noted in the text. (Reprinted with permission from the American College of Obstetricians and Gynecologists. From Ledger, W.J., and Headington, J.T.: Group A beta-hemolytic *Streptococcus:* An important cause of serious infections in obstetrics and gynecology. Obstet. Gynecol., *39*:474, 1972.)

vaginal delivery at arrow 1. At arrow 2, the diagnosis of endomyometritis was made and a blood culture was positive for group A beta-hemolytic *Streptococcus.* The patient was discharged from the hospital at arrow 3.

RETAINED OR INFECTED TISSUE

An uncommon but important cause of early postpartum fever is the infection related to either tissue retained in the uterus or infected tissue secondary to birth trauma. The sequence of delivery causing this complication takes two forms. First, there may have been difficulty with delivery of the placenta that necessitated vigorous intrauterine manipulation in the delivery room. Second, there may have been no recognized problems associated with the delivery, but a soft tissue hematoma formed that became infected. Physical examination, particularly pelvic examination, is important to determine both the site and extent of the infection. If the delivery of the placenta is difficult, curettage is indicated to remove retained tissue after coverage with systemic antibiotics. If a soft tissue mass is found, systemic antibiotics should be administered. Operative intervention may not be necessary unless the mass shows evidence of continued growth.

Onset of Fever 48 Hours After Delivery

Patients who become febrile 48 hours or more after delivery represent the largest segment of those with postpartum infections. Figure 12–2 demonstrates the distribution of patients with postpartum infections and indicates the frequency of this interval.[42] These observations underscore the theoretical problems that can be associated with the widespread practice of early hospital discharge (24 to 48 hours after delivery) of postpartum patients.

URINARY TRACT

A common site of infection is the urinary tract. Diagnosis may be difficult, for the postpartum patients often has trouble collecting a clean-voided urine specimen for culture, and the microscopic examination of the urine of a normal postpartum patient usually reveals red and white blood cells. Significant urinary findings include the presence of bacteria in an unspun urine specimen examined microscopically or a high bacterial colony count from properly obtained urine. If an uncontaminated urine specimen cannot be obtained in the febrile patient with urinary symptoms, I believe it is justified to obtain a urine sample by means of catheterization for culture and microscopic examination.

Prognosis is usually favorable for postpartum patients with urinary tract infections. A high percentage of these infections are caused by gram-negative aerobes, the most commonly recovered being *Escherichia coli.* In postpartum patients, the group B beta-hemolytic *Streptococcus* is the most commonly isolated gram-positive aerobe.[60] In these young healthy women, antibiotic resistance is seldom a problem. In the planning of therapy for urinary tract infection, the policy should be to restrict the administration of powerful antimicrobials. Good clinical results can be obtained with either the sulfas or the nitrofurans. This diminishes the utilization of more powerful systemic agents and prevents the masking of an infection outside the urinary tract. A number of separate factors may cause modifications in this policy. If the patient has a history of urinary tract infections during pregnancy, with many separate regimens of antibiotic treatment, the odds are high that she has a more resistant strain of bacteria than usual. Other agents, such as a broad-spectrum penicillin or an aminoglycoside, may be required for cure. There is little enthusiasm for the use of tetracycline because of the report of Schultz and coworkers on the use of high doses of intravenous tetracycline in pregnant women with urinary tract infections. Doses higher than 2 g a day were administered intravenously to patients, who developed massive fatty infiltration of the liver, manifested clinically by liver failure and death.[61] An important aspect of care of all such patients is to repeat urine cultures after 48 hours of therapy to assess the adequacy of the antibiotic choice for this specific infection.

ENDOMYOMETRITIS

A common cause of postpartum illness during hospitalization is the development of endomyometritis. Patients with this condition usually give a history of a decrease in the amount of lochial flow for 12 to 24 hours prior to the time they first become febrile. On examination, uterine tenderness and a foul-smelling discharge from the endocervical canal are frequently found. The pelvic examination must be done prior to treatment. It helps obstetricians confirm the extent of the clinical infection. An important component of therapy is the establishment of adequate uterine drainage. An entity called lochia block does exist, and removal of a portion of membrane or placenta from the region of the internal os with ring forceps is sometimes the only therapy necessary.

Frequently, patients will remain febrile after examination or there will be evidence on examination of infected beyond the limits of the uterus, for which antibiotics are clearly indicated. A therapeutic dilemma in this condition is the proper choice of antibiotic. These infections are usually multibacterial, with a broad range of susceptibility.

At present, our judgments on treatment have to be based on the clinical outcome. The microorganisms most frequently recovered from the uterus and the bloodstream in these patients include the aerobes *Escherichia coli,* the group B beta-hemolytic *Streptococcus,* the enterococcus, plus the anaerobes, *Peptostreptococcus* and *Bacteroides bivius, B. disiens, B. fragilis,* and *B. melaninogenicus,* and *Chlamydia.* Attempts to cover all these organisms with empirical antibiotic therapy before culture reports are available would require a therapeutic combination of three or four antibiotics. Most physicians justifiably do not like this "shotgun" approach. It rarely is needed and it increases the risk of antibiotic toxicity. Instead, incomplete coverage with the initial therapy is accepted but is focused upon the avoidance of subsequent serious infection. For example, there is less risk of a serious infection following vaginal delivery, especially when the clinical examination shows no evidence of infection beyond the uterus. In this patient population, the use of a single antibiotic such as a broad-spectrum penicillin or a second or third generation cephalosporin is appropriate. The clinical response is usually favorable.

The therapeutic concern for the patient who has had a cesarean section is different. Obstetric surveillance data from the Universities of Michigan[12] and Southern California[9] indicate that endomyometritis is more severe after cesarean section (see Figure 12–6).[9] Based on published results, for these patients the treatment of choice is the combination of clindamycin and gentamicin[33, 62, 63] (Table 12–1). This gives better results than have been noted with ampicillin alone or in combination with an aminoglycoside, penicillin with an aminoglycoside, penicillin

Table 12–1. Therapeutic Results with Two Combination Antibiotic Regimens

	Clindamycin-Gentamicin		Penicillin-Gentamicin		Significance
No. of patients	100		100		N.S.
Therapy completed, no problems	86		64		$p < 0.001$
Poor clinical results:					
No response—third antibiotic	5		29		$p < 0.001$
Abdominal wound infection	8		16		N.S.
Operative drainage only		6		4	N.S.
Prolonged febrile course after drainage		2		12	$p < 0.02$ (Fisher's exact test)
Serious problems:	0		4		$p < 0.06$
Pelvic abscess, total abdominal hysterectomy, bilateral salpingo-oophorectomy	0		1		
Wound evisceration	0		1		
Heparin	0		2		
Reaction during antibiotics:	4		3		N.S.
Rash	2*		2		
Hematuria	0		1†		
Diarrhea	2		0		
Indirect measures of morbidity:					
Hospital days	7.4		8.7		$p < 0.01$ (Mann-Whitney U test)
Fever index in degree hours					
Median	77.3		91.3		$p < 0.02$
Mean	81.2		110.7		
±SD	± 40.6		± 89.6		
±SE	± 4.06		± 9.0		

N.S. = Not significant.
*Drug continued, rash disappeared, one patient.
†Drug continued, hematuria stopped.
(From DiZerega, G., Yonekura, L., Roy, S., Nakamura, R.M., and Ledger, W.J.: A comparison of clindamycin-gentamicin and penicillin-gentamicin in the treatment of post-cesarean endomyometritis. Am. J. Obstet. Gynecol., *134*:238, 1979.)

and tetracycline, or a first generation cephalosporin with an aminoglycoside. The problem for clinicians is that this combination of clindamycin and an aminoglycoside has toxicity. Clindamycin can be associated with diarrhea and less frequently with pseudomembranous enterocolitis, while the aminoglycoside can be toxic to the eighth cranial nerve and the kidneys. In addition, the use of aminoglycosides in postpartum patients requires monitoring of blood levels, because a large percentage of postpartum patients will have subtherapeutic levels despite the use of the recommended dose prescription[61] owing to their excellent renal function. As a result, there has been increasing interest in alternative regimens. To date, studies of second generation cephalosporins such as cefoxitin[65] and cefamandole,[66] third generation cephalosporins such as moxalactam,[67] and the broad spectrum penicillins—ticarcillin,[68] piperacillin,[69] and mezlocillin[70]—have yielded acceptable results. I am not convinced that these single drug regimens are equivalent to combinations in preventing the subsequent development of wound and pelvic infections that require operative drainage, but the collection of a larger number of case studies will answer this question.

Occasionally, patients will remain febrile while receiving these initial treatment regimens. A repeat examination is necessary to be sure there is no evidence of infection beyond the confines of the uterus or that no tissue is retained in the uterus. A ring forceps should be employed at the time of pelvic examination to help evaluate the latter possibility. If there are no abnormal findings, then consideration should be given to the bacteria most frequently isolated from the site of infection not covered by the initial regimen. In the case of the clindamycin-aminoglycoside combination, the main concern should be the enterococcus. I favor the addition of penicillin G in a dose of 20,000,000 U every 24 hours with 5,000,000 U at six hour dosing intervals, but many infectious disease experts will use ampicillin, 8 g a day in four divided doses. I prefer to avoid the combination of clindamycin and ampicillin because each of these drugs has been associated with diarrhea and pseudomembranous enterocolitis. With the newer cephalosporins, I am concerned about coverage of resistant gram-negative anaerobic rods as well as of the enterococci. I stop the cephalosporins and use either clindamycin or metronidazole, plus an aminoglycoside and penicillin. If the newer penicillins are used, my major concerns are the gram-negative anaerobic rods and the coagulase-positive *Staphylococcus.* These can be covered by the use of clindamycin alone or metronidazole plus one of the semisynthetic penicillins such as sodium methicillin (Staphcillin). Obviously, the isolation of a resistant aerobic organism from the bloodstream or the site of infection will modify these choices. If the patient remains febrile for 48 hours after these new antibiotics have been given, a complete reexamination should be performed. If there is no evidence of a wound infection or a pelvic abscess, heparin can be added to the regimen. This indication for treating with heparin rarely occurs today, probably because of the earlier use of antibiotics that are effective against gram-negative anaerobes. If the suspected clinical diagnosis of septic pelvic thrombophlebitis is correct, the patient should become afebrile within 48 hours of the onset of heparin therapy. If the patient becomes afebrile, administration of heparin is continued by constant intravenous perfusion monitored by a partial thromboplastin time (PTT), in addition to antibiotics. The patient is given 10 days of therapy and the drug is then discontinued. Laparotomy for plication of the vena cava and ovarian vein is not performed unless the patient continues to have pulmonary emboli despite laboratory evidence of adequate anticoagulants. I have not had a patient who received an inferior vena caval ligation in the past ten years. More commonly, if the patient remains febrile, serious consideration should be given to the use of an exploratory laparotomy to determine if an abscess or necrotic infected issue is present. A patient requiring operative intervention for a serious postpartum infection represents the exception rather than the rule. In one survey of patients in the 1960s requiring hysterectomy and salpingo-oophorectomy, only six women required this procedure in a period during which there were nearly 10,000 deliveries;[71] we are required to do this even less frequently today.

ABDOMINAL WOUND INFECTION

Another source of postpartum fever is an abdominal wound infection after cesarean section or tubal ligation or an episiotomy infection. Usually, these fevers are discovered the fourth to eighth day after operation, but some develop earlier, particularly when a group A beta-hemolytic *Streptococcus* is the microbiologic entity involved in the infection. On occasion, rapidly spreading synergistic infections, either of the abdominal wound or of the episiotomy, will be seen in the first 48 hours after delivery. The diagnosis should be suspected in any febrile postpartum patient who has an inflamed wound with some purulent exudate from the edges. The key to therapy is wide adequate drainage of the wound. In addition, this operative exploration provides information to the clinician on the status of the fascia. If it is disrupted, further operative care will be necessary to see if the peritoneum is intact and an appropriate repair performed. In most cases, antibiotics are neither indicated nor necessary. However, if there is rapid evidence of spreading wound induration and redness, systemic antibiotics should be used as well as drainage and debridement if necessary. Examination of a smear of the exudate of the infected wound and a properly collected microbiologic specimen may be of great help in the planning of antibiotics for the patient. If only gram-positive cocci are present, the physician should be concerned about the possibility of a synergistic infection with a penicillinase-producing coagulase-positive *Staphylococcus* and an anaerobic *Streptococcus (Peptostreptococcus),* for which a cephalosporin is a good first drug of choice. If gram-positive rods with clubbing are seen, the physician should be concerned about a clostridial infection, and excision of necrotic tissue is indicated as well as administration of systemic antibiotics. The concerns about abdominal wounds also hold true for episiotomy wounds, although infections occur infrequently in episiotomy incisions and usually are not major clinical problems. However, serious problems with synergistic infections causing maternal mortality have been reported.[72–74] The best early sign of these synergistic infections is the anesthesia of the involved area and the lack of bleeding when debridement is begun. Immediate operation and extensive debridement are needed for cure.

ONE DAY FEVER

A small percentage of women will manifest only one elevation of temperature above 100.4° F during their postpartum hospitalization. This fever is often attributed by the house staff to breast engorgement, although it does not parallel the clinical onset of mastitis. Some services have attributed this fever to a lochial block. Obviously, no antibiotics are needed for the cure of these patients. Since there is no way to diagnose absolutely the site of infection causing the fever, I prefer the term one-day fever. If the patient is still febrile four to six hours after the onset of fever, this diagnosis is no longer valid. The physician once again must examine the patient for a source of infection and treat her appropriately with systemic antibiotics.

Late Manifestation of Fever in Postpartum Patients

Although it is not possible to document by comparative study, I believe that more obstetric patients with late postpartum infections are being seen today than 20 years ago. The current popularity of early hospital discharge for obstetric patients may result in the readmission of those who formerly would have had their infections diagnosed and treated during their initial hospitalization. If all patients are routinely discharged on the first, second, or third postoperative day, it is easy to see that some infectious problems can be overlooked (see Figure 12–2).[42] In addition to the variables brought about by changes in the patterns of hospital practice, a number of infections related to delivery can appear for the first time late in the postpartum period.

Urinary Tract

Urinary tract infections occasionally occur late in the postpartum period. There are two different groups of patients involved. In one, a urinary tract infection is noted during the patient's initial hospitalization. The patient responds clinically to the antibacterial agents but returns to the hospital later with either a lower or an upper urinary tract infection. These infections are preventable to a degree. Since simple screening tests for bacteriuria are easy to perform, patients with this type of infection should have cultures repeated after two or three days of therapy to determine if the bacteria have been cleared from the urine. If not, antibiotic susceptibility tests can be done to help in the selection of a more appropriate antibiotic. In the second group, the patient is asymptomatic during initial hospitalization but becomes symptomatic some time after discharge. It is particularly important to obtain a urine culture for all women requiring catheterization or the use of an indwelling catheter during labor or in the postpartum period.

Mastitis or Breast Abscess

Another common cause of late postpartum morbidity is the development of mastitis or breast abscess. Generally, patients who are breast-feeding develop a surface break in the nipple of one or both breasts and note breast redness and tenderness just before coming to see the physician. Evaluation of host carriage of microorganisms indicates that the infant becomes colonized with coagulase-positive *Staphylococcus aureus* that is penicillin-resistant during his or her stay in the nursery. The baby in turn colonizes the mother and provides the bacterial nidus for the initiation of infection when there is a break in the surface integrity of the nipple. The physician caring for patients with mastitis should be aware of high frequency of recovery of the coagulase-positive *Staphylococcus* from this site of infection. I favor the use of cloxacillin orally in the patient with mastitis, but an oral cephalosporin may also be used. One very confusing observation has been the successful treatment of mastitis in which the coagulase-positive *Staphylococcus* has been isolated with antibiotics that were not effective in the laboratory against this organism.[75] The good results in those cases are probably related to host defense mechanisms, for these resistances are due to penicillinase production and are not overcome by higher doses of penicillin. During this treatment phase I allow patients to continue to breast-feed their infants from the unaffected breast and to utilize a breast pump on the infected one. They can discontinue the use of a breast pump and resume feeding when systemic fever and local redness have subsided. Physicians should be aware that ampicillin has no advantage over penicillin in the treatment of infections with penicillinase-producing organisms. If a breast abscess has formed, operative drainage is indicated, along with the administration of appropriate antibiotics, and breast-feeding should be discontinued. Results of smear and culture should be obtained for all patients with mastitis or breast abscess, for other organisms that are not susceptible to semisynthetic penicillin are sometimes involved.

SOFT TISSUE INFECTION

A frequent cause for readmission to the hospital is a soft tissue infection. Some of these patients have had an early discharge with no fever, and some have had infections that seemingly responded to systemic antibiotics during their initial hospitalization. This experience with humans parallels the animal model of mixed peritoneal infection, in which treatment of the aerobic component of the infection diminished the severity of the disease but did not change the number of animals that developed a pelvic abscess later[76] (see Chapter 7). The clinical manifestations of soft tissue infections in postpartum patients take many forms.

A recently reported entity is the late development of an endomyometritis due to *Chlamydia*.[77] These infections occur most frequently in women following vaginal delivery. The organisms are susceptible to both tetracycline and erythromycin, and fortunately the infections are not serious. Patients respond to these antibiotics and do not require operative intervention for cure.

Patients who have undergone a cesarean section can develop a late abdominal wound infection that requires operative drainage. A particularly difficult problem is the infected subfascial hematoma that occurs after a transverse abdominal incision. Some of these seem to dissect endlessly into the retroperitoneal space. Adequate operative drainage is the only way to ensure a cure, and this requires that the patient be managed in the operating room with adequate anesthesia for the exploration.

The patient can have a serious uterine infection after cesarean section that does not respond to antibiotics at the time of readmission. Figures 12–8 and 12–9 illustrate the clinical problems seen. In Figure 12–8, the patient had a cesarean section at another hospital for fetal indications.[71] When she became febrile, she was treated with penicillin and an aminoglycoside. She remained febrile after many days of therapy, and a pelvic abscess was discovered and drained through a colpotomy incision. She continued to have high temperature elevations and was transferred to our hospital at arrow 1. Therapeutic choice was complicated in this patient, for she refused the use of any blood products. She was started on an oral iron preparation. At arrow 2, hyperalimentation was begun and continued until arrow 3. At arrow 4, hysterectomy and bilateral salpingo-oophorectomy were performed because the uterus was grossly infected and the uterine incision had broken down. *Bacteroides fragilis* was isolated. At arrow 5, the patient was started on chloramphenicol. The *Bacteroides fragilis* was susceptible in the laboratory to both clindamycin and chloramphenicol.

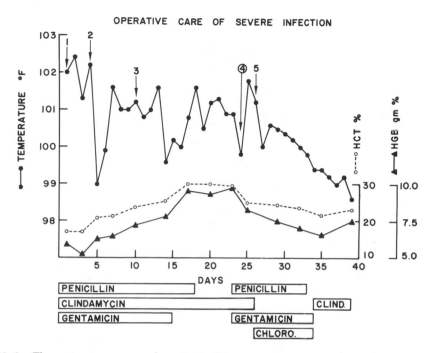

Fig. 12–8. The postpartum course of a patient with a severe postpartum pelvic infection caused by *Bacteroides fragilis*. (From Ledger, W.J., Gassner, C.B., and Gee, C.: Operative care of infections in obstetrics-gynecology. J. Reprod. Med., *13*:128, 1974.)

The next case illustrates a similar clinical problem (see Figure 12–9).[78] A 21-year-old primigravida with no known problems was admitted in active labor with ruptured membranes and the cervix dilated 4 cm. Examination revealed a double footling breech that had not been previously detected. While blood for a possible transfusion was being readied, a fetal electrode was placed on the heel of the baby so that any difficulties that might result from cord compression during contraction would be detected immediately. The fetal heart rate remained normal throughout the period of observation, and the cesarean section was carried out without incident, delivering a healthy term male infant weighing 8 lb, 2 oz with good Apgar scores.

The mother did well for three days. Then she began to run an oral temperature of 100° to 101° F. A complete physical examination was within normal limits, except that the uterus seemed to be a bit more tender than would have been expected. The impression was that it was not as well involuted as it should have been by this time postpartum. A foul-smelling discharge was coming from the cervical os. The diagnosis was postpartum endomyometritis, and the patient was placed on penicillin G, 5,000,000 U IV every six hours, and gentamicin, 80 mg IV every eight hours. Her temperature not only failed to decline but it was higher 72 hours later than at the start of antimicrobial therapy.

Because of concern that anaerobic organisms might be involved, particularly *Bacteroides fragilis, B. bivius,* or *B. disiens,* clindamycin was added. During the next 24 hours the temperature declined but did not become normal, and the patient then began to display spiking temperatures. After another 48 hours, a series of examinations was performed to ascertain whether a pelvic abscess might be present,

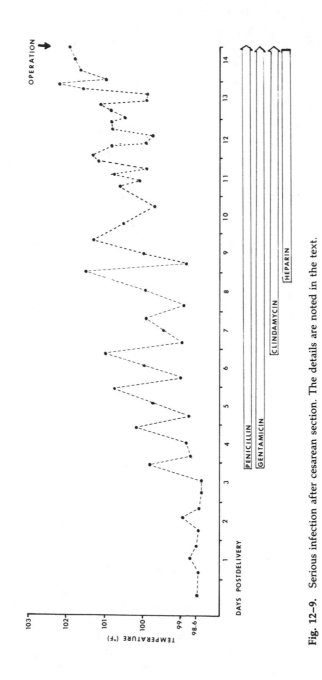

Fig. 12–9. Serious infection after cesarean section. The details are noted in the text.

but no pelvic mass was found. The tentative clinical diagnosis was septic pelvic thrombophlebitis. The patient was placed on intravenous heparin given by infusion pump, 1,000 U per hour, and the antibiotics were continued.

The temperatures eased, but the low-grade fever continued for the next three days, and then the spiking temperature recurred. Examination now suggested that there might be a mass posterior to the uterus and possibly some drainage from the abdominal incision. The patient was accordingly taken to the operating room and the abdominal incision opened. Although no superficial wound infection was found, purulent material was draining through the sutures in the fascia. When these were opened, it was obvious that the drainage was coming from the peritoneal cavity. Opening the peritoneum revealed a uterine incision that had broken down, and an infected uterus was discovered. On further exploration of the abdomen, a tubo-ovarian abscess on the right side was discovered as well as gross inflammation of the opposite adnexa.

A total abdominal hysterectomy and bilateral salpingo-oophorectomy were done. The postoperative course was uncomplicated. Culture of infected material recovered during surgery grew *Escherichia coli,* enterococci, *Peptostreptococcus,* and *Bacteroides fragilis.*

Heparin therapy had been discontinued when the abscess was discovered, but penicillin, clindamycin, and gentamicin were continued until the patient's discharge from the hospital, seven days after the surgery and 21 days after admission. She received oral clindamycin on an outpatient basis to complete 10 days of therapy without fever.

There is a common theme in both of these cases illustrated in Figures 12–8 and 12–9. Both women had a cesarean section performed during labor and both had initial antibiotic therapy that did not provide good coverage of the gram-negative anaerobic rods. When readmitted to the hospital they did not respond to antibiotics effective against gram-negative anaerobic rods, for they had well-established infections that required operative intervention even though the organism recovered from the site of infection were susceptible to antibiotics given preoperatively.

There are other uncommon causes of late infection that should be considered in the postpartum patient. Ovarian abscesses have been seen in women following cesarean section alone or with an associated ovarian biopsy as well as in women who have become febrile following a seemingly normal vaginal delivery.[79] The patients usually have a palpable adnexal mass, a low-grade fever, and do not appear to be acutely ill. The masses and fever usually persist despite antibiotics, and operative removal is needed for cure. Ovarian abscesses are unlike a tubo-ovarian abscess, for the tube is secondarily involved with a perisalpingitis and there is no evidence of an endosalpingitis. An even more uncommon cause of late postpartum morbidity—foreign material—is rarely seen. Figures 12–10 and 12–11 are radiographs of the abdomens of women with persistent postpartum fever. In Figure 12–10, the radiopaque material was recognized as intra-abdominal sponges, which were subsequently removed by elective laparotomy incision. In Figure 12–11, the gas-filled mass proved to be an abdominal pack left at the time of cesarean section three months earlier. In both of these examples, *Clostridium perfringens* was isolated from the retained sponges, and the patients were never seriously ill. The removal of the foreign material resulted in rapid recovery. The abdominal x-ray examinations were important in making the diagnosis.

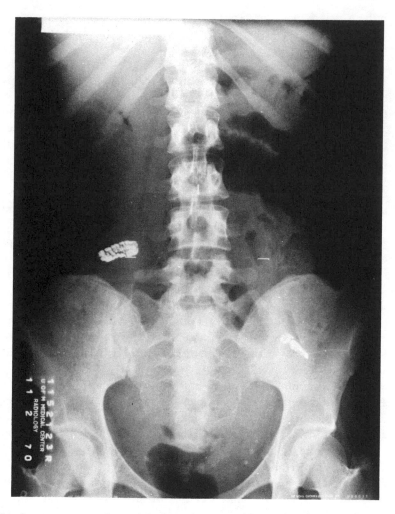

Fig. 12–10. A roentenogram obtained for wound crepitus. Two radiopaque sponges are seen. The sponge count was normal during the operation.

There are other causes of late-developing signs of infection that require hospital readmission for the postpartum patient. If the patient has a history of a sulcus or cervical laceration that required extensive suturing at the time of delivery, or if there was difficulty in achieving hemostasis at the time of cesarean section because of extension into the uterine vessels, an intravenous pyelogram should be ordered. Late onset of fever can be caused by liver toxicity from general anesthesia or be the first sign of hepatitis. Liver function tests should be ordered in these women. Another possible cause of late onset fever is cytomegalovirus infection from blood transfusion received during the initial hospitalization. Blood should be drawn to see if there is an acute phase rise in antibody titer.

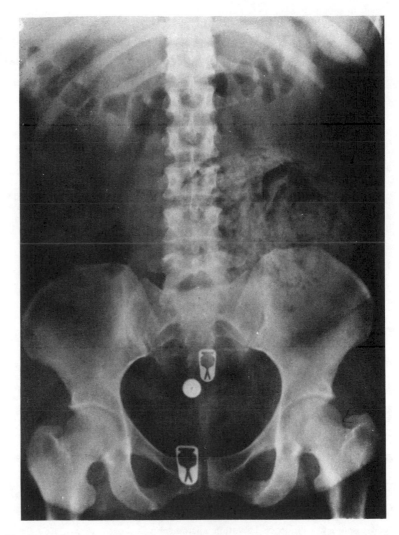

Fig. 12–11. The diffuse gas–filled abdominal mass that on laparotomy was found to be a sponge with no radiopaque marks. *Clostridium perfringens* was recovered from the sponge.

REFERENCES

1. Centers for Disease Control: Abortion surveillance 1979–1980. Atlanta, Ga., May, 1983.
2. Gustavi, B.: First trimester chromosomal analysis of chorionic villi obtained by direct vision technique. Lancet, *2*:507, 1983.
3. Bottoms, S.F., Rosen, M.G., and Sokol, R.J.: The increase in the cesarean birth rate. N. Engl. J. Med., *302*:559, 1980.
4. Binkin, N.J., Schulz, K.F., Grimes, D.A., and Cates, W., Jr.: Urea prostaglandin versus hypertonic saline for instillation abortion. Am. J. Obstet. Gynecol., *146*:947, 1983.
5. Grimes, D.A., Schulz, K.F., Cates, W., Jr., and Tyler, C.W., Jr.: Midtrimester abortion by intra-amniotic prostaglandin $F_{2\alpha}$: Safer than saline? Obstet. Gynecol., *49*:612, 1977.
6. Grimes, D.A., Schulz, K.F., Cates, W., Jr., and Tyler, C.W., Jr.: Midtrimester abortion by dilatation and evacuation: A safe and practical alternative. N. Engl. J. Med., *296*:1141, 1977.
7. Minkoff, H.L., and Schwarz, R.H.: The rising cesarean section rate: Can it safely be reversed? Obstet. Gynecol., *56*:135, 1980.

8. Ledger, W.J., Norman, M., Gee, C., and Lewis, W.: Bacteremia on an obstetric-gynecologic service. Am. J. Obstet. Gynecol., *121*:205, 1975.
9. Ledger, W.J., Kriewall, T.H., and Gee, C.: The fever index: A technique for evaluating the clinical response to bacteremia. Obstet. Gynecol., *45*:603, 1975.
10. Capeless, E.L., and Mann, L.I.: Management of the breech presentation. Mediguide to Ob/Gyn, *3*:Issue 2, 1984.
11. Kubli, F.: Personal communication, 1979.
12. Sweet, R.L., and Ledger, W.J.: Puerperal infectious morbidity: A two year review. Am. J. Obstet. Gynecol., *117*:1093, 1973.
13. Blanco, J.D., Gibbs, R.S., and Castaneda, Y.S.: Bacteremia in obstetrics: Clinical course. Obstet. Gynecol., *58*:621, 1981.
14. Goplerud, C.P., Ohm, M.J., and Galask, R.P.: Aerobic and anaerobic flora of the cervix during pregnancy and the puerperium. Am. J. Obstet. Gynecol., *126*:858, 1976.
15. Sabbagha, R.E., and Hayashi, T.T.: Disseminated intravascular coagulation complicating hysterotomy in elderly gravidas. Obstet. Gynecol., *38*:844, 1971.
16. Stevenson, C.S., Behney, C.A., and Miller, N.F.: Maternal death from puerperal sepsis following cesarean section: A 16 year study in Michigan. Obstet. Gynecol., *29*:181, 1967.
17. Gibbs, R.S., and Weinstein, A.J.: Puerperal infection in the antibiotic era. Am. J. Obstet. Gynecol., *124*:769, 1976.
18. Hagen, D.: Maternal febrile morbidity associated with fetal monitoring and cesarean section. Obstet. Gynecol., *46*:260, 1975.
19. D'Angelo, L.J., and Sokol, R.J.: Time related peripartum determinants of postpartum morbidity. Obstet. Gynecol., *55*:319, 1980.
20. Green, S.L., and Sarubbi, F.A., Jr.: Risk factors associated with post cesarean section febrile morbidity. Obstet. Gynecol., *49*:686, 1977.
21. Gibbs, R.S., Jones, P.M., and Wilder, C.J.Y.: Internal fetal monitoring and maternal infection following cesarean section. Obstet. Gynecol., *52*:193, 1978.
22. Rehu, M., and Nilsson, C.G.: Risk factors for febrile morbidity associated with cesarean section. Obstet. Gynecol., *56*:269, 1980.
23. Nielsen, T.F., and Hokeqard, K.H.: Postoperative cesarean section morbidity: A prospective study. Am. J. Obstet. Gynecol., *146*:911, 1983.
24. Gibbs, R.S., Listwa, H.M., and Read, J.A.: The effect of internal fetal monitoring on maternal infection following cesarean section. Obstet. Gynecol., *48*:653, 1976.
25. Cunningham, F.G., Hauth, J.C., Strong, J.D., and Kappus, S.S.: Infectious morbidity following cesarean section. Obstet. Gynecol., *52*:656, 1978.
26. Perloe, M., and Curet, L.B.: The effect of internal fetal monitoring on cesarean section morbidity. Obstet. Gynecol., *53*:354, 1979.
27. Anstey, J.T., Sheldon, G.W., and Blythe, J.G.: Infectious morbidity after primary cesarean sections in a private institution. Am. J. Obstet. Gynecol., *136*:205, 1980.
28. Iffy, L., Kaminetzky, H.A., Maidman, J.E., Lindsey, J., and Arrata, W.S.M.: Control of perinatal infection in traditional preventive measures. Obstet. Gynecol., *54*:403, 1979.
29. Fara, F.J., Steward, M., Jr. and Standard, J.: Use of unlimited nonsterile vaginal examinations in the conduct of labor. Am. J. Obstet. Gynecol., *72*:1, 1956.
30. Gosselin, O.: Etude de l'invasion microbienne de l'oeuf au cours de travail pour la ponction abdominale du liquide amniotique. Med., *17*:1600, 1937.
31. Lewis, J.F., Johnson, P., and Miller, P.: Evaluation of amniotic fluid for aerobic and anaerobic bacteria. Am. J. Clin. Pathol., *65*:58, 1976.
32. Miller, J.M., Jr., Pupkin, M.J., and Hill, G.B.: Bacterial colonization of amniotic fluid from intact fetal membranes. Am. J. Obstet. Gynecol., *136*:796, 1980.
33. DiZerega, G., Yonekura, L., Roy, S., Nakamura, R.M, and Ledger, W.J.: A comparison of clindamycin-gentamicin and penicillin-gentamicin in the treatment of post-cesarean section endomyometritis. Am. J. Obstet. Gynecol., *134*:238, 1979.
34. Larsen, J.W., Goldkrand, J.W., Hanson, T.M., and Miller, C.R.: Intrauterine infection on an obstetric service. Obstet. Gynecol., *43*:838, 1974.
35. Gassner, C.B., and Ledger, W.J.: The relationship of hospital acquired maternal infection to invasive intrapartum monitoring techniques. Am. J. Obstet. Gynecol., *126*:33, 1976.
36. Blanchette, H.: Elective manual exploration of the uterus after delivery. J. Reprod. Med., *19*:13, 1977.
37. Hibbard, L.T., Snyder, E.N., and McVann, R.M.: Subgluteal and retropsoal infection in obstetric practice. Obstet. Gynecol., *39*:137, 1972.
38. Zlatnick, F.J., and Scott, J.R.: Infection following classical cesarean section: An indication for early hysterectomy. J. Iowa Med. Soc., *69*:52, 1979.
39. Blanco, J.P., and Gibbs, R.S.: Infections following classical cesarean section. Obstet. Gynecol., *55*:167, 1980.

40. Kreutner, A.K., DelBene, V.E., Delamar, D., Bodden, J.L., and Loadholt, C.B.: Perioperative cephalosporin prophylaxis in cesarean section: Effect on endometritis in the high risk patient. Am. J. Obstet. Gynecol., *134*:925, 1979.
41. Lapides, J.: Pathophysiology of urinary tract infections. J. Univ. Michigan Med. Center, *39*:103, 1973.
42. Ledger, W.J., Reite, A.M., and Headington, J.T.: A system for infectious disease surveillance on an obstetric service. Obstet. Gynecol., *37*:769, 1971.
43. Lee, J.H., Jr.: Management of post-partum urinary retention. Obstet. Gynecol., 17:464, 1961.
44. Greenhouse, B.S., Hook, R., and Hehre, F.W.: Aspiration pneumonia following intravenous administration of alcohol during labor. J.A.M.A., *210*:2393, 1969.
45. Taylor, G., and Pryse-Davies, J.: The prophylactic use of antacids in the prevention of the acid pulmonary aspiration syndrome. Lancet, *1*:288, 1966.
46. MacDonald, D., O'Driscoll, M.K., and Geoghegan, F.J.: Intra-amniotic dextrose—a maternal death. J. Obstet. Gynaecol. Br. Commonw., *72*:452, 1965.
47. Goodlin, R.C.: Complications of amnioinfusion with hypertonic saline for mid-trimester abortion. Am. J. Obstet. Gynecol., *110*:885, 1971.
48. Phelan, J.P., Mequiar, T.C., Matey, D., and Newman, C.: Dramatic pyrexic and cardiovascular response to intravaginal prostaglandin E_2. Am. J. Obstet. Gynecol., *132*:28, 1978.
49. Goodlin, R.C., and Chapin, J.W.: Determinants of maternal temperature during labor. Am. J. Obstet. Gynecol., *143*:97, 1982.
50. Tandberg, D., and Sklar, D.: Effect of tachypnea on the estimation of body temperature by an oral thermometer. N. Engl. J. Med., *308*:945, 1983.
51. Bobitt, J.R., and Ledger, W.J.: Amniotic fluid analysis: Its role in maternal and neonatal infection. Obstet. Gynecol., *51*:56, 1978.
52. Nelson, T.E., and Flewellen, E.H.: The malignant hyperthermia syndrome. N. Engl. J. Med., *309*:416, 1983.
53. Dudley, W.R., and Marshall, B.E.: Steroid treatment for acid-aspiration pneumonitis. Anesthesiology, *40*:136, 1974.
54. Bosomworth, P.P., and Hamelberg, W.: The etiologic and therapeutic aspects of aspiration pneumonitis: Experimental study. Surg. Forum, *13*:158, 1962.
55. Bartlett, J.G., Gorbach, S.L., and Finegold, S.M.: The bacteriology of aspiration pneumonia. Am. J. Med., *56*:202, 1974.
56. Bartlett, J.G., and Finegold, S.M.: Anaerobic pleuropulmonary infections. Medicine, *51*:413, 1972.
57. Ledger, W.J.: Anaerobic infections. *In* Communicable and Infectious Diseases. Edited by P.F. Wehrle and F.H. Top, Sr., 9th ed., C.V. Mosby, St. Louis, 1981.
58. Ledger, W.J., and Headington, J.T.: Group A beta-hemolytic *Streptococcus:* An important cause of serious infections in obstetrics and gynecology. Obstet. Gynecol., *39*:474, 1972.
59. Faro, S.: Group B beta-hemolytic streptococci and puerperal infections. Am. J. Obstet. Gynecol., *139*:686, 1981.
60. Mead, P.J., and Harris, R.E.: Incidence of Group B beta-hemolytic *Streptococcus* in antepartum urinary tract infections. Obstet. Gynecol., *51*:412, 1978.
61. Schultz, J.C., Adamson, J.S., Jr., Workman, W.W., and Norman, T.D.: Fatal liver disease after intravenous administration of tetracycline in high dosage. N. Engl. J. Med., *269*:999, 1963.
62. DiZerega, G.S., Yonekura, M.L., Keegan, K., Roy, S., Nakamura, R., and Ledger, W.J.: Bacteremia in post-cesarean section endomyometritis: Differential response to therapy. Obstet. Gynecol., *55*:587, 1980.
63. Sen, P., Apuzzio, J., Reyelt, C., Kaminski, T., Levy, F., Kapila, R., Middleton, J., and Louria, D.: Prospective evaluations of combinations of antimicrobial agents for endometritis after cesarean section. Surg. Gynecol. Obstet., *151*:89, 1980.
64. Zaske, D.E., Cipolle, R.J., Strate, R.G., Malo, J.W., and Koszalka, M.F., Jr.: Rapid gentamicin elimination in obstetric patients. Obstet. Gynecol., *56*:559, 1980.
65. Sweet, R.L., and Ledger, W.J.: Cefoxitin: Single agent treatment of mixed aerobic-anaerobic pelvic infections. Obstet. Gynecol., *54*:193, 1979.
66. Gibbs, R.S., Blanco, J.D., Castaneda, Y.S., and St. Clair, P.J.: A double blind, randomized comparison of clindamycin-gentamicin versus cefamandole for treatment of post-cesarean section endomyometritis. Am. J. Obstet. Gynecol., *144*:261, 1982.
67. Gibbs, R.S., Blanco, J.D., Duff, P., Castaneda, R.N. and St. Clair, P.J.: A double blind randomized comparison of moxalactam versus clindamycin-gentamicin in treatment of endomyometritis after cesarean section delivery. Am. J. Obstet. Gynecol., *146*:769, 1983.
68. Harding, G.K.M., Nicolle, L.E., Haase, D.A., Aoki, F.Y., Stiver, H.G., Blanchard, R.J., and Kirkpatrick, J.R.: Prospective randomized comparative trials in the therapy for intra-abdominal and female genital tract infection. Rev. Infect. Dis., *6*:S283, 1984.
69. Sweet, R.L., Robbie, M.O., Ohm-Smith, M., and Hadly, W.K.: Comparative study of piperacillin versus cefoxitin in the treatment of obstetric and gynecologic infections. Am. J. Obstet. Gynecol., *145*:342, 1983.

70. Sorrell, T.C., Marshall, J.R., Yoshimori, R., and Chow, A.W.: Antimicrobial therapy of postpartum endomyometritis. II. Prospective randomized trial of mezlocillin versus ampicillin. Am. J. Obstet. Gynecol., *141*:246, 1981.
71. Ledger, W.J., Gassner, C.B., and Gee, C.: Operative care of infections in obstetrics-gynecology. J. Reprod. Med., *13*:128, 1974.
72. Borkowf, H.I.: Bacterial gangrene associated with pelvic surgery. Clin. Obstet. Gynecol., *16*:(June) 40, 1973.
73. Golde, S., and Ledger, W.J.: Necrotizing fasciitis in post-partum patients: A report of four cases. Obstet. Gynecol., *50*:670, 1977.
74. Shy, K.K., and Eschenbach, D.A.: Fatal perineal cellulitis from an episiotomy site. Obstet. Gynecol., *54*:292, 1979.
75. Marshall, B.R., Hepper, J.K., and Zirbel, C.C.: Sporadic puerperal mastitis. J.A.M.A., *233*:1377, 1975.
76. Weinstein, W.M., Onderdonk, A.B., Bartlett, J.G., and Gorbach, S.L.: Experimental intra-abdominal abscesses in rats. Development of an experimental model. Infect. Immun., *10*:1250, 1974.
77. Wager, G.P., Martin, D.H., Koutsky, L., Eschenbach, D.A., Daling, J.R., Chiang, W.T., Alexander, E.R., and Holmes, K.K.: Puerperal infectious morbidity: Relationship to route of delivery and to antepartum *Chlamydia trachomatis* infection. Am. J. Obstet. Gynecol., *138*:1028, 1980.
78. Ledger, W.J.: Aftermath of a cesarean. Hosp. Prac., *13*:(Sept.) 41, 1978.
79. Ledger, W.J.: The surgical care of severe infection in obstetric and gynecologic patients. Surg. Gynecol. Obstet., *132*:753, 1973.

INDEX

Anaerobic bacteria (*continued*)
 specimen collection in pelvic infections, 47-49
  aspirate versus swab, 48
  length of time of exposure to oxygen, 48-49
  problems of surface contamination, 47-48
  transport medium in, 49
 susceptibility testing to antibiotics, 61-62
 in vaginal flora, 11
Anemia, aplastic, chloramphenicol causing, 122
Anesthesia
 pneumonia in postpartum period related to, 256
 urinary tract infection in postpartum period related to, 255-256
Antibiotics, 95-122
 in aspiration pneumonia, 260-261
 and bacterial flora, 11
 in *Bacteroides fragilis* infections, 111, 111t
 blood cultures of patients taking, 54
 bolus versus constant infusion, 95-96
 checklist for use, 10t
 colitis associated with, 27
 current recommendations in OB-GYN, 121-122
 disc susceptibility testing, 57-60, 59-60t
  clinical interpretation, 60
  substances interfering with activity, 58, 60t
  technique, 57-58
  zone size interpretation, 58, 59t
 efficacy studies, 88
 in endomyometritis in postpartum period, 266-268, 266t
 historical background, 6-7
 inappropriate usage in OB-GYN, 7
 in infertility therapy, 164
 interactions in intravenous solutions, 96
 intramuscular administration, 97, 99
 intraperitoneal lavage, 118
 intravenous therapy with, 96-97, 98t
 kidney clearance of, 101, 102f, 104
 laboratory testing of, 57-63
  agar dilution testing, 60
  anaerobe susceptibility tests, 61-62
  disc susceptibility tests, 57-60, 59-60t
  limitations of, 57
  serum level determinations, 62-63
  tube dilution tests, 60-61
 and maternal morbidity, 6
 oral administration, 99, 100t
 overuse before infection diagnosis, 85
 pharmacokinetics, 95-104. *See also* Pharmacokinetics
 in postoperative infections
  with fever onset later than 48 hours after operation, 183-188
  with fever onset within 48 hours after operation, 176-183
 in pregnancy, 112-113
  in first trimester, 112-113
  safety to fetus and newborn, 112, 200
  serum levels, 62
 in premature ruptured membranes, 224
 prophylactic use, 113-120
  avoiding agents with important antibacterial spectrum, 119-120
  with bacterial endocarditis risk, 120

 benefits outweighing risks, 120
 efficacy, 116, 175
  laboratory evidence against contaminating organisms, 115-116
 with endogenous bacterial contamination, 115
 in genitourinary tract surgery and instrumentation, 120t
 on-call dose problem, 117-118
 pharmacokinetic considerations, 117-118
 in pregnancy termination, 90
 in premature ruptured membranes, 224
 presence of agent in wound during operation, 117-118
 prolonged use masking postoperative infection, 178, 179f
 research studies on, 87-91
 short-term administration, 117f, 118-119
 significant risk for development of infection related to, 115
 timing of administration and response, 113-114, 114f
  first dose, 118
 trends in, 113
 protein binding
  and clearance by kidney, 101, 102f, 104
  and MIC, 99
 resistance to
  by anaerobes, 61-62
  transfer among different species, 20
 in salpingitis, 150, 150t
  CDC recommendations, 151-152, 152t
  influence on surgical management, 155-158
 serum levels, 62-63
  peak versus trough, 96
  in pregnancy, 62
  in soft tissue pelvic infections, 105-111
 studies in OB-GYN literature, 88-91
  analysis of results, 90
  case control method, 91
  comparability of study population, 89
  double-blind, 88
  method of enrolling patients, 88-89
  multicenter, 89-90
 substances interfering with activity in disc tests, 58, 60t
 susceptibility testing, 57-63. *See also* Antibiotics, laboratory testing of
  periodic reports, 87
  in surveillance, 86
 in urinary tract infections, 104-105. *See also* Urinary tract infection
  postoperative, 184
  in postpartum period, 265
  in pregnancy, 237-239
  pyelonephritis, 238-239
 usage defining existence of infection, 86
 volume of distribution, 96-97
 in wound infections, 186
Antipyretics, 77
Appendicitis, in pregnancy, 243
Arthritis, gonococcal, 160-161
 in pregnancy, 243
Aspiration pneumonia, in postpartum period, 260-261
Atelectasis, in postoperative period, 182

MEFOXIN®

(STERILE CEFOXITIN SODIUM, MSD)

DESCRIPTION

MEFOXIN* (Sterile Cefoxitin Sodium, MSD) is a semi-synthetic, broad-spectrum cepha antibiotic for parenteral administration. It is derived from cephamycin C, which is produced by *Streptomyces lactamdurans*. It is the sodium salt of 3-(hydroxymethyl)-7α-methoxy-8-oxo-7-[2-(2-thienyl)acetamido]-5-thia-1-azabicyclo [4.2.0] oct-2-ene-2-carboxylate carbamate (ester). The empirical formula is $C_{16}H_{16}N_3NaO_7S_2$, and the structural formula is:

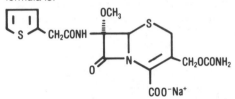

MEFOXIN contains approximately 53.8 mg (2.3 milliequivalents) of sodium per gram of cefoxitin activity. Solutions of MEFOXIN range from clear to light amber in color. The pH of freshly constituted solutions usually ranges from 4.2 to 7.0.

CLINICAL PHARMACOLOGY

Clinical Pharmacology

After intramuscular administration of a 1 gram dose of MEFOXIN to normal volunteers, the mean peak serum concentration was 24 mcg/mL. The peak occurred at 20 to 30 minutes. Following an intravenous dose of 1 gram, serum concentrations were 110 mcg/mL at 5 minutes, declining to less than 1 mcg/mL at 4 hours. The half-life after an intravenous dose is 41 to 59 minutes; after intramuscular administration, the half-life is 64.8 minutes. Approximately 85 percent of cefoxitin is excreted unchanged by the kidneys over a 6-hour period, resulting in high urinary concentrations. Following an intramuscular dose of 1 gram, urinary concentrations greater than 3000 mcg/mL were observed. Probenecid slows tubular excretion and produces higher serum levels and increases the duration of measurable serum concentrations.

Cefoxitin passes into pleural and joint fluids and is detectable in antibacterial concentrations in bile.

Clinical experience has demonstrated that MEFOXIN can be administered to patients who are also receiving carbenicillin, kanamycin, gentamicin, tobramycin, or amikacin (see PRECAUTIONS and ADMINISTRATION).

Microbiology

The bactericidal action of cefoxitin results from inhibition of cell wall synthesis. Cefoxitin has *in vitro* activity against a wide range of gram-positive and gram-negative organisms. The methoxy group in the 7α position provides MEFOXIN with a high degree of stability in the presence of beta-lactamases, both penicillinases and cephalosporinases, of gram-negative bacteria. Cefoxitin is usually active against the following organisms *in vitro* and in clinical infections:

Gram-positive

Staphylococcus aureus, including penicillinase and non-penicillinase producing strains

Staphylococcus epidermidis

Beta-hemolytic and other streptococci (most strains of enterococci, e.g., *Streptococcus faecalis,* are resistant)

Streptococcus pneumoniae (formerly *Diplococcus pneumoniae*)

Gram-negative

Escherichia coli

Klebsiella species (including *K. pneumoniae*)

Hemophilus influenzae

Neisseria gonorrhoeae, including penicillinase and non-penicillinase producing strains

Proteus mirabilis

Morganella morganii (formerly *Proteus morganii*)

Proteus vulgaris

Providencia species, including *Providencia rettgeri* (formerly *Proteus rettgeri*)

Anaerobic organisms

Peptococcus species

Peptostreptococcus species

Clostridium species

Bacteroides species, including the *B. fragilis* group (includes *B. fragilis, B. distasonis, B. ovatus, B. thetaiotaomicron, B. vulgatus*)

MEFOXIN is inactive *in vitro* against most strains of *Pseudomonas aeruginosa* and enterococci and many strains of *Enterobacter cloacae.*

Methicillin-resistant staphylococci are almost uniformly resistant to MEFOXIN.

Susceptibility Tests

For fast-growing aerobic organisms, quantitative methods that require measurements of zone diameters give the most precise estimates of antibiotic susceptibility. One such procedure* has been recommended for use with discs to test susceptibility to cefoxitin. Interpretation involves correlation of the diameters obtained in the disc test with minimal inhibitory concentration (MIC) values for cefoxitin.

Reports from the laboratory giving results of the standardized single disc susceptibility test* using a 30 mcg cefoxitin disc should be interpreted according to the following criteria:

Organisms producing zones of 18 mm or greater are considered susceptible, indicating that the tested organism is likely to respond to therapy.

Organisms of intermediate susceptibility produce zones of 15 to 17 mm, indicating that the tested organism would be susceptible if high dosage is used or if the infection is confined to tissues and fluids (e.g., urine) in which high antibiotic levels are attained.

Resistant organisms produce zones of 14 mm or less, indicating that other therapy should be selected.

The cefoxitin disc should be used for testing cefoxitin susceptibility.

Cefoxitin has been shown by in vitro tests to have activity against certain strains of Enterobacteriaceae found resistant when tested with the cephalosporin class disc. For this reason, the cefoxitin disc should not be used for testing susceptibility to cephalosporins, and cephalosporin discs should not be used for testing susceptibility to cefoxitin.

Dilution methods, preferably the agar plate dilution procedure, are most accurate for susceptibility testing of obligate anaerobes.

A bacterial isolate may be considered susceptible if the MIC value for cefoxitin** is not more than 16 mcg/mL. Organisms are considered resistant if the MIC is greater than 32 mcg/mL.

INDICATIONS AND USAGE

Treatment

MEFOXIN is indicated for the treatment of se-

---

*Bauer, A. W.; Kirby, W.M.M.; Sherris, J.C.; Turck, M.: Antibiotic susceptibility testing by a standardized single disc method, Amer. J. Clin. Path. 45:493-496, Apr. 1966. Standardized disc susceptibility test, Federal Register 37:20527-20529, 1972. National Committee for Clinical Laboratory Standards: Approved Standard: ASM-2, Performance Standards for Antimicrobial Disc Susceptibility Tests, July 1975.

**Determined by the ICS agar dilution method (Ericsson and Sherris, Acta Path. Microbiol. Scand. [B] Suppl. No. 217, 1971) or any other method that has been shown to give equivalent results.

rious infections caused by susceptible strains of the designated microorganisms in the diseases listed below.

(1) **Lower respiratory tract infections,** including pneumonia and lung abscess, caused by Streptococcus pneumoniae (formerly Diplococcus pneumoniae), other streptococci (excluding enterococci, e.g., Streptococcus faecalis), Staphylococcus aureus (penicillinase and non-penicillinase producing), Escherichia coli, Klebsiella species, Hemophilus influenzae, and Bacteroides species.

(2) **Genitourinary infections.** Urinary tract infections caused by Escherichia coli, Klebsiella species, Proteus mirabilis, indole-positive Proteus (i.e., Proteus morganii, rettgeri, and vulgaris), and Providencia species. Uncomplicated gonorrhea due to Neisseria gonorrhoeae (penicillinase and non-penicillinase producing).

(3) **Intra-abdominal infections,** including peritonitis and intra-abdominal abscess, caused by Escherichia coli, Klebsiella species, Bacteroides species including the Bacteroides fragilis group*, and Clostridium species.

(4) **Gynecological infections,** including endometritis, pelvic cellulitis, and pelvic inflammatory disease caused by Escherichia coli, Neisseria gonorrhoeae (penicillinase and non-penicillinase producing), Bacteroides species including the Bacteroides fragilis group*, Clostridium species, Peptococcus species, Peptostreptococcus species, and Group B streptococci.

(5) **Septicemia** caused by Streptococcus pneumoniae (formerly Diplococcus pneumoniae), Staphylococcus aureus (penicillinase and non-penicillinase producing), Escherichia coli, Klebsiella species, and Bacteroides species including the Bacteroides fragilis group.*

(6) **Bone and joint infections** caused by Staphylococcus aureus (penicillinase and non-penicillinase producing).

(7) **Skin and skin structure infections** caused by Staphylococcus aureus (penicillinase and non-penicillinase producing), Staphylococcus epidermidis, streptococci (excluding enterococci, e.g., Streptococcus faecalis), Escherichia coli, Proteus mirabilis, Klebsiella species, Bacteroides species including the Bacteroides fragilis group*, Clostridium species, Peptococcus species, and Peptostreptococcus species.

---

*B. fragilis, B. distasonis, B. ovatus, B. thetaiotaomicron, B. vulgatus.

Appropriate culture and susceptibility studies should be performed to determine the susceptibility of the causative organisms to MEFOXIN. Therapy may be started while awaiting the results of these studies.

In randomized comparative studies, MEFOXIN and cephalothin were comparably safe and effective in the management of infections caused by gram-positive cocci and gram-negative rods susceptible to the cephalosporins. MEFOXIN has a high degree of stability in the presence of bacterial beta-lactamases, both penicillinases and cephalosporinases.

Many infections caused by aerobic and anaerobic gram-negative bacteria resistant to some cephalosporins respond to MEFOXIN. Similarly, many infections caused by aerobic and anaerobic bacteria resistant to some penicillin antibiotics (ampicillin, carbenicillin, penicillin G) respond to treatment with MEFOXIN. Many infections caused by mixtures of susceptible aerobic and anaerobic bacteria respond to treatment with MEFOXIN.

Prevention

When compared to placebo in randomized controlled studies in patients undergoing gastrointestinal surgery, vaginal hysterectomy, abdominal hysterectomy and cesarean section, the prophylactic use of MEFOXIN resulted in a significant reduction in the number of postoperative infections.

The prophylactic administration of MEFOXIN perioperatively (preoperatively, intraoperatively, and postoperatively) may reduce the incidence of certain postoperative infections in patients undergoing surgical procedures (e.g., hysterectomy, gastrointestinal surgery and transurethral prostatectomy) that are classified as contaminated or potentially contaminated.

The perioperative use of MEFOXIN may be effective in surgical patients in whom infection at the operative site would present a serious risk, e.g., prosthetic arthroplasty.

In patients undergoing cesarean section, intraoperative (after clamping the umbilical cord) and postoperative use of MEFOXIN may reduce the incidence of certain postoperative infections.

Effective prophylactic use depends on the time of administration. MEFOXIN usually should be given one-half to one hour before the operation, which is sufficient time to achieve effective levels in the wound during the procedure. Prophylactic administration should usually be stopped within 24 hours since continuing administration of any antibiotic increases the possibility of adverse reactions but, in the majority of surgical procedures, does not reduce the incidence of subsequent infection. However, in patients undergoing prosthetic arthroplasty, it is recommended that MEFOXIN be continued for 72 hours after the surgical procedure.

If there are signs of infection, specimens for culture should be obtained for identification of the causative organism so that appropriate therapy may be instituted.

CONTRAINDICATIONS

MEFOXIN is contraindicated in patients who have shown hypersensitivity to cefoxitin and the cephalosporin group of antibiotics.

WARNINGS

BEFORE THERAPY WITH MEFOXIN IS INSTITUTED, CAREFUL INQUIRY SHOULD BE MADE TO DETERMINE WHETHER THE PATIENT HAS HAD PREVIOUS HYPERSENSITIVITY REACTIONS TO CEFOXITIN, CEPHALOSPORINS, PENICILLINS, OR OTHER DRUGS. THIS PRODUCT SHOULD BE GIVEN WITH CAUTION TO PENICILLIN-SENSITIVE PATIENTS. ANTIBIOTICS SHOULD BE ADMINISTERED WITH CAUTION TO ANY PATIENT WHO HAS DEMONSTRATED SOME FORM OF ALLERGY, PARTICULARLY TO DRUGS. IF AN ALLERGIC REACTION TO MEFOXIN OCCURS, DISCONTINUE THE DRUG. SERIOUS HYPERSENSITIVITY REACTIONS MAY REQUIRE EPINEPHRINE AND OTHER EMERGENCY MEASURES.

Pseudomembranous colitis has been reported with virtually all antibiotics (including cephalosporins); therefore, it is important to consider its diagnosis in patients who develop diarrhea in association with antibiotic use. This colitis may range from mild to life threatening in severity.

Treatment with broad-spectrum antibiotics alters normal flora of the colon and may permit overgrowth of clostridia. Studies indicate a toxin produced by *Clostridium difficile* is one primary cause of antibiotic-associated colitis.

Mild cases of pseudomembranous colitis may respond to drug discontinuance alone. In more severe cases, management may include sigmoidoscopy, appropriate bacteriological studies, fluid, electrolyte and protein supplementation, and the use of a drug such as oral vancomycin as indicated. Isolation of the patient may be advisable. Other causes of colitis should also be considered.

PRECAUTIONS

General

The total daily dose should be reduced when MEFOXIN is administered to patients with transient or persistent reduction of urinary output due to renal insufficiency (see DOSAGE), because high and prolonged serum antibiotic concentrations can occur in such individuals from usual doses.

Antibiotics (including cephalosporins) should be prescribed with caution in individuals with a history of gastrointestinal disease, particularly colitis.

As with other antibiotics, prolonged use of MEFOXIN may result in overgrowth of nonsusceptible organisms. Repeated evaluation of the patient's condition is essential. If superinfection occurs during therapy, appropriate measures should be taken.

Drug Interactions

Increased nephrotoxicity has been reported following concomitant administration of cephalosporins and aminoglycoside antibiotics.

Drug/Laboratory Test Interactions

As with cephalothin, high concentrations of cefoxitin (>100 micrograms/mL) may interfere with measurement of serum and urine creatinine levels by the Jaffé reaction, and produce false increases of modest degree in the levels of creatinine reported. Serum samples from patients treated with cefoxitin should not be analyzed for creatinine if withdrawn within 2 hours of drug administration.

High concentrations of cefoxitin in the urine may interfere with measurement of urinary 17-hydroxy-corticosteroids by the Porter-Silber reaction, and produce false increases of modest degree in the levels reported.

A false-positive reaction for glucose in the urine may occur. This has been observed with CLINITEST* reagent tablets.

Carcinogenesis, Mutagenesis, Impairment of Fertility

Long-term studies in animals have not been performed with cefoxitin to evaluate carcinogenic or mutagenic potential. Studies in rats treated intravenously with 400 mg/kg of cefoxitin (approximately three times the maximum recommended human dose) revealed no effects on fertility or mating ability.

Pregnancy

Pregnancy Category B. Reproduction studies performed in rats and mice at parenteral doses

*Registered trademark of Ames Company, Division of Miles Laboratories, Inc.

of approximately one to seven and one-half times the maximum recommended human dose did not reveal teratogenic or fetal toxic effects, although a slight decrease in fetal weight was observed.

There are, however, no adequate and well-controlled studies in pregnant women. Because animal reproduction studies are not always predictive of human response, this drug should be used during pregnancy only if clearly needed.

In the rabbit, cefoxitin was associated with a high incidence of abortion and maternal death. This was not considered to be a teratogenic effect but an expected consequence of the rabbit's unusual sensitivity to antibiotic-induced changes in the population of the microflora of the intestine.

Nursing Mothers

MEFOXIN is excreted in human milk in low concentrations. Caution should be exercised when MEFOXIN is administered to a nursing woman.

Pediatric Use

Safety and efficacy in infants from birth to three months of age have not yet been established. In children three months of age and older, higher doses of MEFOXIN have been associated with an increased incidence of eosinophilia and elevated SGOT.

ADVERSE REACTIONS

MEFOXIN is generally well tolerated. The most common adverse reactions have been local reactions following intravenous or intramuscular injection. Other adverse reactions have been encountered infrequently.

Local Reactions

Thrombophlebitis has occurred with intravenous administration. Pain, induration, and tenderness after intramuscular injections have been reported.

Allergic Reactions

Rash (including exfoliative dermatitis), pruritus, eosinophilia, fever, and other allergic reactions including anaphylaxis have been noted.

Cardiovascular

Hypotension

Gastrointestinal

Diarrhea, including documented pseudomembranous colitis which can appear during or after antibiotic treatment. Nausea and vomiting have been reported rarely.

Blood

Eosinophilia, leukopenia, including granulocytopenia, neutropenia, anemia, including hemolytic anemia, thrombocytopenia, and bone marrow depression. A positive direct Coombs test may develop in some individuals, especially those with azotemia.

Liver Function

Transient elevations in SGOT, SGPT, serum LDH, and serum alkaline phosphatase have been reported.

Renal Function

Elevations in serum creatinine and/or blood urea nitrogen levels have been observed. As with the cephalosporins, acute renal failure has been reported rarely. The role of MEFOXIN in changes in renal function tests is difficult to assess, since factors predisposing to prerenal azotemia or to impaired renal function usually have been present.

OVERDOSAGE

The acute intravenous LD_{50} in the adult female mouse and rabbit was about 8.0 g/kg and greater than 1.0 g/kg respectively. The acute intraperitoneal LD_{50} in the adult rat was greater than 10.0 g/kg.

DOSAGE

TREATMENT

Adults

The usual adult dosage range is 1 gram to 2 grams every six to eight hours. Dosage and route of administration should be determined by susceptibility of the causative organisms, severity of infection, and the condition of the patient (see Table 1 for dosage guidelines).

Table 1—Guidelines for Dosage of MEFOXIN		
Type of Infection	Daily Dosage	Frequency and Route
Uncomplicated forms* of infections such as pneumonia, urinary tract infection, cutaneous infection	3-4 grams	1 gram every 6-8 hours IV or IM
Moderately severe or severe infections	6-8 grams	1 gram every 4 hours *or* 2 grams every 6-8 hours IV
Infections commonly needing antibiotics in higher dosage (e.g., gas gangrene)	12 grams	2 grams every 4 hours *or* 3 grams every 6 hours IV
*Including patients in whom bacteremia is absent or unlikely.		

In adults with renal insufficiency, an initial loading dose of 1 gram to 2 grams may be given. After a loading dose, the recommendations for *maintenance dosage* (Table 2) may be used as a guide.

When only the serum creatinine level is available, the following formula (based on sex, weight, and age of the patient) may be used to convert this value into creatinine clearance. The serum creatinine should represent a steady state of renal function.

$$\text{Males:} \quad \frac{\text{Weight (kg)} \times (140 - \text{age})}{72 \times \text{serum creatinine (mg/100 mL)}}$$

Females: $0.85 \times$ above value

MEFOXIN may be used in patients with reduced renal function with the following dosage adjustments:

Table 2—Maintenance Dosage of MEFOXIN in Adults with Reduced Renal Function			
Renal Function	Creatinine Clearance (mL/min)	Dose (grams)	Frequency
Mild impairment	50-30	1-2	every 8-12 hours
Moderate impairment	29-10	1-2	every 12-24 hours
Severe impairment	9-5	0.5-1	every 12-24 hours
Essentially no function	<5	0.5-1	every 24-48 hours

In patients undergoing hemodialysis, the loading dose of 1 to 2 grams should be given after each hemodialysis, and the maintenance dose should be given as indicated in Table 2.

Antibiotic therapy for group A beta-hemolytic streptococcal infections should be maintained for at least 10 days to guard against the risk of rheumatic fever or glomerulonephritis. In staphylococcal and other infections involving a collection of pus, surgical drainage should be carried out where indicated.

The recommended dosage of MEFOXIN **for uncomplicated gonorrhea** is 2 grams intramuscularly, with 1 gram of BENEMID* (Probenecid, MSD) given by mouth at the same time or up to ½ hour before MEFOXIN.

Infants and Children

The recommended dosage in children three months of age and older is 80 to 160 mg/kg of body weight per day divided into four to six equal doses. The higher dosages should be used for more severe or serious infections. The total daily dosage should not exceed 12 grams.

At this time no recommendation is made for children from birth to three months of age (See PRECAUTIONS).

In children with renal insufficiency the dosage and frequency of dosage should be modified consistent with the recommendations for adults (see Table 2).

*Registered trademark of MERCK & CO., INC.

MEFOXIN®
(Sterile Cefoxitin Sodium, MSD)

PREVENTION

For prophylactic use, the following doses are recommended:

Adults:

(1) 2 grams administered intravenously or intramuscularly just prior to surgery (approximately one-half to one hour before the initial incision).

(2) 2 grams every 6 hours after the first dose for no more than 24 hours (continued for 72 hours after prosthetic arthroplasty).

Children (3 months and older):

30 to 40 mg/kg doses may be given at the times designated above.

Cesarean section patients:

The first dose of 2.0 grams is administered intravenously as soon as the umbilical cord is clamped. The second and third doses should be given as 2.0 grams intravenously or intramuscularly 4 hours and 8 hours after the first dose. Subsequent doses may be given every 6 hours for no more than 24 hours.

Transurethral prostatectomy patients:

One gram administered just prior to surgery; 1 gram every 8 hours for up to five days.

PREPARATION OF SOLUTION

Table 3 is provided for convenience in constituting MEFOXIN for both intravenous and intramuscular administration.

For intravenous use, 1 gram should be constituted with at least 10 mL of Sterile Water for

Table 3—Preparation of Solution			
Strength	Amount of Diluent to be Added (mL)*	Approximate Withdrawable Volume (mL)	Approximate Average Concentration (mg/mL)
1 gram Vial	2 (Intramuscular)	2.5	400
2 gram Vial	4 (Intramuscular)	5	400
1 gram Vial	10 (IV)	10.5	95
2 gram Vial	10 or 20 (IV)	11.1 or 21.0	180 or 95
1 gram Infusion Bottle	50 or 100 (IV)	50 or 100	20 or 10
2 gram Infusion Bottle	50 or 100 (IV)	50 or 100	40 or 20
10 gram Bulk	50 or 100 (IV)	55 or 105	180 or 95
*Shake to dissolve and let stand until clear.			

Injection, and 2 grams, with 10 or 20 mL. The 10 gram bulk package should be constituted with 50 or 100 mL of Sterile Water for Injection or any of the solutions listed under the *Intravenous* portion of the COMPATIBILITY AND STABILITY section. CAUTION: NOT FOR DIRECT INFUSION. One or 2 grams of MEFOXIN for infusion may be constituted with 50 or 100 mL of 0.9 percent Sodium Chloride Injection, 5 percent or 10 percent Dextrose Injection, or any of the solutions listed under the *Intravenous* portion of the COMPATIBILITY AND STABILITY section.

Benzyl alcohol as a preservative has been associated with toxicity in neonates. While toxicity has not been demonstrated in infants greater than three months of age, in whom use of MEFOXIN may be indicated, small infants in this age range may also be at risk for benzyl alcohol toxicity. Therefore, diluent containing benzyl alcohol should not be used when MEFOXIN is constituted for administration to infants.

For intramuscular use, each gram of MEFOXIN may be constituted with 2 mL of Sterile Water for Injection, *or*—

For intramuscular use ONLY: each gram of MEFOXIN may be constituted with 2 mL of 0.5 percent lidocaine hydrochloride solution* (without epinephrine) to minimize the discomfort of intramuscular injection.

ADMINISTRATION

MEFOXIN may be administered intravenously or intramuscularly after constitution.

Parenteral drug products should be inspected visually for particulate matter and discoloration prior to administration whenever solution and container permit.

Intravenous Administration

The intravenous route is preferable for patients with bacteremia, bacterial septicemia, or other severe or life-threatening infections, or for patients who may be poor risks because of lowered resistance resulting from such debilitating conditions as malnutrition, trauma, surgery, diabetes, heart failure, or malignancy, particularly if shock is present or impending.

For intermittent intravenous administration, a solution containing 1 gram or 2 grams in 10 mL of Sterile Water for Injection can be injected over a period of three to five minutes. Using an infusion system, it may also be given over a longer period of time through the tubing system by which the patient may be receiving other intra-

*See package circular of manufacturer for detailed information concerning contraindications, warnings, precautions, and adverse reactions.

MEFOXIN®
(Sterile Cefoxitin Sodium, MSD)

venous solutions. However, during infusion of the solution containing MEFOXIN, it is advisable to temporarily discontinue administration of any other solutions at the same site.

For the administration of higher doses by continuous intravenous infusion, a solution of MEFOXIN may be added to an intravenous bottle containing 5 percent Dextrose Injection, 0.9 percent Sodium Chloride Injection, 5 percent Dextrose and 0.9 percent Sodium Chloride Injection, or 5 percent Dextrose Injection with 0.02 percent sodium bicarbonate solution. BUTTERFLY* or scalp vein-type needles are preferred for this type of infusion.

Solutions of MEFOXIN, like those of most beta-lactam antibiotics, should not be added to aminoglycoside solutions (e.g., gentamicin sulfate, tobramycin sulfate, amikacin sulfate) because of potential interaction. However, MEFOXIN and aminoglycosides may be administered separately to the same patient.

Intramuscular Administration

As with all intramuscular preparations, MEFOXIN should be injected well within the body of a relatively large muscle such as the upper outer quadrant of the buttock (i.e., gluteus maximus); aspiration is necessary to avoid inadvertent injection into a blood vessel.

COMPATIBILITY AND STABILITY

Intravenous

MEFOXIN, as supplied in vials or the bulk package and constituted to 1 gram/10 mL with Sterile Water for Injection, Bacteriostatic Water for Injection, (see PREPARATION OF SOLUTION), 0.9 percent Sodium Chloride Injection, or 5 percent Dextrose Injection, maintains satisfactory potency for 24 hours at room temperature, for one week under refrigeration (below 5°C), and for at least 30 weeks in the frozen state.

These primary solutions may be futher diluted in 50 to 1000 mL of the following solutions and maintain potency for 24 hours at room temperature and at least 48 hours under refrigeration:

Sterile Water for Injection†
0.9 percent Sodium Chloride Injection
5 percent or 10 percent Dextrose Injection†
5 percent Dextrose and 0.9 percent Sodium Chloride Injection
5 percent Dextrose Injection with 0.02 percent sodium bicarbonate solution

*Registered trademark of Abbott Laboratories.
†In these solutions, MEFOXIN has been found to be stable for a period of one week under refrigeration.

MEFOXIN®
(Sterile Cefoxitin Sodium, MSD)

5 percent Dextrose Injection with 0.2 percent or 0.45 percent saline solution
Ringer's Injection
Lactated Ringer's Injection†
5 percent Dextrose in Lactated Ringer's Injection†
5 percent or 10 percent invert sugar in water
10 percent invert sugar in saline solution
5 percent Sodium Bicarbonate Injection
Neut (sodium bicarbonate)*†
M/6 sodium lactate solution
AMINOSOL* 5 percent Solution
NORMOSOL-M in D5-W*†
IONOSOL B w/Dextrose 5 percent*†
POLYONIC M 56 in 5 percent Dextrose**
Mannitol 5% and 2.5%
Mannitol 10%†
ISOLYTE*** E
ISOLYTE*** E with 5% Dextrose

MEFOXIN, as supplied in infusion bottles and constituted with 50 to 100 mL of 0.9 percent Sodium Chloride Injection, or 5 percent or 10 percent Dextrose Injection, maintains satisfactory potency for 24 hours at room temperature or for 1 week under refrigeration (below 5°C).

Limited studies with solutions of MEFOXIN in 0.9 percent Sodium Chloride Injection, Lactated Ringer's Injection, and 5 percent Dextrose Injection in VIAFLEX**** intravenous bags show stability for 24 hours at room temperature, 48 hours under refrigeration, 26 weeks in the frozen state, and 24 hours at room temperature thereafter. Also, solutions of MEFOXIN in 0.9 percent Sodium Chloride Injection show similar stability in plastic tubing, drip chambers, and volume control devices of common intravenous infusion sets.

After constitution with Sterile Water for Injection and subsequent storage in disposable plastic syringes, MEFOXIN is stable for 24 hours at room temperature and 48 hours under refrigeration.

After the periods mentioned above, any unused solutions or frozen material should be discarded. Do not refreeze.

Intramuscular

MEFOXIN, as constituted with Sterile Water for Injection, Bacteriostatic Water for Injection, or 0.5 percent or 1 percent lidocaine hydro-

*Registered trademark of Abbott Laboratories.
**Registered trademark of Cutter Laboratories, Inc.
***Registered trademark of American Hospital Supply Corporation.
****Registered trademark of Travenol Laboratories, Inc.
†In these solutions, MEFOXIN has been found to be stable for a period of one week under refrigeration.

MEFOXIN®
(Sterile Cefoxitin Sodium, MSD)

chloride solution (without epinephrine), maintains satisfactory potency for 24 hours at room temperature, for one week under refrigeration (below 5°C), and for at least 30 weeks in the frozen state.

After the periods mentioned above, any unused solutions or frozen material should be discarded. Do not refreeze.

MEFOXIN has also been found compatible when admixed in intravenous infusions with the following:

Heparin 0.1 units/mL at room temperature—8 hours

Heparin 100 units/mL at room temperature—24 hours.

M.V.I.* concentrate at room temperature 24 hours; under refrigeration 48 hours

BEROCCA** C-500 at room temperature 24 hours; under refrigeration 48 hours

Insulin in Normal Saline at room temperature 24 hours; under refrigeration 48 hours

Insulin in 10% invert sugar at room temperature 24 hours; under refrigeration 48 hours

HOW SUPPLIED

Sterile MEFOXIN is a dry white to off-white powder supplied in vials and infusion bottles containing cefoxitin sodium as follows:

No. 3356—1 gram cefoxitin equivalent
NDC 0006-3356-71 in trays of 10 vials.
NDC 0006-3356-45 in trays of 25 vials.
No. 3368—1 gram cefoxitin equivalent
NDC 0006-3368-71 in trays of 10 infusion bottles.
No. 3357—2 gram cefoxitin equivalent
NDC 0006-3357-73 in trays of 10 vials.
NDC 0006-3357-53 in trays of 25 vials.
No. 3369—2 gram cefoxitin equivalent
NDC 0006-3369-73 in trays of 10 infusion bottles.
No. 3388—10 gram cefoxitin equivalent
NDC 0006-3388-10 in bulk bottles.

Special storage instructions

MEFOXIN in the dry state should be stored below 30°C. Avoid exposure to temperatures above 50°C. The dry material as well as solutions tend to darken, depending on storage conditions; product potency, however, is not adversely affected.

A.H.F.S. Category: 8:12.28
Issued July 1985   DC 7057120

INJECTION

PRIMAXIN®
(IMIPENEM-CILASTATIN SODIUM, MSD)

DESCRIPTION

PRIMAXIN† (Imipenem-Cilastatin Sodium, MSD) is a formulation of imipenem, a thienamycin antibiotic, and cilastatin sodium, the inhibitor of the renal dipeptidase, dehydropeptidase I, with sodium bicarbonate added as a buffer. PRIMAXIN is a potent broad spectrum antibacterial agent for intravenous administration.

Imipenem (N-formimidoylthienamycin monohydrate) is a crystalline derivative of thienamycin, which is produced by *Streptomyces cattleya*. Its chemical name is [5R-[5α, 6α (R*)]]-6-(1-hydroxyethyl)-3-[[2-[(iminomethyl)amino] ethyl]thio]-7-oxo-1-azabicyclo [3.2.0] hept-2-ene-2-carboxylic acid monohydrate. It is an off-white, non-hygroscopic crystalline compound with a molecular weight of 317.37. It is sparingly soluble in water, and slightly soluble in methanol. Its empirical formula is $C_{12}H_{17}N_3O_4S \cdot H_2O$, and its structural formula is:

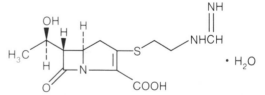

Cilastatin sodium is the sodium salt of a derivatized heptenoic acid. Its chemical name is [Z, 7(R),2(S)]-7-[(2-amino-2-carboxyethyl)thio]-2-[[(2,2-dimethyl-cyclopropyl)carbonyl]amino]-2-heptenoic acid monosodium salt. It is an off-white to yellowish-white, hygroscopic, amorphous compound with a molecular weight of 380.43. It is very soluble in water and in methanol. Its empirical formula is $C_{16}H_{25}N_2O_5S$ Na, and its structural formula is:

PRIMAXIN®
(Imipenem-Cilastatin Sodium, MSD)

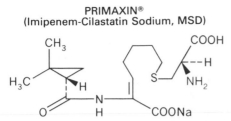

PRIMAXIN is buffered to provide solutions in the pH range of 6.5 to 7.5. There is no significant change in pH when solutions are prepared and used as directed. (See COMPATIBILITY AND STABILITY.) PRIMAXIN 250 contains 18.8 mg of sodium (0.8 mEq) and PRIMAXIN 500 contains 37.5 mg of sodium (1.6 mEq). Solutions of PRIMAXIN range from colorless to yellow. Variations of color within this range do not affect the potency of the product.

CLINICAL PHARMACOLOGY

Intravenous Administration

Intravenous infusion of PRIMAXIN over 20 minutes results in peak plasma levels of imipenem antimicrobial activity that range from 14 to 24 mcg/mL for the 250 mg dose, from 21 to 58 mcg/mL for the 500 mg dose and from 41 to 83 mcg/mL for the 1000 mg dose. At these doses, plasma levels of imipenem antimicrobial activity decline to below 1 mcg/mL or less in 4 to 6 hours. Peak plasma levels of cilastatin following a 20-minute intravenous infusion of PRIMAXIN, range from 15 to 25 mcg/mL for the 250 mg dose, from 31 to 49 mcg/mL for the 500 mg dose and from 56 to 88 mcg/mL for the 1000 mg dose.

General

The plasma half-life of each component is approximately 1 hour. The binding of imipenem to human serum proteins is approximately 20% and that of cilastatin is approximately 40%. Approximately 70% of the administered imipenem is recovered in the urine within 10 hours after which no further urinary excretion is detectable. Urine concentrations of imipenem in excess of 10 mcg/mL can be maintained for up to 8 hours with PRIMAXIN at the 500 mg dose. Approximately 70% of the cilastatin sodium dose is recovered in the urine within 10 hours of administration of PRIMAXIN.

No accumulation of PRIMAXIN in plasma or urine is observed with regimens administered as frequently as every 6 hours in patients with normal renal function.

Imipenem, when administered alone, is metabolized in the kidneys by dehydropep-

tidase I resulting in relatively low levels in urine. Cilastatin sodium, an inhibitor of this enzyme, effectively prevents renal metabolism of imipenem so that when imipenem and cilastatin sodium are given concomitantly fully adequate antibacterial levels of imipenem are achieved in the urine.

After a 1 gram dose, the following average levels of imipenem were measured (usually at 1 hour post-dose) in the tissues and fluids listed:

sputum	2.1 mcg/mL
pleural	22.0 mcg/mL
peritoneal	3.9 mcg/mL
bile	2.5 mcg/mL
aqueous humor	1.8 mcg/mL
interstitial fluid	16.0 mcg/mL
CSF (uninflamed meninges)	0.8 mcg/mL
reproductive organs	4.3 mcg/g (2½ hours post-dose)
bone	2.4 mcg/g

Microbiology

The bactericidal activity of imipenem results from the inhibition of cell wall synthesis. Its greatest affinity is for penicillin binding proteins (PBP) 1A, 1B, 2, 4, 5, and 6 of *Escherichia coli,* and 1A, 1B, 2, 4 and 5 of *Pseudomonas aeruginosa.* The lethal effect is related to binding to PBP 2 and PBP 1B. Imipenem has *in vitro* activity against a wide range of gram-positive and gram-negative organisms.

Imipenem has a high degree of stability in the presence of beta-lactamases, both penicillinases and cephalosporinases produced by gram-negative and gram-positive bacteria. It is a potent inhibitor of beta-lactamases from certain gram-negative bacteria which are inherently resistant to most beta-lactam antibiotics, e.g., *Pseudomonas aeruginosa, Serratia* spp., and *Enterobacter* spp.

In vitro, imipenem is active against most strains of clinical isolates of the following microorganisms:

Gram-positive:

Group D streptococci (including enterococci e.g., *Streptococcus faecalis*)
    NOTE: Imipenem is inactive against *Streptococcus faecium.*
Streptococcus pyogenes (Group A streptococci)
Streptococcus agalactiae (Group B streptococci)
Group C streptococci

Group G streptococci
Viridans streptococci
Streptococcus pneumoniae (formerly *Diplococcus pneumoniae*)
Staphylococcus aureus including penicillinase producing strains
Staphylococcus epidermidis including penicillinase producing strains

> NOTE: Many strains of methicillin-resistant staphylococci are resistant to imipenem.

Gram-negative:
  Escherichia coli
  Proteus mirabilis
  Proteus vulgaris
  Morganella morganii
  Providencia rettgeri
  Providencia stuartii
  Citrobacter spp.
  Klebsièlla spp. including *K. pneumoniae* and *K. oxytoca*
  Enterobacter spp.
  Hafnia spp. including *H. alvei*
  Serratia marcescens
  Serratia spp. including *S. liquefaciens*
  Haemophilus parainfluenzae
  H. influenzae
  Gardnerella vaginalis
  Acinetobacter spp.
  Pseudomonas aeruginosa

> NOTE: Imipenem is inactive against *P. maltophilia* and some strains of *P. cepacia*

Anaerobes:
  Bacteroides spp. including *Bacteroides bivius, Bacteroides fragilis, Bacteroides melaninogenicus*
  Clostridium spp. including *C. perfringens*
  Eubacterium spp.
  Fusobacterium spp.
  Peptococcus spp.
  Peptostreptococcus spp.
  Propionibacterium spp. including *P. acnes*
  Actinomyces spp.
  Veillonella spp.

Imipenem has been shown to be active *in vitro* against the following microorganisms; however, clinical efficacy has not yet been established.

Gram-positive:
  Listeria monocytogenes
  Nocardia spp.
Gram-negative:
  Salmonella spp.
  Shigella spp.

Yersinia spp. including *Yersinia enterocolitica, Yersinia pseudotuberculosis*
Bordetella bronchiseptica
Campylobacter spp.
Achromobacter spp.
Alcaligenes spp.
Moraxella spp.
Pasteurella multocida
Aeromonas hydrophila
Plesiomonas shigelloides
Neisseria gonorrhoeae (including penicillinase-producing strains)
Anaerobes:
  Bacteroides asaccharolyticus
  Bacteroides disiens
  Bacteroides distasonis
  Bacteroides ovatus
  Bacteroides thetaiotaomicron
  Bacteroides vulgatus

In vitro tests show imipenem to act synergistically with aminoglycoside antibiotics against some isolates of *Pseudomonas aeruginosa.*

Susceptibility Testing

Quantitative methods that require measurement of zone diameters give the most precise estimate of antibiotic susceptibility. One such procedure has been recommended for use with discs to test susceptibility to imipenem.

Reports from the laboratory giving results of the standard single-disc susceptibility test with a 10 mcg imipenem disc should be interpreted according to the following criteria.

Susceptible organisms produce zones of 16 mm or greater, indicating that the test organism is likely to respond to therapy.

Organisms that produce zones of 14 to 15 mm are expected to be susceptible if high dosage is used or if the infection is confined to tissues and fluids in which high antibiotic levels are attained.

Resistant organisms produce zones of 13 mm or less, indicating that other therapy should be selected.

A bacterial isolate may be considered susceptible if the MIC value for imipenem is equal to or less than 8 mcg/mL. Organisms are considered resistant if the MIC is equal to or greater than 16 mcg/mL.

The standardized quality control procedure requires use of control organisms. The 10 mcg imipenem disc should give the zone diameters listed below for the quality control strains.

Organism	ATCC	Zone Size Range
E. coli	25922	27-31 mm
Ps. aeruginosa	27853	20-28 mm

Dilution susceptibility tests should give MICs between the ranges listed below for the quality control strains.

Organism	ATCC	MIC (mcg/mL)
E. coli	25922	0.06-0.25
S. aureus	29213	0.008-0.03
S. faecalis	29212	0.25-1.0
Ps. aeruginosa	27853	1.0-4.0

Based on blood levels of imipenem achieved in man, breakpoint criteria have been established for imipenem.

Category	Zone Diameter (mm)	Recommended MIC Breakpoint (mcg/mL)
Susceptible	≥16	≤8
Moderately Susceptible	14-15	
Resistant	≤13	≥16

INDICATIONS AND USAGE

PRIMAXIN is indicated for the treatment of serious infections caused by susceptible strains of the designated microorganisms in the diseases listed below:

(1) **Lower respiratory tract infections.** *Staphylococcus aureus* (penicillinase producing strains)*, *Escherichia coli, Klebsiella* species, *Enterobacter* species, *Haemophilus influenzae, Haemophilus parainfluenzae*, *Acinetobacter* species*, *Serratia marcescens*.

(2) **Urinary tract infections** (Complicated and uncomplicated). *Staphylococcus aureus* (penicillinase producing strains)*, Group D streptococci (enterococci), *Escherichia coli, Klebsiella* species, *Enterobacter* species, *Proteus vulgaris*, *Providencia rettgeri*, *Morganella morganii*, *Pseudomonas aeruginosa*.

(3) **Intra-abdominal infections.** *Staphylococcus aureus* (penicillinase producing strains)*, *Staphylococcus epidermidis*, Group D streptococci (enterococci), *Escherichia coli, Klebsiella* species, *Enterobacter* species, *Proteus* species (indole positive and indole negative), *Morganella morganii*, *Pseudomonas aeruginosa, Citrobacter* species*, *Clostridium* species, Gram-positive anaerobes, including *Peptococcus* species*, *Peptostreptococcus* species*, *Eubacterium* species, *Propionibacterium* species*, *Bifidobacterium* species, *Bacteroides* species, including *B. fragilis, Fusobacterium* species*.

---
*Efficacy for this organism in this organ system was demonstrated in less than 10 infections.

(4) **Gynecologic infections.** *Staphylococcus aureus* (penicillinase producing strains)*, *Staphylococcus epidermidis,* Group B streptococci, Group D streptococci (enterococci), *Escherichia coli, Klebsiella* species*, *Proteus* species (indole positive and indole negative)*, *Enterobacter* species*, Gram-positive anaerobes, including *Peptococcus* species*, *Peptostreptococcus* species*, *Propionibacterium* species*, *Bifidobacterium* species*, *Bacteroides* species, *B. fragilis*, *Gardnerella vaginalis*.

(5) **Bacterial septicemia.** *Staphylococcus aureus* (penicillinase producing strains), Group D streptococci (enterococci)*, *Escherichia coli, Klebsiella* species*, *Pseudomonas aeruginosa*, *Serratia* species*, *Enterobacter* species*, *Bacteroides* species, *B. fragilis*.

(6) **Bone and joint infections.** *Staphylococcus aureus* (penicillinase producing strains), *Staphylococcus epidermidis*, Group D streptococci (enterococci)*, *Enterobacter* species*, *Pseudomonas aeruginosa*.

(7) **Skin and skin structure infections.** *Staphylococcus aureus* (penicillinase producing strains), *Staphylococcus epidermidis,* Group D streptococci (enterococci), *Escherichia coli, Klebsiella* species, *Enterobacter* species, *Proteus vulgaris*, *Providencia rettgeri*, *Morganella morganii, Pseudomonas aeruginosa, Serratia* species, *Citrobacter* species*, *Acinetobacter* species*, Gram-positive anaerobes, including *Peptococcus* species and *Peptostreptococcus* species, *Bacteroides* species, including *B. fragilis, Fusobacterium* species*.

(8) **Endocarditis.** *Staphylococcus aureus* (penicillinase producing strains).

(9) **Polymicrobic infections.** PRIMAXIN is indicated for polymicrobic infections including those in which *S. pneumoniae* (pneumonia, septicemia), Group A beta-hemolytic streptococcus (skin and skin structure), or nonpenicillinase-producing *S. aureus* is one of the causative organisms. However monobacterial infections due to these organisms are usually treated with narrower spectrum antibiotics, such as penicillin G.

Although clinical improvement has been observed in patients with cystic fibrosis,

---
*Efficacy for this organism in this organ system was demonstrated in less than 10 infections.

PRIMAXIN®
(Imipenem-Cilastatin Sodium, MSD)

chronic pulmonary disease, and lower respiratory tract infections caused by *Pseudomonas aeruginosa,* bacterial eradication may not necessarily be achieved.

As with other beta-lactam antibiotics, some strains of *Pseudomonas aeruginosa* may develop resistance fairly rapidly on treatment with PRIMAXIN. When clinically appropriate during therapy of *Pseudomonas aeruginosa* infections, periodic susceptibility testing should be done.

Infections resistant to other antibiotics, for example, cephalosporins, penicillin, and aminoglycosides, have been shown to respond to treatment with PRIMAXIN.

CONTRAINDICATIONS

PRIMAXIN is contraindicated in patients who have shown hypersensitivity to any component of this product.

WARNINGS

SERIOUS AND OCCASIONALLY FATAL HYPERSENSITIVITY (anaphylactic) REACTIONS HAVE BEEN REPORTED IN PATIENTS RECEIVING THERAPY WITH BETA-LACTAMS. THESE REACTIONS ARE MORE APT TO OCCUR IN PERSONS WITH A HISTORY OF SENSITIVITY TO MULTIPLE ALLERGENS.

THERE HAVE BEEN REPORTS OF PATIENTS WITH A HISTORY OF PENICILLIN HYPERSENSITIVITY WHO HAVE EXPERIENCED SEVERE HYPERSENSITIVITY REACTIONS WHEN TREATED WITH ANOTHER BETA-LACTAM. BEFORE INITIATING THERAPY WITH PRIMAXIN, CAREFUL INQUIRY SHOULD BE MADE CONCERNING PREVIOUS HYPERSENSITIVITY REACTIONS TO PENICILLINS, CEPHALOSPORINS, OTHER BETA-LACTAMS, AND OTHER ALLERGENS. IF AN ALLERGIC REACTION TO PRIMAXIN OCCURS, DISCONTINUE THE DRUG. SERIOUS HYPERSENSITIVITY REACTIONS MAY REQUIRE EPINEPHRINE AND OTHER EMERGENCY MEASURES.

Pseudomembranous colitis has been reported with virtually all antibiotics, including PRIMAXIN; therefore it is important to consider its diagnosis in patients who develop diarrhea in association with antibiotic use. This colitis may range in severity from mild to life threatening.

Mild cases of pseudomembranous colitis may respond to drug discontinuance alone. In more severe cases, management may include sigmoidoscopy, appropriate bacteriological studies, fluid, electrolyte and protein supplementation, and the use of a drug such as oral vancomycin, as indicated. Isolation of the patient may be advisable. Other causes of colitis should also be considered.

PRECAUTIONS
General

CNS adverse experiences such as myoclonic activity, confusional states, or seizures have been reported with PRIMAXIN. These experiences have occurred most commonly in patients with CNS disorders (e.g., brain lesions or history of seizures) who also have compromised renal function. However, there were rare reports in which there was no recognized or documented underlying CNS disorder. Close adherence to recommended dosage schedules is urged especially in patients with known factors that predispose to seizures (see DOSAGE AND ADMINISTRATION). Anticonvulsant therapy should be continued in patients with a known seizure disorder. If focal tremors, myoclonus, or seizures occur, patients should be placed on anticonvulsant therapy. If CNS symptoms continue, the dosage of PRIMAXIN should be decreased or discontinued.

As with other antibiotics, prolonged use of PRIMAXIN may result in overgrowth of nonsusceptible organisms. Repeated evaluation of the patient's condition is essential. If superinfection occurs during therapy, appropriate measures should be taken.

While PRIMAXIN possesses the characteristic low toxicity of the beta-lactam group of antibiotics, periodic assessment of organ system function during prolonged therapy is advisable.
Drug Interactions

Since concomitant administration of PRIMAXIN and probenecid results in only minimal increases in plasma levels of imipenem and plasma half-life, it is not recommended that probenecid be given with PRIMAXIN.

PRIMAXIN should not be mixed with or physically added to other antibiotics. However, PRIMAXIN may be administered concomitantly with other antibiotics, such as aminoglycosides.
Carcinogenesis, Mutagenesis, Impairment of Fertility

Gene toxicity studies were performed in a

variety of bacterial and mammalian tests *in vivo* and *in vitro*. The tests were: V79 mammalian cell mutation assay (PRIMAXIN alone and imipenem alone), Ames test (cilastatin sodium alone), unscheduled DNA synthesis assay (PRIMAXIN) and *in vivo* mouse cytogenicity test (PRIMAXIN). None of these tests showed any evidence of genetic damage.

Reproduction tests in male and female rats were performed with PRIMAXIN at dosage levels up to 8 times the usual human dose. Slight decreases in live fetal body weight were restricted to the highest dosage level. No other adverse effects were observed on fertility, reproductive performance, fetal viability, growth or postnatal development of pups. Similarly, no adverse effects on the fetus or on lactation were observed when PRIMAXIN was administered to rats late in gestation.

Pregnancy

Pregnancy Category C. Teratogenicity studies with cilastatin sodium in rabbits and rats at 10 and 33 times the usual human dose, respectively, showed no evidence of adverse effect on the fetus. No evidence of teratogenicity or adverse effect on postnatal growth or behavior was observed in rats given imipenem at dosage levels up to 30 times the usual human dose. Similarly, no evidence of adverse effect on the fetus was observed in teratology studies in rabbits with imipenem at dosage levels at the usual human dose.

Teratology studies with PRIMAXIN at doses up to 11 times the usual human dose in pregnant mice and rats during the period of major organogenesis revealed no evidence of teratogenicity.

Data from preliminary studies suggests an apparent intolerance to PRIMAXIN (including emesis, inappetence, body weight loss, diarrhea and death) at doses equivalent to the average human dose in pregnant rabbits and cynomolgus monkeys that is not seen in non-pregnant animals in these or other species. In other studies, PRIMAXIN was well tolerated in equivalent or higher doses (up to 11 times the average human dose) in pregnant rats and mice. Further studies are underway to evaluate these findings.

There are, however, no adequate and well-controlled studies in pregnant women. PRIMAXIN should be used during pregnancy only if the potential benefit justifies the potential risk to the fetus.

Nursing Mothers

It is not known whether this drug is excreted in human milk. Because many drugs are excreted in human milk, caution should be exercised when PRIMAXIN is administered to a nursing woman.

Pediatric Use

Safety and effectiveness in infants and children below 12 years of age have not yet been established.

ADVERSE REACTIONS

PRIMAXIN is generally well tolerated. Many of the 1,723 patients treated in clinical trials were severely ill and had multiple background diseases and physiological impairments, making it difficult to determine causal relationship of adverse experiences to therapy with PRIMAXIN.

Local Adverse Reactions

Adverse local clinical reactions that were reported as possibly, probably or definitely related to therapy with PRIMAXIN were:

Phlebitis/thrombophlebitis—3.1%
Pain at the injection site—0.7%
Erythema at the injection site—0.4%
Vein induration—0.2%
Infused vein infection—0.1%

Systemic Adverse Reactions

The most frequently reported systemic adverse clinical reactions that were reported as possibly, probably, or definitely related to PRIMAXIN were nausea (2.0%), diarrhea (1.8%), vomiting (1.5%), rash (0.9%), fever (0.5%), hypotension (0.4%), seizures (0.4%) (see *PRECAUTIONS*), dizziness (0.3%), pruritus (0.3%), urticaria (0.2%), somnolence (0.2%).

Additional adverse systemic clinical reactions reported as possibly, probably or definitely drug related occurring in less than 0.2% of the patients are listed within each body system in order of decreasing severity: *Gastrointestinal*—pseudomembranous colitis (see WARNINGS), hemorrhagic colitis, gastroenteritis, abdominal pain, glossitis, tongue papillar hypertrophy, heartburn, pharyngeal pain, increased salivation; *CNS*—encephalopathy, confusion, myoclonus, paresthesia, vertigo, headache; *Special Senses*—transient hearing loss in patients with impaired hearing, tinnitus; *Respiratory*—chest discomfort, dyspnea, hyperventilation, thoracic spine pain; *Cardiovascular*—palpitations, tachycardia; *Renal*—oliguria/anuria, polyuria; *Skin*—erythema multiforme, facial edema, flushing, cyanosis, hyperhidrosis, skin texture changes, candidiasis, pruritis vulvae; *Body as a whole*—polyarthralgia, asthenia/weakness.

Adverse Laboratory Changes

Adverse laboratory changes without regard to drug relationship that were reported during clinical trials were:

Hepatic: Increased SGPT, SGOT, alkaline phosphatase, bilirubin and LDH.

Hemic: Increased eosinophils, positive Coombs test, decreased WBC and neutrophils, increased WBC, increased platelets, decreased platelets, decreased hemoglobin and hematocrit, increased monocytes, abnormal prothrombin time, increased lymphocytes, increased basophils.

Electrolytes: Decreased serum sodium, increased potassium, increased chloride.

Renal: Increased BUN, creatinine.

Urinalysis: Presence of urine protein, urine red blood cells, urine white blood cells, urine casts, urine bilirubin, and urine urobilinogen.

OVERDOSAGE

The intravenous LD_{50} of imipenem is greater than 2000 mg/kg in the rat and approximately 1500 mg/kg in the mouse.

The intravenous LD_{50} of cilastatin sodium is approximately 5000 mg/kg in the rat and approximately 8700 mg/kg in the mouse.

The intravenous LD_{50} of PRIMAXIN is approximately 1000 mg/kg/day in the rat and approximately 1100 mg/kg/day in the mouse.

Information on overdosage in humans is not available.

DOSAGE AND ADMINISTRATION

The dosage recommendations for PRIMAXIN represent the quantity of imipenem to be administered. An equivalent amount of cilastatin is also present in the solution.

Initially, the total daily dosage for PRIMAXIN should be based on the type or severity of infection and given in equally divided doses. Subsequent dosing must be based on consideration of severity of illness, degree of susceptibility of the pathogen(s), age, weight, and creatinine clearance.

Serum creatinine alone may not be a suffi-

ciently accurate measure of renal function. Creatinine clearance (T_{cc}) may be estimated from the following equation:

$$T_{cc} \text{ (Males)} = \frac{(\text{wt. in kg}) (140 - \text{age})}{(72) (\text{creatinine in mg/dL})}$$

$$T_{cc} \text{ (Female)} = 0.85 \text{ x above value}$$

Each 250 mg or 500 mg dose should be given by intravenous infusion over twenty to thirty minutes. Each 1000 mg dose should be infused over forty to sixty minutes. In patients who develop nausea during the infusion, the rate of infusion may be slowed.

INTRAVENOUS DOSING SCHEDULE FOR ADULTS WITH NORMAL RENAL FUNCTION

Type or severity of infection	Gram-positive organisms Anaerobes Highly susceptible gram-negative organisms	Other gram-negative organisms
Mild	250 mg q6h	500 mg q6h
Moderate	500 mg q8h- 500 mg q6h	500 mg q6h- 1 g q8h
Severe, life threatening	500 mg q6h	1 g q8h- 1 g q6h
Uncomplicated urinary tract infection	250 mg q6h	250 mg q6h
Complicated urinary tract infection	500 mg q6h	500 mg q6h

Due to the high antimicrobial activity of PRIMAXIN, it is recommended that the maximum total daily dosage not exceed 50 mg/kg/day or 4.0g/day, whichever is lower. There is no evidence that higher doses provide greater efficacy.

INTRAVENOUS DOSING SCHEDULE FOR ADULTS WITH IMPAIRED RENAL FUNCTION

Patients with creatinine clearance of $\leq$ 70 mL/min/1.73 m^2 require adjustment of the dosage of PRIMAXIN as indicated in the table below. Doses cited are in every case the imipenem component of a 1:1 ratio of imipenem:cilastatin Na and are based on a body weight of 70 kg. Proportionate reduction in dose administered should be made for patients with reduced body weight.

PRIMAXIN®
(Imipenem-Cilastatin Sodium, MSD)

Intravenous Dosage of PRIMAXIN in Adults With Impaired Renal Function

Creatinine Clearance (mL/min/ 1.73 m2)	Renal Function	Less Severe Infections or Presence of Highly Susceptible Organisms	Life Threatening Infections— Maximum Dosage
30-70	Mild Impairment	500 mg q8h	500 mg q6h
20-30	Moderate Impairment	500 mg q12h	500 mg q8h
5-20	Severe to Marked Impairment	250 mg q12h	500 mg q12h
0-5	None, but on hemodialysis	250 mg q12h	500 mg q12h

PRIMAXIN is cleared by hemodialysis. In patients undergoing hemodialysis, a supplemental dose of PRIMAXIN should be given after hemodialysis unless the next dose is scheduled within four hours. The benefits versus the risks should be considered in patients on hemodialysis. Dialysis patients, especially those with CNS background diseases, should be carefully monitored (see PRECAUTIONS).

PREPARATION OF SOLUTION

120 mL Infusion Bottles

Contents of the 120 mL infusion bottles of PRIMAXIN Powder should be restored with 100 mL of diluent (see list of diluents under COMPATIBILITY AND STABILITY) and shaken until a clear solution is obtained.

13 mL Vials

Contents of the 13 mL vials must be suspended and transferred to 100 mL of an appropriate infusion solution.

A suggested procedure is to add approximately 10 mL from the appropriate infusion solution (see list of diluents under COMPATIBILITY AND STABILITY) to the vial. Shake well and transfer the resulting suspension to the infusion solution container. CAUTION: THE SUSPENSION IS NOT FOR DIRECT INFUSION.

Repeat with an additional 10 mL of infusion solution to ensure complete transfer of vial contents to the infusion solution. **The resulting mixture should be agitated until clear.**

COMPATIBILITY AND STABILITY

Before reconstitution:

The dry powder should be stored at a temperature below 30°C.

Reconstituted solutions:

Solutions of PRIMAXIN range from colorless to yellow. Variations of color within this range do not affect the potency of the product.

PRIMAXIN, as supplied in infusion bottles and vials and reconstituted as above with the following diluents, maintains satisfactory potency for four hours at room temperature and for 24 hours under refrigeration (4°C) (note exception below). Solutions of PRIMAXIN should not be frozen.

0.9% Sodium Chloride Injection*

5% or 10% Dextrose Injection

5% Dextrose Injection with 0.02% sodium bicarbonate solution

5% Dextrose and 0.9% Sodium Chloride Injection

5% Dextrose Injection with 0.225% or 0.45% saline solution

NORMOSOL† – M in D5-W

5% Dextrose Injection with 0.15% potassium chloride solution

Mannitol 2.5%, 5% and 10%

PRIMAXIN should not be mixed with or physically added to other antibiotics. However, PRIMAXIN may be administered concomitantly with other antibiotics, such as aminoglycosides.

HOW SUPPLIED

PRIMAXIN is supplied as a sterile powder mixture in vials and infusion bottles containing imipenem (anhydrous equivalent) and cilastatin sodium as follows:

No. 3514—250 mg imipenem equivalent and 250 mg cilastatin equivalent and 10 mg sodium bicarbonate as a buffer

NDC 0006-3514-74 in trays of 10 vials.

No. 3516—500 mg imipenem equivalent and 500 mg cilastatin equivalent and 20 mg sodium bicarbonate as a buffer

NDC 0006-3516-75 in trays of 10 vials.

No. 3515—250 mg imipenem equivalent and 250 mg cilastatin equivalent and 10 mg sodium bicarbonate as a buffer

NDC 0006-3515-74 in trays of 10 infusion bottles.

No. 3517—500 mg imipenem equivalent and 500 mg cilastatin equivalent and 20 mg sodium bicarbonate as a buffer

NDC 0006-3517-75 in trays of 10 infusion bottles.

*PRIMAXIN has been found to be stable in 0.9% Sodium Chloride Injection for 10 hours at room temperature and 48 hours under refrigeration.
†Registered trademark of Abbott Laboratories, Inc.

MERCK SHARP & DOHME, Division of Merck & Co., INC. West Point, Pa. 19486

A.H.F.S. Category: 8:12.28

Issued November 1985   DC 7362400

PRIMAXIN®
(Imipenem-Cilastatin Sodium, MSD)